Relaxation Techniques

For Elsevier:

Senior Commissioning Editor: Sarena Wolfaard
Associate Editor: Dinah Thom
Project Manager: Gail Wright
Senior Designer: Judith Wright
Illustration Manager: Bruce Hogarth

Relaxation Techniques

A Practical Handbook for the Health Care Professional

THIRD EDITION

Rosemary A. Payne BSc(Psychology) MCSP

Chartered physiotherapist and tutor in relaxation training, Cardiff, UK

Foreword by

Marie Donaghy PhD BA(Hons) FCSP ILTM

Associate Dean and Head of School of Health Sciences, Faculty of Health and Social Science,
Queen Margaret University College, Edinburgh, UK;
President of the Association of Chartered Physiotherapists in Mental Healthcare

Photographs by

Keith Bellamy MSc MIMI RMIP

Director/Clinical Director of the Media Resources Centre, University of Wales College of Medicine, Cardiff, UK

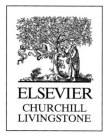

ELSEVIER
CHURCHILL
LIVINGSTONE

EDINBURGH LONDON NEW YORK OXFORD PHILADELPHIA ST LOUIS SYDNEY TORONTO 2005

ELSEVIER
CHURCHILL
LIVINGSTONE

First edition 1995
Second edition 2000
Third edition 2005

ISBN 0 443 07447 X

British Library Cataloguing in Publication Data
A catalogue record for this book is available from the British Library

Library of Congress Cataloging in Publication Data
A catalog record for this book is available from the Library of Congress

Notice
Knowledge and best practice in this field are constantly changing. As new research and experience broaden our knowledge, changes in practice, treatment and drug therapy may become necessary or appropriate. Readers are advised to check the most current information provided (i) on procedures featured or (ii) by the manufacturer of each product to be administered, to verify the recommended dose or formula, the method and duration of administration, and contraindications. It is the responsibility of the practitioner, relying on their own experience and knowledge of the patient, to make diagnoses, to determine dosages and the best treatment for each individual patient, and to take all appropriate safety precautions. To the fullest extent of the law, neither the publisher nor the author assumes any liability for any injury and/or damage.

The Publisher

 ELSEVIER your source for books, journals and multimedia in the health sciences

www.elsevierhealth.com

The Publisher's policy is to use **paper manufactured from sustainable forests**

Printed in China

Contents

Foreword

Relaxation is a word that is commonly used across many different cultures to describe a range of feelings, emotions and behaviour. It is associated with feelings of pleasure, control and self-assurance; emotions of laughter, calmness and tranquillity; activities such as resting, exercise, massage, bathing, listening to music, eating, drinking alcohol and relaxation training. Health professionals and lay people alike are regularly informed by articles in the popular press, texts and scientific journals of the benefits of relaxation for health; however, there is often uncertainty about what is meant by relaxation, which technique to choose and how to go about it.

The need for relaxation as a therapeutic intervention is evidenced through the links between stress and illness; when undertaken as part of our everyday activities, relaxation can provide a mechanism for lowering stress and thus offer some protection against stress-related problems. Health care professionals such as psychologists, nurses, physiotherapists, occupational therapists, speech and language therapists, social workers, GPs and professionals such as coaches and sport and exercise scientists working in the health and leisure industries may all be involved in teaching relaxation techniques.

The third edition of this popular textbook retains its eclectic and practical approach, presenting a number of additional relaxation techniques along with those previously included, all of which can be successfully self-taught or taught by health care personnel. The text is well illustrated and this is helpful for gaining an understanding of the various techniques and putting them into practice. The layout of the content is such that specific techniques can be readily accessed as stand-alone chapters; however, for health care students and health professionals to benefit fully from the knowledge carefully and systematically brought together by the author, the text should be read in full.

The book is presented in a logical sequence starting with a review of stress as a concept that can be explained by various physiological, endocrinological and psychological theories. The rationale for the techniques presented in subsequent chapters highlights the theoretical links where these are explicit and identifies where techniques are based on principles that may not fit or may overlap with more than one of these existing theoretical positions. As well as the underpinning rationale, a summary of the research evidence to support each technique is discussed. The importance of reviewing the evidence to inform decisions in practice is reiterated in Chapter 27, which includes a useful discussion on issues around current research, on strengths to date and on future directions. This chapter also contains an interesting discussion around selection of techniques. Chapter 23, highlighting 'on-the-spot' techniques, is crucial for putting into practice a shortened version of what has previously been learned.

Relaxation Techniques will continue to provide a useful guide for health professionals, students and lay people who wish to increase their understanding of stress, its causes and its impact on health. It also provides a concise and detailed summary of measurement strategies that can be used to evaluate the outcome of interventions designed to reduce or alleviate the effects of stress. The book is eclectic, with no one method being presented more favourably than another, the author acknowledging that in practice, physical and cognitive methods are often presented together. For students, this single volume provides theoretical underpinning, evidence from current research and practical application of many different techniques of relaxation. In this regard it is a unique and useful text. For clinicians, this is a useful bench text with opportunity to extend existing practice through the introduction and application of additional approaches which are informed by both current research and current practice. Techniques are presented with an explanation of why they are useful, how to use them, where they have been evaluated, where they can be used interchangeably, and what needs to be done to ensure that the best techniques can be selected for the right situation. For lay people, this book raises awareness of relaxation as a strategy to improve physical and psychological health; and for readers wishing to teach themselves a method of relaxation, there is plenty of choice.

This book provides essential information that will be useful to those involved in training others in relaxation techniques and to individuals who wish to teach themselves skills of relaxation, irrespective of the level of prior knowledge of the topic or practical experience. This third edition is an exciting addition to the current literature, bringing further techniques and greater indepth discussion and critique to the topic. Read on; you will find the direction given by the author to be practical, meaningful and stimulating, with new points of debate emerging.

Marie Donaghy

Preface to the third edition

Since the preface to the first edition of *Relaxation Techniques* was written, developments in the health care scene have created a new emphasis on evidence of effectiveness. This has led to the need for an additional chapter on the results of research. New evidence has also been incorporated into the individual chapters and may be found in their sections on evaluation.

The chapter on exercise (Ch. 14) has been rewritten to take account of developments in that field; it also contains an expanded section on the psychological effects of physical activity.

Chapter 26 now carries a passage relating to audit, in acknowledgement of the importance of this topic, although the contribution made here is no more than an introduction to what has become a major subject.

This third edition contains two new chapters, one on cognitive behavioural approaches, reflecting their increasingly dominant position (Ch. 22); the other on techniques which did not appear in earlier editions (Ch. 24). There is also a glossary and a table (Appendix 3) suggesting certain techniques for specific conditions.

Particular thanks are offered to Marie Donaghy who has been through the whole manuscript making useful suggestions and contributing many of the ideas which appear in this edition. Her advice has been invaluable and I am again greatly indebted to her. The people who so kindly helped with the first and second editions are also remembered for their valued assistance, with a special appreciation in respect of Margaret Polden and June Tiley, who have sadly since died. I would also like to acknowledge the guidance I have received from the publishers, Elsevier, and to thank them for the way they have presented the work.

This edition focuses on the same techniques as the first one, i.e. techniques which are easily learned and which can be readily applied in the stressful situation, wherever it arises. It is hoped that the work in its present form will provide the reader with useful additions. In essence, it remains the same book in an expanded and updated form.

Rosemary Payne
Cardiff 2004

Preface to the first edition

A few years ago, when giving a talk on relaxation techniques, I was asked by a social worker if the techniques I was describing could all be found in one publication. I said I knew of no book which contained them all. Since then, other health care professionals have, on different occasions, put similar questions to me. Is there a book which focuses on the practical side of relaxation training? Can the detail of the methods be found under one cover?

Many books mention relaxation techniques but tend not to present them in any depth, unless the entire work is devoted to a single method. It seemed that there was a gap which needed to be filled.

It is estimated that 80% of modern diseases have their beginnings in stress (Powell & Enright 1990) and that stress-related illness accounts for at least 75% of GP consultations (Looker & Gregson 1989). As concern about the safety, efficacy and cost of psychotropic drugs grows (Sibbald et al 1993), there is increasing interest in non-drug treatments, of which relaxation training is an example.

The book is addressed to health care professionals such as nurses, occupational therapists, physiotherapists, speech and language therapists and social workers; GPs and psychologists also may find it useful. It can equally be used by lay people since it is written in a jargon-free style.

Factors of practicality have governed the selection of methods. Thus, techniques which require expensive equipment or specialized expertise are not included, while the methods chosen are those which lend themselves to presentation in small group settings.

The book begins with a review of some of the theory surrounding stress and relaxation. This is followed by a chapter on general procedure which is applicable to all methods. Chapter 3 discusses stress, beginning with a further passage of theory and moving on to consider a variety of practical coping skills. The following 19 chapters deal with specific techniques: 12 chapters are, broadly speaking, concerned with physical or muscular techniques and seven deal with mental or psychological methods. There follows a chapter concerning 'on-the-spot' techniques for dealing with stressful situations, using skills drawn from earlier lessons. Relaxation in the antenatal context is the subject of Chapter 25*, and is included because of the prominent role that relaxation plays in the field of obstetrics. Assessment is addressed in Chapter 26, and the final chapter takes a look at a few topics not so far discussed: the relation between the approaches themselves, some ways in which they can be combined, and a brief reference to approaches which are not included. Physical and psychiatric disorders are not within the scope of this work.

Techniques whose main purpose is to promote relaxation are termed primary. The 'muscular' methods belong in this category, as does autogenic training. Where relaxation is not the main purpose, the technique can be seen as secondary: visualization, meditation and the Alexander technique fall

---

* To avoid confusion, the chapter numbers have been changed to match the chapter numbers in the third edition rather than the first.

into this category. Other approaches which enhance relaxation may be still further removed. These include cognitive techniques such as uncovering irrational assumptions and modifying automatic thoughts. Here, relaxation can be seen as a side-effect rather than a goal (Fanning 1988).

It is not intended that health care professionals should, on the strength of reading this book, consider themselves teachers of autogenics and the Alexander technique. These two methods are included to indicate their contribution to the field; they are described for interest and for the applicability of their central ideas. For example, images of warmth and heaviness (autogenics) are relaxing in any context, as also is postural advice (Alexander technique). Such concepts have universal value.

Indications of the effectiveness of the techniques are included but the book does not set out to review the evidence from the scientific literature. Other works do that, for example Lichstein (1988). Pitfalls associated with some methods are listed at the end of the relevant chapters.

The word 'relaxation' is used in two ways here as it is in other works: first, in a general sense where it signifies a global state of rest; and second, as a technique such as progressive relaxation. It is difficult to avoid both meanings in a book of this sort; however, efforts are made throughout the work to distinguish the meanings wherever ambiguity arises.

The author is aware of the implications of gender-weighted language. She is also aware of the cumbersome phrasing that can result from a determination to avoid sexist forms of speech. In an attempt to avoid both traps and for the sake of clarity, it has been decided to refer throughout the book to the trainer as female. The trainee is referred to as male in Chapters 2–15 and as female in Chapters 16–28.

The words 'trainer' and 'instructor' are both used, the choice being largely determined by the nature of the method: for example, in autogenics, progressive relaxation and behavioural relaxation training the word 'trainer' is often used, while in imagery, meditation, Alexander technique and Mitchell's approach, the word 'instructor' seems more appropriate. The word 'therapist' is also used where it seems fitting.

A number of people have helped in the making of this book. One important contributor is Keith Bellamy, whose photographs have done so much to make the book what it is, not forgetting Sarah McDermott, who acted as the model. With regard to the text, Ian Hughes has given invaluable help in his careful reading and refining of the chapter on measurement. I would also like to mention those who have read other chapters and to whom I am indebted for their helpful suggestions. Alexandra Hough, Wendy Mair, Margaret Polden and Jim Robinson have all been kind enough to do this, and Christopher Rowland Payne undertook to read the whole manuscript. Thanks also go to Michael Adams, Joyce Gibbs, Olga Gregson, Andrzej Kokoszka, Brenda MacLachland, Pat Miller, Alison Ough, Stuart Skyte, Dinah Thom, June Tiley and Elizabeth Valentine. Finally, a word of appreciation for the members of all the groups with whom I have worked. Without them, this book would never have been written.

Rosemary Payne
Cardiff 1994

SECTION 1

Introduction

SECTION CONTENTS

Chapter 1

Theoretical background

It could be said that relaxation is doing nothing (Beck 1984). In spite of this, many people say they find it difficult to relax. Doing nothing, it seems, is not as easy as it sounds, and the existence of a wealth of relaxation techniques appears to endorse this view.

'Relaxation' is often used with reference to muscles, where it signifies release of tension and the lengthening of muscle fibres, as opposed to the shortening which accompanies muscular tension, or contraction. Such a definition could be applied to the methods described in the earlier chapters of this book. However, since relaxation has a mental, as well as a physical dimension, this definition is too restricted for our purposes.

A more comprehensive view comes from Ryman (1995), who defines relaxation as 'a state of consciousness characterized by feelings of peace, and release from tension, anxiety and fear'. This emphasizes psychological aspects of the relaxation experience, such as the pleasant sensation and absence of stressful or uncomfortable thoughts.

Thus, the word 'relaxed' is used to refer either to lax muscles or to peaceful thoughts. It is assumed that a link exists between them since an apparently general state of relaxation can be induced by using either physical or psychological methods.

Relaxation can be said to have three aims (Titlebaum 1988):

1. As a preventive measure, to protect body organs from unnecessary wear, and in particular, the organs involved in stress-related disease (Selye 1956, 1974).

2. As a treatment, to help relieve stress in conditions such as essential hypertension (Patel & Marmot 1988), tension headache (Spinhoven et al 1992), insomnia (Lichstein 1983), asthma (Henry et al 1993), immune deficiency (Antoni et al 1991), panic (Öst 1988) and many others. Relaxation strategies may help to make the body's innate healing mechanisms more available.

3. As a coping skill, to calm the mind and allow thinking to become clearer and more effective. Stress can impair people mentally; relaxation can help to restore clarity of thought. It has been found that positive information in memory becomes more accessible when a person is relaxed (Peveler & Johnston 1986).

Mechanisms thought to be responsible for bringing about the state of relaxation have been explored, giving rise to a number of theories. Some of these emphasize physiological aspects, such as autonomic activity and muscle tension, while others focus on psychological elements such as attitudes towards the self. The major theories are briefly described below.

PHYSIOLOGICAL THEORIES

Body systems associated with the states of stress and relaxation include:

- the autonomic nervous system
- the endocrine system and
- the skeletal musculature.

The autonomic nervous system

Physiological arousal is governed by the autonomic nervous system. This has two branches: the sympathetic, which increases arousal when the organism is under threat, and the parasympathetic, which restores the body to a resting state. Their actions are involuntary and designed to enable the organism to survive (Fig. 1.1).

In a situation of challenge, excitement or danger the sympathetic nervous system increases the activity of the heart and redistributes blood from the viscera to the voluntary muscles. Blood pressure and respiratory rate are increased; sensory awareness is heightened, and there is a mechanism for losing excess heat. These factors enable the

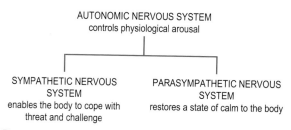

Figure 1.1   The autonomic nervous system.

individual to make a physical response. The changes are collectively known as the 'fight–flight response' which is characterized by an increase in:

- heart rate
- blood pressure
- blood coagulation rate
- blood flow to voluntary muscles
- glucose content of the blood
- respiratory rate
- acuity of the senses
- sweat gland activity

and a decrease of:

- activity in the digestive tract.

In the absence of challenge or excitement, these actions are reversed: the sympathetic nervous system loses its dominance and the parasympathetic assumes control. The actions of these systems are shown in greater detail in Figures 1.2 and 1.3.

Some of the changes which occur as a result of sympathetic stimulation produce noticeable symptoms, such as an increased respiratory rate, stomach cramps and cold sweat. States such as fear and anger illustrate this and underline the association between the emotions and the internal organs. When the changes are pronounced and occur frequently, the organs concerned can become fatigued and this has given rise to the concept of psychosomatic illness (p. 27). The relaxation response method of Benson aims to counteract the effects of sympathetic activity by promoting the action of the parasympathetic nervous system (Ch. 21), thereby exploiting the reciprocal nature of the two parts of the autonomic nervous system.

However, activity of the parasympathetic system is not always benign (Poppen 1988). Asthma is exacerbated by bronchial constriction and gastric ulcers by acid secretion. Both bronchial constriction

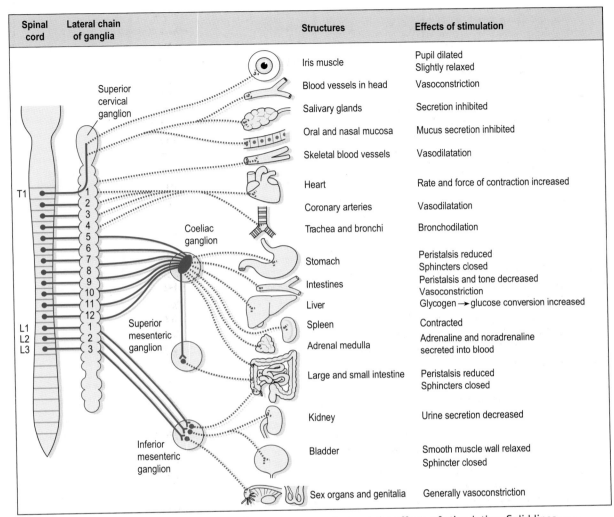

Spinal cord	Lateral chain of ganglia	Structures	Effects of stimulation
		Iris muscle	Pupil dilated / Slightly relaxed
		Blood vessels in head	Vasoconstriction
		Salivary glands	Secretion inhibited
		Oral and nasal mucosa	Mucus secretion inhibited
		Skeletal blood vessels	Vasodilatation
		Heart	Rate and force of contraction increased
		Coronary arteries	Vasodilatation
		Trachea and bronchi	Bronchodilation
		Stomach	Peristalsis reduced / Sphincters closed
		Intestines	Peristalsis and tone decreased / Vasoconstriction
		Liver	Glycogen → glucose conversion increased
		Spleen	Contracted
		Adrenal medulla	Adrenaline and noradrenaline secreted into blood
		Large and small intestine	Peristalsis reduced / Sphincters closed
		Kidney	Urine secretion decreased
		Bladder	Smooth muscle wall relaxed / Sphincter closed
		Sex organs and genitalia	Generally vasoconstriction

Superior cervical ganglion

Coeliac ganglion

Superior mesenteric ganglion

Inferior mesenteric ganglion

T1 1 2 3 4 5 6 7 8 9 10 11 12

L1 L2 L3 1 2 3

Figure 1.2 The sympathetic outflow, the main structures supplied and the effects of stimulation. Solid lines ——, preganglionic fibres; broken lines ---, postganglionic fibres. (From Waugh & Grant 2001.)

and acid secretion are associated with parasympathetic dominance, yet the conditions of asthma and gastric ulcer are often relieved by relaxation and aggravated by stress. The theory is not consistent regarding these conditions (Ch. 27, p. 232).

The endocrine system

Closely associated with the autonomic nervous system are the endocrine system and the adrenal glands. These are situated above the kidneys (Fig. 1.4) and consist of medulla and cortex (Fig. 1.5). Their function is to produce hormones which modify

the action of the internal organs in response to environmental stimuli.

When a situation is perceived to be stressful the brain immediately responds by stimulating the adrenal medulla to release the catecholamines adrenaline and noradrenaline. The function of these neurotransmitters is to prepare the organs for action by, for example, increasing alertness and redistributing the blood. Acting in the longer term, the pituitary gland releases the adrenocorticotrophic hormone (ACTH). This stimulates the adrenal cortex to produce mineralocorticoids and glucocorticoids, the most important of which is cortisol, which

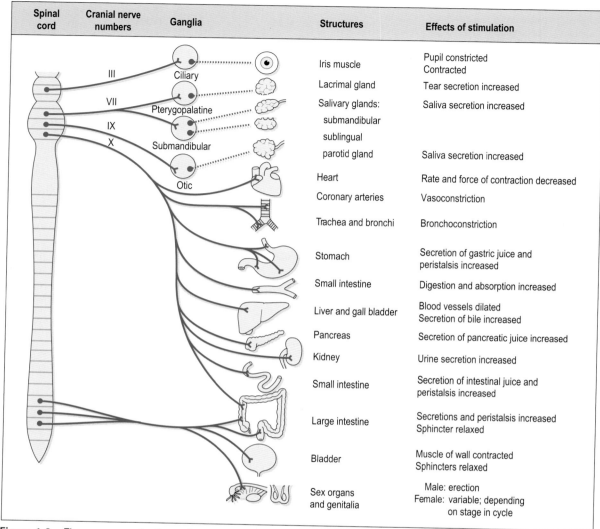

Spinal cord	Cranial nerve numbers	Ganglia	Structures	Effects of stimulation
	III	Ciliary	Iris muscle	Pupil constricted Contracted
	VII	Pterygopalatine	Lacrimal gland	Tear secretion increased
	IX		Salivary glands: submandibular sublingual	Saliva secretion increased
	X	Submandibular	parotid gland	Saliva secretion increased
		Otic	Heart	Rate and force of contraction decreased
			Coronary arteries	Vasoconstriction
			Trachea and bronchi	Bronchoconstriction
			Stomach	Secretion of gastric juice and peristalsis increased
			Small intestine	Digestion and absorption increased
			Liver and gall bladder	Blood vessels dilated Secretion of bile increased
			Pancreas	Secretion of pancreatic juice increased
			Kidney	Urine secretion increased
			Small intestine	Secretion of intestinal juice and peristalsis increased
			Large intestine	Secretions and peristalsis increased Sphincter relaxed
			Bladder	Muscle of wall contracted Sphincters relaxed
			Sex organs and genitalia	Male: erection Female: variable; depending on stage in cycle

Figure 1.3 The parasympathetic outflow, the main structures supplied and the effects of stimulation. Solid lines ——, preganglionic fibres; broken lines ---, postganglionic fibres. (From Waugh & Grant 2001.)

helps to maintain the fuel supply to the muscles. In this way it supports the action of the cate-cholamines (Waugh & Grant 2001) (Fig. 1.6). There is also evidence suggesting that the stimulation of normal levels of cortisol enhances the immune system (Looker & Gregson 1989, Jefferies 1991). High levels of cortisol, such as those created by prolonged stress or by pharmacological doses are, however, associated with a suppressed immune system.

Under challenge, all the above hormones are released. When the situation of challenge passes,

and the stress response is no longer needed, the neurotransmitter acetylcholine is released to restore a state of balance in the autonomic nervous system. The organs which were previously stimulated now weaken their hold and their actions subside.

The skeletal musculature

Jacobson (1938) proposed that the release of tension in the skeletal musculature had the effect of calming the mind. The neuromuscular system is thus

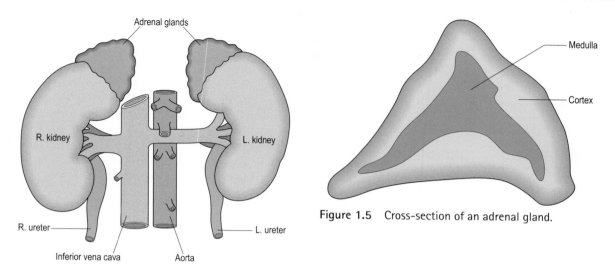

Figure 1.5 Cross-section of an adrenal gland.

Figure 1.4 The positions of the adrenal glands and some of their associated structures. (From Wilson 1990.)

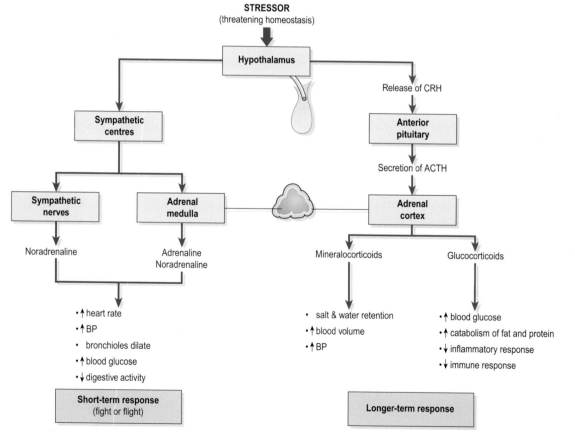

Figure 1.6 Responses to stressors that threaten homeostasis. CRH, corticotrophin releasing hormone; ACTH, adrenocorticotrophic hormone. (From Waugh & Grant 2001.)

seen as a mediator in the relief of stress and anxiety. Jacobson's method, progressive relaxation, consists of tense–release techniques designed to cultivate awareness of muscular sensations. This awareness allows the individual to develop the skill of consciously releasing tension (Ch. 4).

PSYCHOLOGICAL THEORIES

Three types of psychological theory concerning relaxation are discussed in this section:

- cognitive
- behaviour
- cognitive behaviour.

Cognitive theories

'Our thoughts define our universe' writes Piero Ferrucci in *What We May Be* (1982). The way we view what happens to us determines how we feel about it. This idea epitomizes the cognitive approach, which sees feeling as a function of thought. Interpretations, perceptions, assumptions and conclusions will all give rise to particular feelings, which in their turn govern our behaviour. This means that our experience of stress and anxiety is related to the way we interpret events in our lives: we may, for example, appraise situations in ways which make them appear unnecessarily threatening (Lazarus & Folkman 1984).

Ellis (1962, 1976), a psychotherapist, attributes much anxiety to the irrational responses made by individuals, and cites the following example:

> If person X puts me off, it must mean she doesn't like me, and if she doesn't like me it's probably because I'm unlikeable.

In this example the individual is basing his view of himself on one isolated event. Ellis also indicates that such a person tends to think in terms of absolutes, for example: 'I must be liked by everyone, otherwise I'll feel worthless'. An individual locked into this pattern of thinking is doomed to disappointment and anxiety because of the impossible standards he has set for himself.

Treatment consists in identifying the irrational beliefs, challenging them and considering more rational alternatives. These ideas form the basis of Ellis's rational emotive therapy.

Beck (1984), a contemporary psychiatrist, also sees anxiety (and depression) as stemming from wrong thinking. To Beck, the distress is created by faulty thinking patterns which allow the individual to have a distorted view of events. For example:

- An individual blames himself whenever something goes wrong although he is not responsible.
- He feels he is unemployable after one job rejection.
- He blows up a minor mistake into a catastrophe: accidentally scratching his car, he sees it as irredeemably damaged.

Such a person tends to magnify his weaknesses and to see his minor mistakes as disasters; he dwells on his failures and dismisses his achievements. The first step in therapy is to identify the automatic thoughts that make up the faulty thinking patterns. This is done by keeping a diary of anxiety-related events together with the thoughts and fantasies which accompany them. These thoughts are then tested against reality by asking what evidence there is to justify them. Are they plausible? Does it matter if what he fears happens? If the automatic thoughts do not stand up to reality testing, he will need to modify them. Some thought patterns may need to become more positive and less negative, but the principal aim is to help the individual adopt a more realistic view of himself, his world and his future (Beck 1976).

Recognition of the value of Beck's cognitive therapy is increasing. Its effects have been compared with those of pharmacological treatments, behaviour therapy, supportive non-directive therapy and anxiety management, and found to be either superior or of equal efficacy (Beck et al 1979, Durham & Turvey 1987, Blackburn & Davidson 1990).

Both Ellis and Beck see the individual as having control over his thoughts, and thus having the power to modify his feelings and his behaviour if he wants to. Their models are respectively concerned with challenging irrational thoughts and questioning faulty thinking patterns. Such approaches belong to the area of cognitive restructuring, i.e. the combatting of 'self-defeating thought patterns by reordering the client's perceptions, values and attitudes' (Lichstein 1988). Although their theories are similar in many ways, their styles of therapy differ; Ellis adopts a confrontational approach while Beck is more collaborative (Neimeyer 1985).

While cognitive theory is referred to several times in this book, the theories of Beck and Ellis are particularly relevant to the chapters on stress (Ch. 3), goal-directed visualization (Ch. 18) and cognitive behavioural therapy (Ch. 22).

Also influential in this field is Kelly (1955, 1969), whose theory of personal constructs offers a different approach. To Kelly, interpretations are not irrational or illogical, so much as the product of the way each individual construes the world. If the individual has problems, Kelly helps him work out alternative ways of looking at the world, and he does this by attempting to enter the individual's frame of reference (Neimeyer 1985). His approach is thus essentially explorative.

While sharing the view that the interpretation of events can be as important as the events themselves, Kelly has rejected the label 'cognitive theorist'. Such a label has, in the past, implied that cognitions and emotions could be studied separately, while to Kelly they are components of a single psychological entity. The climate has, however, changed in recent decades, as cognitive theorists in general have come to see emotion and cognition as 'intricately and intimately intertwined' (Strongman 1987).

A further researcher whose work has been influential in the cognitive field is Seligman (1975). He focused on the degree of control which a person perceived himself to have over his environment. People who lacked this kind of control were subject to a state he termed 'learned helplessness' which predisposed them to depression.

Cognitive methods may be seen to include most approaches involving the mind. Thus, self-talk and mental diversion are cognitive, as are other techniques which aim to restructure the thoughts. Some of these, however, are less amenable to scientific investigation than the structured approach of Beck.

Behaviour theory

Behaviour theory, by contrast, is concerned with observable actions. Discounting what goes on in the mind, it sees behaviour as conditioned by environmental events. Such events are seen as leading the individual to act in predictable ways. In the case of classical conditioning, behaviour is governed by associations; for example, Pavlov's dog learned to salivate at the sound of a bell because the bell was linked with the smell of food. In the case of operant conditioning, behaviour is governed by a system of reinforcement (Skinner 1938). Positive reinforcement refers to action which increases the likelihood of a certain behaviour, for example, giving a dog a biscuit every time it brings back a thrown ball. Negative reinforcement refers to the withdrawal of certain action, in order to extinguish a behaviour, for example, no biscuit, no retrieval of ball. Together, these two concepts can be used to shape behaviour.

Since these theories were first propounded, behaviour theory has developed in ways which take it away from its original reductionist models. However, it still retains its central principle, that observable behaviour is more worthy of investigation than behaviour which is only inferred, i.e. mental processes.

Behavioural approaches include muscular relaxation, distraction, graded exposure and social skills training. Muscular relaxation is described in the early chapters of this book; distraction consists of activity which diverts the attention; graded exposure offers a step-by-step approach towards mastery over a feared object or situation; and social skills training concerns interpersonal communication and covers verbal and non-verbal behaviour. Assertiveness techniques, developed in the 1970s by Alberti & Emmons, are a central component of social skills training. These writers define the concept as behaviour where people are acting in their best interests without experiencing undue anxiety and without denying the rights of others (Alberti & Emmons 1982). Topics included in assertiveness training are:

- exercising personal rights
- setting personal priorities
- expressing views
- making requests
- refusing requests
- countering manipulative behaviour in others
- allowing oneself to make mistakes.

Behaviour styles can range from aggressive to submissive, but the style of choice in most situations is the assertive one. Knowing when and how to use it is one of the social skills.

It can be seen from the above items that assertiveness training contains a strong cognitive element and that there is a certain overlap between cognitive and behavioural methods. This has led some researchers to combine the two approaches.

Cognitive behaviour theory

A belief that behaviourism as a general theory was incomplete led to the formal integration of cognitive and behaviourist principles (Reber & Reber 2001). Early proponents of this integration were Meichenbaum & Cameron (1974) whose aim was to promote behavioural change through the restructuring of conscious thoughts and to weave these into the behaviourist approach. Behaviour was seen as largely governed by the 'self-talk' in which we engage. This is the internal dialogue we conduct with ourselves in order to interpret the world. If the self-talk is positive, the outcome of a given task tends to be viewed in positive terms; if the self-talk is negative, the outcome tends to be viewed in negative terms. Positive self-talk leads to goal achievement and increased confidence; negative self-talk to feelings of defeat. The approach was designed to give the individual a feeling of greater control over his life and a protection against unnecessary stress.

In this, and in a later publication (Meichenbaum & Cameron 1983), three phases were planned. Phase one was educative and aimed at developing awareness of thoughts, feelings, sensations and behaviours; the individual identified his self-talk. In phase two he restructured his self-talk, converting responses from negative to positive, while other coping skills such as problem solving, relaxation, assertiveness and distraction were learned and practised. Finally, in phase three, these new responses and skills were applied to events through mental rehearsal, role play and graded exposure.

The approach has been taken up and developed by Beck who has carried it forward in a series of publications over the years. Research has shown it to be at least as effective as medication in a wide range of anxiety disorders (Blackburn & Twaddle 1996, Davis et al 2000).

Cognitive behavioural principles are described in Chapter 22. They also underlie some of the stress-relieving strategies in Chapter 3 and feature in the goal-directed visualizations in Chapter 18.

THE 'SPECIFIC EFFECTS' HYPOTHESIS AND UNITARY THEORIES

Anxiety can express itself in any of three modes: the somatic (physiological), the cognitive (psychological) and the behavioural (observable actions). It has been proposed that the pattern of changes produced by cognitive techniques will be different from those produced by physiological techniques, so that an anxiety which expresses itself in a physiological mode will require a different approach from one which expresses itself in a cognitive mode. This is the 'specific effects' hypothesis (Davidson & Schwartz 1976) and it states that benefit can be derived from matching the treatment to the problem. For example, tension headache will be more likely to respond to a somatic approach, such as releasing muscle tension, than to a cognitive one, such as correcting faulty thinking patterns (Lehrer 1996, Yung et al 2001). Thus training in one mode is inappropriate if anxiety manifests itself in another. Table 1.1 groups relaxation methods according to the presenting mode of anxiety. It is only a rough classification since some approaches, e.g. autogenics, operate in more than one mode. Even the pre-eminently somatic method of progressive relaxation contains cognitive elements, by virtue of the attention that is focused on muscle sensations (Ch. 4).

In contrast, unitary models propose a nonspecific relaxation effect resulting from any one method. Benson's 'relaxation response' (Benson et al 1974) is such a one, based on the hypothesis that all relaxation techniques evoke a common integrated response of reduced sympathetic arousal (Ch. 21). There is no separation of body and mind. Jacobson's (1938) progressive relaxation method is also based on unitary theory, in that the release of muscle tension is seen as creating a generalized and non-specific state of relaxation (Ch. 4).

Table 1.1 Modes of anxiety and appropriate relaxation methods according to the 'specific effects' hypothesis (Adapted from Davidson & Schwartz 1976)

Somatic	Progressive relaxation
	Applied relaxation
	Mitchell's relaxation
	Breathing
Cognitive	Cognitive restructuring
	Imagery
	Self-statements
	Meditation
Behavioural	Behavioural relaxation training
	Social skills
Cognitive and somatic	Autogenics

The gulf between the 'specific effects' and 'generalized' theories narrowed somewhat when it was proposed that the specific effects themselves might be superimposed on a general relaxation response, i.e. that any relaxation technique, to some extent, created a general effect, on which was superimposed a specific pattern of changes elicited by the particular technique employed (Schwartz et al 1978).

Current thinking favours a model in which interactions occur between somatic and cognitive processes; for example, a painful joint is not simply a physical symptom but one which also involves psychological factors such as worry. This view constitutes the transactional model (Lazarus & Folkman 1984).

The mechanism underpinning these models, however, is far from being fully understood. Smith et al (1996) suggest that one problem lies in the tendency for relaxation to be seen exclusively in terms of arousal reduction. They point to a variety of cognitive and spiritual elements which also feature in the experience and which lead them to conclude that relaxation is a richly differentiated state, far more complex than the simple reduction of arousal. In their model (the Attentional Behavioural Cognitive relaxation model), 15 relaxation state categories are identified (Smith 2001). These are: sleepiness, disengagement, physical relaxation, mental quiet, rested/refreshed, at ease/peace, positive detachment, energized, joy, thankfulness

and love, mystery, awe and wonder, prayerfulness, timeless/boundless/infinite, aware. Smith and colleagues propose that each relaxation technique evokes its own characteristic responses or combination of responses from the above list. Their work raises questions such as what clients understand by the word 'relax', and what trainers mean when they ask people to relax.

CASE SCENARIOS

Two examples will serve to illustrate how theory can inform practice. The first concerns a 55-year-old male office worker with tension headaches associated with pain in his neck and shoulders. The second relates to a 35-year-old housewife with agoraphobia. They would each benefit from a course of relaxation training but, whereas the first is a relatively straightforward problem, the second has more complex requirements.

Tension headache

This is a condition of physiological origin involving the neck and shoulder muscles. A muscular relaxation technique, such as progressive relaxation (Chs 4–8), would have the effect of relaxing his neck and shoulder region, which might relieve pressure on the nerves causing the headache. Seen in this light, the relaxation technique is having a specific effect on the factor causing the headache. However, since progressive relaxation is based on a unitary theory whereby a generalized effect extends from a single technique, a degree of mental relaxation would also be expected to occur which might additionally help to relieve the tension headache. Progress could be charted by electromyography.

Agoraphobia

In contrast with the above is the case of the woman suffering from agoraphobia. The condition dates from a visit to the local supermarket 8 months previously when she accidentally knocked over a stand of tins. The incident attracted the attention of management and shoppers and she felt acutely embarrassed. Since that occasion she has not been back and has become increasingly tied to the house.

This problem calls for a more elaborate programme featuring a cognitive approach. Beck's work has much to offer here. He proposes that her condition stems from faulty patterns of thinking, such as believing that the incident is bound to happen again or that her apprehension heralds a heart attack. She is asked whether she thinks such thoughts are justified and to make a point of testing them against reality. For example, it is very unlikely that she will knock over a second stand, and what does it matter if she does? Or, what evidence is there that she has a weak heart? She is encouraged to collect her unrealistic, negative thoughts in a diary and subject them one-by-one to a challenging process. This leads to a cognitive restructuring.

Behavioural strategies, such as graded exposure to the feared situation, can be incorporated into the cognitive programme. However, since real-life exposure initially creates a sense of high threat, visualizations and relaxation training can provide a useful preliminary (Ch. 18).

Having experienced success in her visualizations, the client could then be introduced to the situation in real life. This is often done in stages, with intermediate goals. She might on the first occasion simply step out into the street; on subsequent occasions she would travel ever nearer to the supermarket, and eventually go through the check-out. Whereas in the early stages she is accompanied, later stages will see her coping on her own. Her progress throughout could be charted on the Hospital Anxiety and Depression Scale (Ch. 24).

As this case has a strong psychological component, treatment could be linked with the work of the clinical psychologist or the community mental health team.

STRESS MANAGEMENT

Relaxation training is often viewed as one component of a more comprehensive package, variously referred to as stress management, anxiety management or stress inoculation (Powell & Enright 1990, Keable 1997). What, however, *is* stress management? There is no precise definition because it is not a specific treatment and there is no one standard method. Rather, it is a general approach which offers coping skills.

However, the varying methods do contain common threads, delineated by Lichstein (1988). There is always some element of each of the following:

- Cognitive restructuring: modifying conscious thought patterns in order to promote more successful behaviours.
- Relaxation for reducing physiological arousal.
- Social skills and assertiveness training to enhance interpersonal communication.
- Self-monitoring. This consists of recognizing the items which cause stress, recording their occurrence and noting the level of stress which they generate. Self-monitoring encourages an individual to take a more objective view of himself as well as charting his progress. It has been found that the very fact of monitoring increases the likelihood of desired behaviour occurring and decreases the likelihood of undesired behaviour occurring, in a phenomenon known as the 'reactivity of monitoring' (Hiebert & Fox 1981).

TYPES OF RELAXATION TECHNIQUE

Thus, relaxation is only one component of stress management. The present work focuses on that component, setting out a variety of methods and techniques. These techniques are drawn from recognized sources and appear in slightly paraphrased versions of the originals. One chapter is devoted to each method which is described and presented in a step-by-step manner. Rationale is contained in a short paragraph near the beginning and the chapter ends with a section on evidence relating to the effectiveness of the method. However, evidence to support the techniques is limited and cannot in all cases be used to inform the rationale. For this reason, the rationale has been kept separate from the research. In each chapter the reader is directed to available research, but it is beyond the scope of this book to provide a systematic review of the literature. In this connection, the reader is referred to the critical review of Kerr (2000) whose paper covered progressive relaxation, Mitchell's method, massage, the Alexander technique, Benson's method and Hatha Yoga. Appendix 4 contains a table of existing reviews from which it can be seen that not all techniques have been systematically reviewed and this limits the drawing of conclusions in this field.

The purpose of the book is to provide a compendium of different relaxation techniques and to describe them in relation to their underpinning rationales. The range is not comprehensive: methods which require specialized training such as hypnosis and advanced autogenics, or elaborate apparatus such as biofeedback, are left out. In general, choice has been governed by factors of practicality such as the following, that the method should:

- be easily learned and applied
- not require specialized expertise on the part of the trainer
- not require elaborate equipment
- be convenient for use with small groups
- be suitable for all ages.

'DEEP' AND 'BRIEF' RELAXATION

Lichstein (1988) distinguishes between methods which create 'deep relaxation' and those which create 'brief relaxation'. Deep relaxation refers to procedures which induce an effect of large magnitude, and which are carried out in a calm environment with the trainee lying down, e.g. progressive relaxation and autogenic training. Brief relaxation refers to techniques (often contracted versions of the above) which produce immediate effects and can be used when the individual is faced with stressful events; the object here is the rapid release of excess tension. Thus, whereas deep relaxation refers to a full process of total-body relaxation, brief relaxation applies these procedures in everyday life.

SOMATIC AND COGNITIVE TECHNIQUES

Most methods, whether deep or brief, fall roughly into one of the two broad categories: somatic and cognitive. The somatic methods presented in this book are:

- Jacobson's progressive relaxation (1938)
- Bernstein & Borkovec's modified version (1973)

- Everly & Rosenfeld's passive relaxation (1981)
- Madders' release-only (1981)
- Öst's applied relaxation (1987)
- Poppen's behavioural relaxation training (1988)
- the Mitchell method (1987)
- the Alexander technique (1932)
- differential relaxation
- stretchings
- exercise
- breathing methods.

The cognitive methods are:

- self-awareness
- imagery
- goal-directed visualization
- autogenic training (Schultz & Luthe 1969)
- meditation
- Benson's relaxation response (1976)
- cognitive behavioural approaches.

A table summarizing the principles of each method and suggesting applications for its use may be found in Appendix 3.

SKILL ACQUISITION AND MOTOR LEARNING THEORY

Relaxation training involves the learning of skills. As a number of relaxation techniques are somatic in nature, i.e. focusing on muscles rather than thoughts, the principles of motor learning apply. Here, learning is defined as having stages, of which Schmidt (1998) delineates three: a verbal-cognitive one, a motor one and an autonomous one. In the verbal-cognitive one the individual learns how to perform the motor task; he repeatedly talks himself through the action, imagining the task without actually performing it. In the motor stage the individual learns how to perform the physical action as the mentally rehearsed material is converted into muscular activity. The autonomous stage sees a refining of the newly acquired skill, as execution of the movement becomes automatic. Wishart et al (2000) condense the stages into two: a cognitive and an automatic one.

The learning process is aided by a system of feedback, both intrinsic and extrinsic, which helps the individual to make necessary corrections, while motivation is maintained by record-keeping. Practice is an essential feature of motor learning and must be carried out daily if mastery of the skill is to be achieved.

Further reading

Physiological and psychological background

Smith E E, Nolen-Hoeksema S, Fredrickson B 2002 Atkinson & Hilgard's introduction to psychology, 13th edn. Harcourt Brace, Fort Worth

Waugh A, Grant A 2001 Ross & Wilson anatomy and physiology in health and illness, 9th edn. Elsevier Science, Edinburgh, Ch 9

Relaxation and stress management

Payne R A 2004 Relaxation techniques. In: Kolt G, Andersen M (eds) Psychology in the physical and manual therapies. Churchill Livingstone, Edinburgh, Ch 9

Powell T J, Enright S J 1990 Anxiety and stress management. Routledge, London

Reilly C M 2002 Relaxation: a concept analysis. Graduate Research in Nursing 2(1): 1–12

Chapter 2

General aspects of relaxation training

CHAPTER CONTENTS

Aspects of relaxation training which apply to all approaches are discussed here and include setting, confidentiality, position, introductory remarks, delivery, termination, number of sessions, homework, the therapist, supervisory back-up and pitfalls. Working with groups is then considered.

ASPECTS OF PROCEDURE

SETTING

Most authors advise a quiet, warm setting, free from disturbance. However, others favour one that bears more resemblance to the normal environment, on the grounds that the relaxation skills learned will be more readily transferred to real life, and also that too heavy a silence is artificial, or even anxiety-inducing. For these reasons a background which includes faint external sounds may be deliberately sought.

ESTABLISHING CONFIDENTIALITY

In the case of group work, confidentiality must be established at the outset and re-established each time a new member joins. Confidentiality in this context means that nothing of a self-disclosing nature made by any member of the group is referred to outside the session. Topics can be discussed outside but only in a general sense.

POSITION

For deep relaxation lying is preferable to sitting, since a totally supported body will more readily lose its tension. However, some people, for different reasons, do not like lying. Another drawback of the lying position is a tendency on the part of the trainee to fall asleep (p. 21). In defence of sitting, however, it can be argued that the skill of relaxing transfers to everyday situations more effectively if it is taught in a position in which stress is more likely to occur, i.e. sitting rather than lying. Thus it can be seen that both positions have value and may be used on different occasions during tuition.

Various starting positions will be mentioned in later chapters. Mitchell (p. 84) lists three: lying supine, sitting and leaning forward with the arms and head supported on a high surface, and sitting with the back and head supported (1987). Jacobson (1938) mentions two: lying and sitting (p. 34); Bernstein & Borkovec (1973) favour a reclining chair or an easy chair with a footstool (p. 45), as also does Poppen (1988) (p. 76). When lying on the floor, participants may find it comfortable to place a pillow under the knees as well as the head.

Many groups meet in public buildings, such as schools or church halls, where the floors are wooden or tiled. These are hard, but a length of foam or a beach mattress provides a suitably softer surface and can be supplied at very little cost by the participant himself. Women will find trousers more comfortable than a skirt for most of the exercises.

Whether the eyes are open or closed is determined by the nature of the approach and the preference of the trainee.

INTRODUCING THE METHOD TO PARTICIPANTS

A short introduction will help to put the client at his ease.

> Injury and illness can create stress, I think you'll agree. Stress is uncomfortable. It also interferes with the body's healing mechanisms because energy is diverted from the healing process to the maintenance of a state of high alert. To reduce this state of high alert we need to promote a calm body and mind. Relaxation techniques can help to

> achieve this. There are different kinds of relaxation technique. Some involve the muscles and breathing pattern while others involve the thoughts in the head. Often both are involved.

When presenting any particular method it is believed that clients want to know two things above all others: that the approach is well established and that it works (Lichstein 1988). A short rationale addressed to the client is therefore appropriate. In addition, for the benefit of any trainees who fear that they are going to be hypnotized, Hendler & Redd (1986) suggest adding a disclaimer to reassure participants that such is not the purpose. It can also reduce the possibility of unintentional trance induction.

A sample introduction might be:

> This relaxation procedure is one that has been practised for x [number of] years. It has been studied by researchers and found to be effective. You will feel very relaxed and calm as a result. It is not the same as hypnosis, neither will you lose consciousness at any point.

As some techniques involve the musculature, the concept of muscle action could be described, as in the paragraph below.

Muscle action

> When a muscle contracts, its fibres shorten, making the muscle fat. On relaxing, the muscle returns to a resting state in which the fibres are by comparison long and thin. A contracting muscle feels hard to the touch. You can illustrate this by taking your thumb across the palm of your hand and, using the fingers of the other hand, feel the muscle below the thumb getting hard. Now, relax the thumb, and feel the muscle below it become soft.
>
> This exercise demonstrates that the relaxation, as well as the contraction of skeletal muscles, is under the control of the will.

The introductory passages above need only be stated once; however, one of the two following passages may be used every time a session begins. These are used to help create the mood for relaxation by gently leading the trainee into a calm frame of mind. The first approach is called 'sinking' and the second 'imaginary bubble'. It is not necessary to use both.

Sinking

> Make yourself as comfortable as you can ... become aware of the surface underneath you ... let your body settle into it ... notice how it supports you ... notice the points of contact between you and the floor: your head ... shoulders ... spine ... ribs ... hips ... heels ... elbows ... forearms and hands ... feel your body sinking into the surface you are lying on ... feel the tension leaving it ... your body getting heavier as the tension ebbs away ... feel at peace ... Take one good breath and as you let it out, feel it carrying all your tensions away ... then let your breathing settle into a gentle rhythm ...

Imaginary bubble

> As you lie or sit, reflect on the idea that you are going to give the next half-hour to yourself. No telephone can ring for you; no doorbell disturb you; no-one will call your name. You may hear sounds around you: voices, horns, sirens, bangs and revs ... think of them as being outside your world. With these thoughts in mind, draw an imaginary circle around yourself, about three feet from the centre. Create an imaginary bubble ... think of the interior as *your* space ... your own private space. Feel how safe it is ... safe to get in touch with yourself. Turn your thoughts inwards.

DELIVERY

Any relaxation procedure calls for a tone of voice that is quiet and calm. That does not imply that it should be hypnotic. Bernstein & Borkovec suggest that the tone should be conversational to begin with, but that the volume and pace of speech should be gradually reduced as the session wears on. They advise a tone which is, 'smooth and quiet, perhaps even monotonous, but not purposely hypnotic' (Bernstein & Borkovec 1973).

The pauses between instructions should always be long to give the trainees time to carry out the action or to evoke the image. Dots in the text indicate these pauses.

The 'live' voice is more effective at inducing relaxation than the taped voice (Paul & Trimble 1970, Beiman et al 1978, Hillenberg & Collins 1982). Tapes are not recommended for teaching (Lichstein 1988). They may, however, have value; for example, a trainee might learn initially from the live voice, then continue at home with a tape (preferably one containing the trainer's voice) until he knows the technique (Borkovec & Sides 1979). A disadvantage of tapes is that the individual may become dependent on them and unable to relax without them. Any advantage that tapes have in controlling the verbal aspect of the instruction is more relevant to research than to therapy.

TERMINATION

All deep relaxation procedures should be brought to a gradual end, allowing the participant to make a slow return to the alert state. A variety of methods are described throughout this book. Some practitioners use a counting process; others, a simple sentence such as: 'When you feel ready, please open your eyes and sit up'. Some teachers recommend bending and stretching the limbs, while others advise sitting quietly for a few minutes. Most of the relaxation approaches mentioned in this book carry their own form of termination. The following is a sample procedure:

> I am going to bring this relaxation session to an end ... I'd like you gradually to become aware of your surroundings ... feel the floor/chair underneath you ... in your own time open your eyes ... give your limbs a few gentle stretches ... make a few fists to stir up the circulation ... have the feeling that you are alert and ready to carry on with your life ...

Termination is sometimes referred to as 'arousal' or 'return to everyday activity'. In autogenic training it is called a cancellation.

DEBRIEFING

At the end of a relaxation session there is a debriefing process, the object being twofold: to make the experience more satisfying for the client and to provide the therapist with feedback. The therapist might open the discussion with questions such as: 'How did you find that experience?',

'Did it make you feel more relaxed?', 'Did you find the technique easy to follow?', 'Was anything about it confusing?', 'Were you able to relate to the different body parts?'. Plenty of time should be allotted to the debriefing section to give the client opportunity to express his reactions or confide his experiences, all of which help the therapist to understand her client better. Information gathered in this way helps to increase the success of the following session.

HOMEWORK

Emphasis is placed on homework in every method of relaxation training as it leads to greater skill in using the technique. Skill is important because stress-related behaviour patterns tend to be resistant to change. Experienced use of the technique therefore increases its effectiveness.

Skill is built up by practice (see Ch. 1, Motor learning theory). Only by regular and frequent practice will behavioural change take place. The need to practise, therefore, is paramount, a point that needs bringing out as trainees do not always appreciate its need. Investigating this topic in 1983, Hillenberg & Collins found significant levels of non-compliance in the home practice component of their study.

One way of increasing motivation is by introducing the record sheet or diary as a form of self-monitoring (see Ch. 1, Stress management). Regular, time-recorded entries of homework sessions and their outcomes are made on the sheet by the trainee and these provide feedback and encourage the trainee to continue. As it is important that these practice sessions fit in with the trainee's daily routine, convenient times can be discussed at the outset of treatment. Figure 8.3 (p. 71) offers a useful model.

The frequency and duration of homework are conventionally set at two periods a day, each lasting 15 minutes (Bernstein & Borkovec 1973). Whether or not this should be carried out soon after meals has been debated, the above researchers pointing to the benefits of postprandial low arousal. Others, however, favour avoidance of that time: Benson (1976) suggests that the process of digestion interferes with the physiological changes associated with meditation (Ch. 21).

Lichstein (1988), however, advises trainees to experiment and find the times that best suit them.

When the tuition course has come to an end, trainees are urged to continue practising, perhaps in some less frequent form, so that the benefits of training are not lost.

NUMBER OF SESSIONS

It is possible to learn most methods in about six sessions, assuming that attention is given to home practice. Transcendental meditation can be taught in six, and progressive relaxation in five to ten sessions (Lichstein 1988). Many relaxation courses, however, cover several methods, and may do more than simply teach relaxation. They may include group discussion, topics (see p. 27), mutual support and other concerns, thus extending the duration of the course beyond six sessions.

THE TRAINER/INSTRUCTOR/THERAPIST

On the thorny question of training, Luthe (1970), referring to autogenics, insists that only medically qualified practitioners are equipped to teach. Lichstein (1988) has viewed this position as untenable, believing that health care professionals have much to offer, provided they use their judgement and recognize the limits of their training. He feels that the interests of society are best served by allowing and even encouraging such individuals to teach relaxation methods.

The requirements for therapists who wish to teach relaxation methods include:

1. basic training as a health care professional
2. professional experience with the type of group with whom they are working
3. arrangements for supervision on a regular basis (see below)
4. recognition that relaxation therapy is not a panacea, while it can be a powerful tool.

A therapist is further advised to carry out three measures (Lichstein 1988):

1. to study beforehand the method she plans to use
2. to experience the method herself, as a trainee
3. to practise the method on friends, relatives or colleagues in order to build up a skilful presentation.

Today, however, there are validated courses on relaxation techniques which interested therapists are strongly advised to attend and, as relaxation training, in some form or other, has traditionally featured in the core training of many health care professionals, the therapy clinic becomes an appropriate setting for such work with clients (Potter & Grove 1999).

SUPERVISORY BACK-UP

Essential to both group and individual relaxation therapy is the provision of supervisory back-up for the therapist. Its main purpose is to strengthen and maintain her skills, which in turn ensure the value of the treatment received by the client.

Supervision also helps to protect the therapist from emotional fatigue by providing an opportunity for her to release her own tensions, thereby guarding against the state of burn-out or exhausted empathy. Supervision performs another function, namely, in helping the therapist to handle her reactions if old wounds are re-opened during treatment, as they can be when past emotional experiences are stirred by listening to other people recounting theirs. Contact with a more experienced colleague is useful for resolving these and other problems which may arise in the course of work.

Finding a supervisor is the responsibility of the therapist.

PITFALLS

Relaxation training includes techniques which can have powerful effects. It therefore needs to be handled responsibly and with due regard to the attendant pitfalls. These are discussed in the relevant chapters. It is essential, before taking up any method, to become aware of its pitfalls.

MEASUREMENT

Measurement, both physiological and psychological, plays an essential role and is discussed in Chapter 26.

AUTONOMY OF THE INDIVIDUAL

A central feature of relaxation training is that the individual is seen as a self-determining being.

Throughout all procedures he remains self-aware and free of control by outside forces. The state of relaxation he achieves is his own making. In so doing he assumes ownership of this state and responsibility for the progress he makes. Relaxation training is firmly rooted in this principle.

WORKING WITH GROUPS

The material in the succeeding chapters may be used with individuals or with groups of people. As group work is a subject on its own, a short summary will be relevant. Groups, in this context, may be of three kinds.

Led. Here a leader offers a previously prepared programme. Although it is presented in a systematic way, the leader displays flexibility when appropriate.

Facilitated. Responsibility for the group is taken by a particular individual who, at the same time, imposes no strict format. The facilitator helps to steer the group in the way the members have decided it shall go, but she avoids telling them what to do. Her role is to suggest possibilities. If problems arise, however, she is responsible for dealing with them.

Self-help. There is no designated leader or facilitator. The style is informal but the members are usually highly committed, attending as they do for mutual help and support. Relevant information is collected for circulation among them and their experiences are shared. A role of acting facilitator is often rotated.

Lichstein (1988) considers that the group format is an effective way of delivering relaxation. The led group particularly lends itself to this function since an entire course can be worked out in advance. Relaxation training also occurs in facilitated and self-help groups; however, since the facilitators may not have had relevant training and experience, extra care should be taken in observing the pitfalls.

ORGANIZATION

Starting a group is one matter, but keeping it going can be more difficult. In order to build up and maintain group bonding, certain points need attention.

1. *Establishing and maintaining confidentiality.* The need for confidentiality was mentioned above. It is repeated here as it cannot be overstated.

2. *Course programme.*   A knowledge of what to expect enables members to make plans. Dates should be supplied in advance together with, in the case of a formal course, a syllabus.

Some classes offer relaxation alone; others begin each session with a topic related to the needs of the participants (p. 27), before moving into the area of relaxation itself.

3. *Client choice.*   The sense of belonging to the group is enhanced if members are given some choice in the way it is run. How much choice depends on the nature of the group: in the formal led group, less choice may be appropriate than in the informal self-help group. However, choice can still be introduced into the formal group by finding out from the members at the outset why they joined and what they hope to get out of the meetings. This strategy helps the instructor to meet their needs and provides the participants with a more rewarding experience.

A system of paper slips can be used to collect the written answers. The alternative is to ask members directly. However, many people find it threatening to have to voice their private thoughts in front of strangers; such an approach may also be non-productive if it draws false replies. In the author's experience, people prefer not to be asked such questions in front of a group, but respond more favourably to the paper slip system (Payne 1989).

4. *Ice-breakers.*   These are strategies for relaxing the atmosphere. Their essential characteristic is that the members physically participate. Some are designed for use in pairs while others involve the whole group. An example of the first is seen when one member of each pair tells the other about something pleasant that happened in the previous week; then they switch over. Another example of working in pairs is when person A talks to person B for two minutes, telling him who she is and what she does. Then B talks to A.

Whole group activities are particularly useful for learning people's names. Remocker & Storch (1992) suggest a game in which each member wears a name tag. The aim is to collect everyone's name in the shortest time.

5. *Discussion.*   Exchanging information and sharing experiences are features of the group debriefing period and give the session an extra dimension. The therapist now occupies the role of facilitator, maintaining the focus of the group and seeing that all members who wish to, get a chance to express their views. Clients tend to enjoy the discussion and normally display an eagerness to take part. There may, however, be a short period before clients have learned to trust each other when a natural reticence holds them back from disclosing personal information. This can cause the discussion to dry up. It can be revived by adopting the strategy of 'circular questions' (Powell & Enright 1990). This entails drawing one participant into conversation with another, for example: 'Peter, you've been in this situation. What would you say to Jenny who is going through the same experience?'. In most circumstances, however, the discussion period helps to hold the group together.

Although the discussion period has value, participants should not feel under any obligation to take part. The voluntary principle, which states that pressure should never be exerted on individuals, must be upheld (Heron 1977).

6. *Handouts.*   Printed material setting out the points made in the session acts as an aide-memoire for participants (Ley & Spelman 1967). Handouts should relate to the topic currently being discussed: the information loses its relevance if it is produced a week later.

7. *Sharing the time.*   Inevitably, some people talk more than others. Trainers are glad to have 'talkers' in the group: they liven it up. At the same time, it is part of the trainer's responsibility to see that the quiet ones have an opportunity to speak. Thus, the trainer may feel that she sometimes has to intervene. A tactful way of doing it is the following: 'I don't want to dismiss what you are saying, but I wonder what X thinks about it?'.

8. *Friction-dispelling techniques.*   Occasionally, friction arises; a member may consistently disagree

with the way the group is run. Calmly facing such a person and asking how she would like things changed, then putting it to the rest of the group, often resolves the matter.

FALLING ASLEEP

There is a tendency in group work for some members to fall asleep during the session. This is discouraged by most therapists. Bernstein & Borkovec (1973) take the view that it interferes with the learning of a skill and suggest strategies for preventing or dealing with it:

- regularly asking for signals in the form of requests such as 'lift your index finger if you are beginning to feel relaxed'
- directing the voice towards any sleeping trainee

- avoiding the early afternoon for teaching sessions.

Keable (1997) suggests informing participants at the outset that they will be awakened with a light tap if they fall asleep. Others suggest that people who are inclined to fall asleep should sit in a chair rather than lie down, since making people less comfortable reduces their tendency to fall asleep (Lichstein 1988). Kokoszka (1992) refers to the effectiveness of focusing attention on a repetitive stimulus, e.g. counting the breaths, for keeping people awake.

Thus, falling asleep tends to be seen in negative terms. Fanning (1988), however, takes the view that if people have come purely for respite from stress, they should be allowed to sleep.

Further reading

Ernst S, Barnes B, Hyde K 1999 An introduction to group-work. Palgrave, Basingstoke

Payne R A 1986 Health education for small groups. Physiotherapy 72: 56–57

Chapter 3

Stress

THEORIES OF STRESS

The concept of stress in the living organism was studied by Selye (1956). His work showed that when a body is subjected to a challenging stimulus, a characteristic response occurs. Selye identified three stages (Fig. 3.1):

- alarm
- resistance
- exhaustion.

Exposure to the stimulus results in the release of hormones and chemicals whose purpose is to create appropriate physiological changes. This is the alarm reaction. It is cancelled as soon as the stressor is withdrawn. If exposure to the stressor persists,

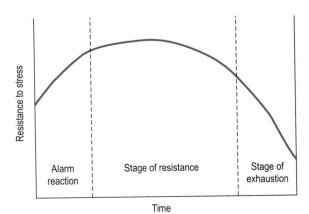

Figure 3.1   The 'general adaptation syndrome'. (Adapted from Cox T. 1978 Stress. Reproduced with kind permission of the author and Palgrave Macmillan, London.)

the body will adapt by developing a resistance which serves it well at the time. Such resistance, however, takes a toll of the organism's resources and the stage will not last indefinitely. As body resources become depleted, a stage of exhaustion takes over. Together these stages make up the 'general adaptation syndrome' (Selye 1956).

Selye, whose concern was centred on physiological aspects, viewed stress as the non-specific response of the body to any demand made on it. (By non-specific, he meant that the same response would occur irrespective of the nature of the stimulus.) Twenty years later, the psychologists Cox & Mackay (1976) defined stress as 'a perceptual phenomenon arising from a comparison between the demand on the person and his ability to cope. An imbalance ... gives rise to the experience of stress and to the stress response'. The emphasis here is on the individual's perceptions, on the subjective nature of stress and on its psychological dimension. Selye, in 1956, had ignored the role of psychological processes (Cox 1978).

Cox & Mackay's model introduces the idea of perceived coping powers as a factor governing the resulting stress. If an individual perceives his ability to cope as weak, and sees environmental demands as heavy, the level of stress he experiences will be high. If his self-perceived coping powers are strong, then those same demands may be readily tolerated and the level of stress experienced will be comparatively low. The environmental demands may, however, be too low, so low that stress arises from boredom. When the individual's perception of environmental demand is matched by his perceived coping ability, a state of balance can be said to exist.

It is clearly desirable for the individual to operate in situations where demands and coping skills are balanced. Establishing and maintaining that balance may involve regulating his exposure to the stressor. Alternatively he could reduce his anxiety levels and increase his coping ability.

This is a model which allows for variation among individuals as well as for changing perceptions over time in the same person. The ideas enshrined in it have led to the concept of the 'human performance curve' which is based on the relationship between demands placed on the individual and his coping ability (Fig. 3.2). Moderate levels of demand are associated with efficient

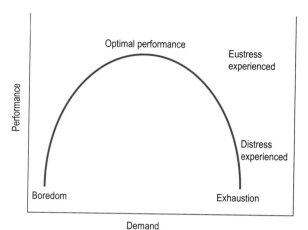

Figure 3.2   Human performance curve.

performance. When demands are perceived as too heavy, the overtaxed individual begins to experience fatigue; when they are too low, boredom results from understimulation. Distress is experienced in both events (Looker & Gregson 1989).

At the top of the curve is the zone of high performance. Here the individual is operating at levels of demand which match his coping skills. Daily variation may result in one slightly outweighing the other: for example, sometimes he feels that he has more capacity than he is being called upon to use, which gives him a feeling of confidence and control; other times he may feel that environmental demands are mildly drawing on untapped inner resources, creating the rewarding experience of being pleasantly stretched. These feelings are collectively referred to as 'eustress' or 'good' stress.

Lower down the curve, on either side, the individual's performance gradually declines as the curve runs through transition zones of moderate stress and, ultimately, into zones of deep distress.

Thus, while distress erodes his quality of life, eustress enhances it. Working at levels of arousal that feel comfortable promotes not only the efficiency of the individual's output, but also his mental well-being.

SYMPTOMS OF STRESS

Stress is associated with physiological symptoms, characteristic of sympathetic nervous system activity. These symptoms relate to the fight/flight response (p. 4) and are summarized below, together with the psychological symptoms of stress, both the subjective (how a person feels) and the behavioural (how a person acts), although there is considerable overlap in these areas.

The symptoms vary among individuals because of the differing sensitivities of organs to the experience of stress.

Physiological symptoms

As mentioned in Chapter 1, these comprise:

- raised heart rate
- increased blood pressure
- sweating
- raised blood coagulation rate
- increased ventilation
- raised blood glucose level.

Subjective symptoms

These include:

- tiredness and/or difficulty in sleeping
- muscle tension particularly in neck and shoulder muscles
- indigestion, constipation, diarrhoea
- palpitations
- headache
- difficulty in concentrating and a tendency to worry
- impatience; feeling irritable and easily roused to anger.

Behavioural symptoms

Behavioural symptoms include:

- increased consumption of alcohol, tobacco, food, etc.
- loss of appetite or excessive eating
- restlessness
- loss of sexual interest
- a tendency to experience accidents.

MEASURING STRESS

A physiological assessment of stress would include such measurements as heart rate, blood pressure, respiratory rate and skin conductance. Psychological as well as physiological attempts have been made to measure stress. One which has had particular influence is the Social Re-adjustment Rating Scale (SRRS) of Holmes & Rahe (1967). These researchers compiled a table of life events ranging from minor violations of the law to the death of a spouse, rating each one in terms of the mental readjustment it demanded. A high score in one year was associated with a high risk of developing a stress-related illness. But the SRRS has its critics: whereas Holmes & Rahe had proposed that any change in a person's circumstances, positive or negative, contributed to the risk, other researchers (Lazarus et al 1980) argued that positive experiences could moderate the effects of negative life events, making them less damaging to the immune system. For example, a broken bone is easier to tolerate if it coincides with the announcement of good exam results.

Another point of discussion raised by the SRRS is whether the stress caused by a series of minor adverse events is more harmful than one major adverse event. Lazarus believes it can be, and has devised a tool for measuring small, day-to-day problems, calling it the Hassles Scale (Kanner et al 1981).

The meaning that an event has for the individual also needs to be considered: moving house, for example, can be a pleasant form of stress if you choose to move, but a source of deep distress if you are forced to do so. Our interpretation of an event thus determines the nature and intensity of our response (Lazarus 1991).

In spite of these and other criticisms, the SRRS has been highly influential as a tool for measuring the effects of stress. Changing social values have, however, rendered some of the ratings out-of-date and created a need for additional items. As a result, the original scale has been succeeded by a new instrument, the Recent Life Changes Questionnaire (Rahe 1975), which has itself been rescaled (Miller & Rahe 1997) (Appendix 5).

SOURCES OF STRESS

Stress can arise from a multitude of sources. Broadly speaking, these sources can be categorized as those in the environment and those within the individual (Powell & Enright 1990).

STRESS IN THE ENVIRONMENT

The work environment

Conditions may be such that the levels of noise are excessively high; it may be too hot or too cold; the atmosphere may be polluted by tobacco smoke or exhaust fumes.

The individual may be suffering from work overload in the form of unrealistic deadlines, long hours or a feeling that the job is beyond his competence. On the other hand, the job may lack stimulation causing him to feel bored; or it may lack opportunity for him to demonstrate his ability.

There may be uncertainty as to the boundaries of his responsibility and the work objectives may be inadequately defined. Relationships with colleagues and superiors may be strained. He may be obliged to move to other departments or to other geographical locations; he may be declared redundant or be forced to retire before he wants to (Powell & Enright 1990).

The social environment

Social ties seem to play a large part in determining the way in which we cope with negative events. These ties include partners, relatives, friends and acquaintances and they act as a buffer between the event itself and the individual's reaction to it. The support may take the form of moral support or material aid. Among the many researchers to demonstrate this association are Cohen & Wills (1985), who have shown that stress-related illnesses are less likely to occur among people with strong social support, and Pennebaker (1990), who shows the protective value of having a confidant.

STRESS IN THE INDIVIDUAL

Personality types

Friedman & Rosenman (1974) described a personality type particularly associated with coronary heart disease. This type was characterized by a tendency for the individual to:

- drive himself to achieve goals one after another
- have a spirit of fierce competitiveness
- create a programme filled with deadlines
- perform activities as fast as possible

- be excessively alert
- have a constant need to be recognized.

Individuals who displayed these tendencies were referred to as 'Type A' personalities, while those with the opposite characteristics were described as 'Type B'. Type B individuals were found to be almost immune to coronary heart disease. Type A characteristics are seen as negative insofar as they may lead to stress-related illness. However, they also lead to high achievement which is to be valued. Cooper (1981) suggests emphasizing the need to *manage* Type A behaviour rather than extinguish it. This may mean slowing down, resetting goals, regularly taking five minutes off and recording the occasions when this is performed. It may also mean seeking alternative ways of gaining rewards.

Kobasa (1982) described what he called the 'hardy' personality. Such a person was seen as being relatively resistant to stress by virtue of possessing three qualities: a sense of control over his life; a feeling of being committed to his work, hobby or family; and a sense of challenge in which change was viewed as an opportunity to develop himself rather than a threat to his equilibrium. Individuals who do not possess these qualities are more likely to suffer from stress-related disease than those who do.

Personality traits are, however, not set in stone. The genetic predispositions we are born with are subject to external influences, particularly in early life, resulting in some traits being emphasized while others are diminished (Cassidy 1999). Personality can be seen as a shifting entity (Apter 2003) and since our actions are governed less by trait than by contingency (Dawes 1994), stress levels and associated behaviour in the individual can vary.

Locus of control

Locus of control is a phrase which refers to the individual's perception of the degree of control he has over the environment (Rotter 1966). If he feels he has influence over most situations in his life, he is said to have an internal locus of control. If, on the other hand, he believes that his life is largely controlled by factors such as fate or other people, his locus is said to be external.

Locus of control is a feature which has been studied in various contexts, one of which is stress where low vulnerability to stress seems to be related to internal locus and high vulnerability to external locus. Thus the more influence an individual believes he has over his environment, the less likely he will be to experience stress.

Other stressors of internal origin

Beck (1984) refers to stressors within the individual, such as the tendency to interpret events in a consistently negative way. Ellis (1962) points to the maladaptive effect of holding unrealistic belief systems, for instance believing one has to be right every time in order to be a worthwhile person (p. 8). Other maladaptive styles include:

- Having unclear goals; a lot of effort can be wasted if people do not know where they are going.

- Failing to make decisions; unmade decisions can so preoccupy the individual that he cannot get on with his life. The unresolved matter continues to claim his attention and eventually wears him out.

- Bottling up emotions; anxiety and anger are examples of emotions that people often keep to themselves, allowing the feelings to grow out of proportion.

- Having low self-esteem; a feeling that one lacks the rights that are accorded to others. Such a person may allow himself to be overruled on every side.

A CLASSIFICATION OF SOURCES OF STRESS

Skelly (2003) presents the sources of stress in four categories:

1. Social stressors. These relate to the interpersonal environment of the individual but also include states such as poverty, isolation and disability. Social stressors are considered to be the dominant causes of mental stress (Goldberg & Huxley 1992).
2. Psychological stressors, such as certain personality traits and cultural beliefs.
3. Chemical stressors. These include additives in food and pollutants in the air and water.

4. Physical stressors, in the form of excessive load demands experienced in the work environment.

On the whole, a crisis perceived to be solvable and of short-term duration seems to be less harmful than a long-lasting succession of small hassles which the individual feels he is unable to control (Stevens & Price 1996).

STRESS–RELATED TOPICS AS A COMPONENT OF RELAXATION TRAINING

When offering relaxation training sessions to a group of people, the health care professional may wish to include certain topics and a discussion. The topics will relate to those conditions from which group members are suffering and may include some of the following:

- anxiety, panic
- depression
- substance dependency, e.g. tobacco, alcohol, tranquillizers
- life crises, e.g. bereavement
- life changes, e.g. menopause
- eating disorders, e.g. bulimia, anorexia
- insomnia
- hyperventilation
- stress-related physical disorders.

Stress has been associated with a number of medical conditions such as bronchial asthma, essential hypertension, peptic ulcer, ulcerative colitis, neurodermatitis, rheumatoid arthritis and thyrotoxicosis. These conditions have been described as psychosomatic illnesses. The concept of psychosomatic illness has, however, been extended in recent years from the original few illnesses for which the term was coined to include many more, as it has come to be realized that psychosocial elements are present in the aetiology of a wide variety of medical conditions (J. O. Robinson 1994, personal communication).

(Relaxation should not be seen as a substitute for medical help. However, insofar as stress is an acknowledged component of any particular condition, health care professionals may find themselves being asked to help alleviate it.)

It is assumed that the instructor has knowledge concerning the problems from which her group members are suffering, and is in a position to provide material about the topic. This can in turn lead into a discussion. The relaxation method subsequently offered can, where possible, be linked to it: for example, slow breathing can be offered in the case of hyperventilation (p. 134), smoking cessation imagery for people quitting smoking (p. 166), and eye exercises in cases of insomnia (p. 38).

In a study investigating the components of stress management, Powell (1987) reports that information and group support were rated the most helpful components of the treatment package. The present author, however, found that participants rated relaxation as the most helpful element, in a small study conducted on self-referred members of a led group featuring topic, discussion and relaxation (Payne 1989).

The topic can revolve around coping skills as well as causes of stress.

COPING

The word 'coping' refers to the efforts made by individuals to manage the demands placed on them (Lazarus & Folkman 1984). Some coping strategies focus on the problem itself; others on the emotion it arouses. The first kind seek to alter the situation in some way to make it less challenging; the second kind aim to reduce the emotional response to the problem. In most situations, however, people use a combination of problem-focused and emotion-focused approaches (Lazarus & Folkman 1984).

Listed below are examples of coping skills which could feature as topics for discussion in group meetings.

1. Getting as much control over the stressor as circumstances allow. While accepting the restrictions of the situation, there may be areas of freedom which a person can develop.

2. If control is not possible or expedient, a person can change the way he thinks about the stressor: for example, instead of being irritated by traffic queues, he could see the time as an opportunity to play music tapes.

3. Training oneself to predict stressful situations in order to weaken their impact.

4. Being task-oriented and not letting emotions take over. Emotions fuddle the mind and interfere with problem solving. If the emotion is strong, it can first be acknowledged then separated from the issue, which can then be judged dispassionately.

5. Avoidance of blaming; the latter tends to arouse anger. A more constructive attitude is to see mistakes as the result of a series of events which simply happened.

6. Dealing with anger. Some anger may serve a useful purpose; much anger, however, is purely destructive. The energy that goes into its arousal could often be more profitably spent in solving the problem. Ways in which anger can be controlled include:

- Reinterpreting the stimulus in a more positive light; many situations contain ambiguities which allow reinterpretations to be made.
- Being realistic in one's expectations of other people.
- Modifying one's internal dialogue to include self-statements such as 'I am easygoing' or 'I keep my cool'.
- Focusing on the issue rather than the personality.

7. Giving oneself permission to make a mistake. It is part of being human to make mistakes occasionally.

8. Distancing oneself. If circumstances seem to be overwhelming, one can try stepping back mentally to get a more objective view (pp 155 and 164). It is sometimes useful to visualize another person coping with the same problem.

9. Introducing humour at suitable moments. When a person smiles and laughs the relaxation response takes over (p. 215).

10. Managing time efficiently. Priorities need to be established and time allotted to tasks proportionately. If time is short, inessentials can be cut out and tasks delegated. It is sometimes possible to say 'No' to demands when time is restricted.

11. Having someone to confide in.

12. Rewarding himself if one has done a job well.

13. Living in the present. This means savouring the moment; enjoying the journey as well as the arrival. It is useful to remember that the future is to a large extent determined by the way we handle the present. A lot of stress arises from dwelling on

the past with its regrets or on the future with its uncertainties.

14. Establishing good relationships. The support derived from both intimate relationships and the wider social network acts as a buffer to protect the individual from the full effects of stressful events (Ganster & Victor 1988). Relationships, however, whether at work or at home, demand time and attention.

15. Taking exercise (Ch. 14).

16. Learning to become more assertive.

Table 3.1 sets out some stress-evoking factors alongside appropriate coping strategies.

Table 3.1 Stress-evoking factors and related coping strategies

Stress–evoking factor	Coping strategy
Faulty belief system	Cognitive restructuring
Unclear goals	Goal setting
Unmade decisions	Decision making
Low self-esteem	Building positive self-image
Bottling up feelings	Confiding, assertiveness
Deadlines and time constraints	Restructuring time
Deteriorating relationships	Enhancing personal interaction

Further reading

Gatchel R J 1996 The bio-psycho-social model. In: Gatchel R J, Turk D C (eds) Psychological approaches to pain management: a practitioner's handbook. Guilford Press, New York, pp 33–52

Payne R A, Rowland Payne C M E, Marks R 1985 Stress does not worsen psoriasis? A controlled study of 32 patients. Clinical and Experimental Dermatology 10: 239–245

Skelly M 2003 Stress and mental health. In: Everett T, Donaghy M, Feaver S (eds) Interventions for mental health. Butterworth-Heinemann, Oxford

Smith E E, Nolen-Hoeksema S, Fredrickson B 2002 Atkinson & Hilgard's introduction to psychology, 13th edn. Harcourt Brace, Fort Worth, Ch 14

SECTION 2

Somatic methods of relaxation

Chapter 4

Progressive relaxation

HISTORY AND DESCRIPTION

To many people, relaxation training means learning techniques such as 'tense–release', i.e. the tightening and letting-go of specific muscle groups. Tense–release is an active process in the sense that the individual is working his muscles. Some muscle relaxation methods, however, are concerned only with the 'release' part of the sequence, and these could be described as passive muscular approaches.

This chapter introduces the work of Edmund Jacobson, a pioneer in this field. His work lays the foundation of both the tense–release and the passive approaches, which are described here and developed in Chapters 5–8.

Working as a physiologist-physician in the 1930s, Jacobson was investigating the startle reaction that follows a sudden loud noise. He noticed that people who were able to fully relax their muscles made no start. Thus, the state of the muscle influenced the magnitude of the reflex. He invented a technique for measuring the electrical activity in muscles and nerves which became known as electromyography (EMG), and which allowed him to study hitherto unexplored aspects of physiology. Arising out of this new technology, he was able to demonstrate that thinking was related to muscle state and that mental images, particularly those associated with movement, were accompanied by small but detectable levels of activity in the muscles concerned (Jacobson 1938).

This integrated activity between the mind and the muscles led him to view the brain centres and the voluntary muscles as working together 'in one effort circuit' (Jacobson 1970); a neuromuscular circuit, since it was composed of both neural and muscular tissue. Just as a calm mind would be reflected in a tension-free body, so, Jacobson proposed, a relaxed musculature would be accompanied by the quietening of thoughts and the reduction of sympathetic activity, notions that would have relevance in the treatment of anxiety and associated conditions. The task facing Jacobson, therefore, was to find a way of inducing the skeletal muscles to lose their tension.

Muscle activity is accompanied by sensations so faint that we do not normally notice them. To promote awareness of tension, Jacobson emphasized the need to concentrate on those sensations, cultivating what he called 'learned awareness'. Once tension had been recognized, it would be easier to release it. If relaxation were then achieved, however, how deep would it be?

It is traditionally held that, in the waking state, healthy muscle, even during rest, is in a state of sustained, slight contraction. This is called muscle tone. Jacobson's EMG studies (1938) did not, however, support this notion. He found that voluntary muscle could achieve a state of complete relaxation during rest. He consequently formed the view that the aim of relaxation training should be to eliminate *all* tension; and relaxation could only be called complete if it proceeded 'to the zero point of tonus for the part or parts involved' (Jacobson 1938). Any tension that remained while resting a muscle was called 'residual', and it was this residual tension that Jacobson sought to eliminate in deep relaxation. 'Doing away with residual tension is … the essential feature of the present method' (Jacobson 1976).

Defining relaxation as the cessation of activity in the skeletal (voluntary) muscles, Jacobson devised a technique which he called progressive relaxation. It consisted of systematically working through the major skeletal muscle groups, creating and releasing tension. As a result, the trainee learned how to recognize muscle tension. Only one muscle action was carried out in each session and it was repeated twice. The rest of the time was spent releasing tension.

Jacobson (1938) insisted that his method be regarded as a skill to be learned. Unlike most other approaches, the use of suggestion was discouraged. Trainers were urged to avoid planting ideas of the kind: 'Your limbs are heavy/limp/relaxed', or even 'Notice how your limbs are feeling heavy/limp/relaxed'. Jacobson wanted the learner to make his own discoveries.

RATIONALE

Progressive relaxation (PR) is based on the idea that people think more clearly when they are relaxed and this helps them to solve their emotional problems (Lehrer 1982). Jacobson proposed that relaxation of the musculature offered a means to that end, since he further proposed that a relaxed musculature exerted a calming influence on the whole organism including the mind. The effect was non-specific. Its generalizing nature places his method in the category of a unitary theory (Ch. 1). The approach is a physiologically oriented one since its procedures are concerned with physical organs, i.e. muscles and nerves, although the act of focusing on muscular sensations gives it also a cognitive slant.

PRESENTING PROGRESSIVE RELAXATION

CONDITIONS

Ideal conditions for presenting progressive relaxation include the following:

- A room that is quiet.
- Somewhere to lie down. A large room with a carpeted floor is suitable for a group. Trainees may be asked to bring a beach mattress or the equivalent to lie on, and a small pillow for the head. Lying is the position of choice; however, it is possible to learn progressive relaxation in the sitting position.

INTRODUCING THE METHOD

Before starting the training proper, the relaxation method must be introduced. With the trainees seated, the trainer describes the rationale of progressive relaxation on the following lines:

> Knowing how to rest the body enables body energy to be used more efficiently. It can also help to protect us from illness. This is a method of relaxing that involves the muscles. By creating and releasing tension you will learn to tune into subtle feelings in the muscles, to recognize different levels of tension and to release that tension.
>
> Muscle tension is believed to be closely associated with your state of mind: it is believed that muscles which are unnecessarily tense reflect their tension in the mind. If that muscle tension can be released, you will feel mentally calmer.
>
> Your internal organs will also benefit in that pulse rate and blood pressure will be lowered while you are relaxing.
>
> The method we are using is called progressive relaxation. It is not possible to learn it in one lesson. However, every bit as important as the lessons is the practice that you put in between them. Like any skill, the more you practise it, the more proficient you will become, and the more you will benefit from its effects, in this case relaxation.

The muscle action to be taught is then demonstrated, after which trainees are asked to lie down, face upwards, with arms resting on either side of the body, legs uncrossed. The eyes are open to begin with, but after three or four minutes trainees are asked to close them and to spend a few minutes quietly unwinding.

PROCEDURE

First session: wrist-bending backwards

A first session would take the following form. The trainee is asked to extend the left wrist (bend it back) and to hold it in that position for one minute (Fig. 4.1). He then releases the tension, letting go all at once, and continues to relax the arm for three minutes during which any residual tension is also released. This action is then repeated twice. The instruction might run as follows:

> Would you please bend the left hand back at the wrist. Do this steadily without seesawing ... and avoid raising the forearm ... continue to hold the

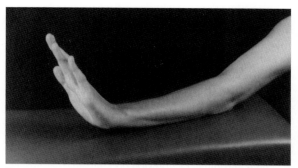

Figure 4.1   Wrist-bending backwards.

> hand back for a full minute, noticing the different sensations you get from doing it.

Using Jacobson's technique, it is not suggested to the trainee what these sensations might be; the idea is that the trainee should discover them for himself. However, in this case they would include tension in the working muscles situated along the top of the forearm and across the back of the hand, together with some sensations of strain in the wrist joint and skin-stretching in the palm. Of these, it is the muscle sensations that the trainee should learn to focus on.

> As you continue to bend your wrist back, distinguish between the various feelings you are experiencing ... pick out particularly those related to the muscles ... concentrate on the sensation of tenseness ... keeping the action sustained until the minute is up ...
>
> And now, discontinue the action ... allow the hand to fall by its own weight. Let it flop down. Avoid lowering it slowly or in any way controlling its descent.
>
> Although you have let go as completely as you could, there may still be some tension there. Give it plenty of time to disappear ... give it at least three minutes as you focus on the sensation in the muscles ...
>
> Now, bend the wrist back a second time ... feel the effort ... if you are finding difficulty in sorting out the feelings in the arm, allow the hand to fall down and try the following: with your right hand, pick up the left hand and gently press it back as if it didn't belong to you ... continue to press for about half a minute. Make sure the right hand does all the

work. The feelings you're getting are coming from the wrist and from the palm. With your left hand still bent back, take away your right hand and as you do, transfer the power to your left arm. You are now using muscles in the left forearm to hold the left wrist back. Notice the new feelings you are getting... these are the feelings you are asked to concentrate on... continue to hold the wrist back for about a minute...

Now, cease the action and allow the hand to fall down, letting all the tension go... letting the muscle go negative... concentrating on the feelings you are getting from it... continue in that direction for the next three minutes...

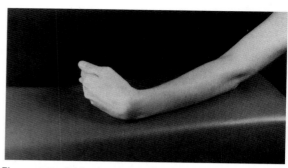

Figure 4.2 Wrist-bending forwards.

The trainee is not asked to 'relax', which Jacobson felt might create tensions on its own account, but to 'discontinue', 'cease to bend' or 'go negative'. Relaxation occurs on its own as the learner releases tension.

One further repetition is carried out before the trainee adopts a state of continuous rest for the remainder of the hour when the session comes to an end.

Second session: wrist–bending forwards

At the following session a new action is introduced: wrist flexion (bending forwards). This action follows the same pattern as the previous one except that the wrist is bent forwards instead of backwards (Fig. 4.2).

I'd like you to bend the left hand forward at the wrist... hold the position steadily... locate the feeling of tenseness (the underside of the forearm)... and... (when the minute is up)... discontinue the action... let the hand fall back... continue letting go any remaining tension over the next few minutes... tuning in to the feelings in the muscle in the forearm...

Two repetitions are carried out, after which the trainee rests. That marks the end of session number two.

Third and subsequent sessions

The third session does not contain any tensing component. Instead, the time is entirely devoted to releasing tension. Subsequent sessions are spent addressing other actions and may cover many

weeks. The protocol is outlined below and laid out in full in Table 4.1.

Arms. Five items for each arm; tensing and releasing of arm and hand muscles.

Legs. Seven items for each leg; tensing and releasing of thigh, leg and foot muscles.

Trunk. Seven items; tensing and releasing of back, abdomen and shoulder muscles.

Neck. Four items; tensing and relaxing of muscles around the neck.

Eye area. Eight items; tensing and relaxing the muscles of the forehead and the eyes.

Visualization. Six items; imagining different objects, moving and stationary.

Speech area. Fifteen items; tensing and relaxing muscles associated with speech; counting and reciting, first in a normal voice, then gradually getting fainter.

Only one or two new actions are introduced at each period of tuition, and the whole programme takes about 50 sessions. In addition, an hour a day is devoted to home practice.

'DIMINISHING TENSIONS'

Jacobson avoided using the word 'exercise' to describe the actions, since exercise, designed as it is to strengthen muscles, implies increasing effort. The wrist bending and other actions in progressive relaxation are introduced simply to teach awareness of the different sensations that arise in activated muscle tissue. Learning to recognize these sensations requires differing levels of muscle tension. Of these, the lower levels are the most useful for picking up residual tension as it is here that sensitivity to small fluctuations is greatest

Table 4.1   Progressive relaxation: schedule of items (Adapted from Jacobson 1964)

Arms	Extend wrist (bend hand back) Flex wrist (bend hand forward) Relax only Flex (bend) elbow Extend elbow (straighten arm) Relax only Stiffen whole arm	Eye area (*contd*)	Close eyes tightly Look left with eyes closed Relax only Look right with eyes closed Look up with eyes closed Relax only Look down with eyes closed Look forward with eyes closed Relax only
Legs	Dorsiflex foot (bend foot up at ankle joint) Plantarflex foot (bend foot down at ankle joint) Relax only Extend (straighten) knee from a bent position Flex (bend) knee dragging foot along floor Relax only Flex hip (raise bent knee towards chest) Extend hip (press thigh down into the supporting surface) Relax only Stiffen entire leg	Visual imagination	Imagine a pen moving slowly, then fast Imagine a train passing, a person walking by Relax eyes Imagine a bird flying and stationary Imagine a ball rolling, the Houses of Parliament Relax eyes Imagine a horse grazing, a reel of cotton Imagine the Prime Minister Relax eyes

Trunk	Contract (pull in) abdomen
	Extend spine (arch back slightly)
	Relax only
	Observe the action of breathing
	Brace shoulders back
	Relax only
	Flex shoulder joint (bring bent arm across chest)
	Repeat with other arm
	Relax only
	Raise (hunch) shoulders
		Jaw, voice,
		and auditory
		imagination
			Close jaws firmly
			Open jaws
			Relax only
			Bare teeth
			Pout
			Relax only
			Press tongue against teeth
			Pull tongue backwards
			Relax only
			Count aloud up to 10
			Count half as loudly up to 10
			Relax only
			Count softly up to 10
			Count under your breath up to 10
			Relax only
			Imagine you are counting
			Imagine you are reciting the alphabet
			Relax only
			Imagine saying:
			    your name three times
			    your address three times
			    the Prime Minister's name three times

Neck	Press head back into pillow/headrest Raise head off pillow Relax only Bend head to right Bend head to left Relax only		
Eye area	Raise eyebrows Frown Relax only *(contd on right column)*		

(Jacobson 1970 p. 45, Lehrer et al 1988). Thus, the actions require an ever-*decreasing* intensity of contraction to fulfil their purpose. To help the trainee become sensitized to low levels of tension, Jacobson devised a technique called 'diminishing tensions'.

It is introduced as the learner becomes proficient in recognizing the sensation of tension.

Returning to the action of wrist bending, the trainee would be instructed in the following way:

> Bend your wrist back, but this time using only half as much effort as you did the first time. Hold it back for about a minute, noticing the sensations you're getting from the muscle ... and at the end of the minute ... cease holding it back. Go negative ... feel the tension leaving ... allow plenty of time for the remaining tension to disappear ... allow three minutes ... then bend the wrist back again, this time tensing the muscle half as much as last time ... hold it for about a minute, tuning in to the sensations ... then release the tension ... release it further ... and further still ... allow three minutes ... now, raise the wrist the smallest amount possible ... hold it there ... for one minute ... discontinue ... allow three minutes ... and finally, make the action just a thought ... hold the thought for one minute ... go negative ... spend three minutes continuing to go negative...

These progressively diminishing tensions train the individual to recognize differing levels, thus increasing his control over the voluntary musculature.

Jacobson's assigning of every third session exclusively to passive relaxation is evidence of the high value he placed on the relaxation phase and the relatively low value he gave to the contraction phase, using it simply as a means of cultivating sensitivity to the tension sensation. Many of his successors have, by contrast, attached great importance to the contraction, claiming that it leads to a deepening of the subsequent relaxation. Jacobson argued that the reverse may be the case, namely, that tensions which build up during the contraction phase would continue to persist for some time, thus hindering relaxation. In untrained participants he showed that muscle tension continues to remain elevated for up to several minutes following a contraction, even when the participant is cooperating with appeals to 'go negative' (Jacobson 1934). Thus, deliberate muscle tensing may, in the short term at least, actually obstruct the relaxation process.

The issue of tense–release versus a release-only approach has not been satisfactorily resolved. It has been common in clinical practice to favour tense–release. However, the results of a study in 1991 (Lucic et al) support the view that initial tensing is detrimental to relaxation, and this finding may have strengthened interest in passive approaches.

EYE MOVEMENTS

The procedures for the eye and forehead and for the area of the speech muscles differ somewhat from those of the trunk and limbs. Consequently they are presented in more detail.

Although Jacobson (1938) indicated that only one or two actions should be carried out in each session, it is customary today to work through all the eye actions in a single session. Plenty of time should still be allowed for 'going negative'.

Jacobson's studies had demonstrated the effectiveness of progressive relaxation in reducing muscle tension. He had also been able to show that a relaxed musculature had a calming effect on the mind (Jacobson 1938). Muscle relaxation could thus be seen as a mental relaxant. But Jacobson went further: he claimed that in deep relaxation, thought itself disappeared. In the totally relaxed body, the mind would be a blank.

The eye muscles were considered by him to be particularly closely related to thought, since thinking created mental images which were accompanied by a sense of tension around the eyes. Releasing tension from the eyes, Jacobson believed, had the effect of cancelling those images. The following sequences are adapted from Jacobson (1970). Time should be allowed between the items for the trainee to absorb the message:

> With your eyes open, raise your eyebrows ... feel the tension ... and release it ... frown ... feel the tension ... and discontinue ... shut your eyes tightly ... feel the tension ... and let it go ... with your eyes still closed, spend a few minutes releasing tension in this part of your face...
>
> Moving on to the eyes themselves (they are still closed) ... without moving your head, turn your eyes upwards as if you were looking at the ceiling. As you do so, notice the sensation you get in the eye region ... next, turn your eyes downwards as if you were looking at your feet, again taking note of the feelings around the eyes ... repeat that several times, until you become familiar with the sensation in the eye muscles ... then discontinue, going negative for a

minute or so ... still with your eyes closed, turn your eyes to the left for a few moments ... now to the right ... repeat this a few times to experience the transient sensations in the muscles ... then, cease the action ... do nothing for a few minutes ...

Would you now, still with your eyes closed, *imagine* you are looking at the ceiling and the floor; do not actively look up and down, but simply think of looking up and down ... notice the feelings (that is, the same sensations as when you deliberately turned your eyes up and down, although to a much lesser degree) ... when you have identified the feeling, let your eye muscles go negative ... notice what happens to the images ... rest for a few minutes ...

Now, imagine that you see the wall on your left ... and the wall on your right ... imagine seeing one after the other, noticing that slight tensions accompany the images ... now, let your eyes go ... and notice what happens to the images ...

Similar effects can be created by imagining objects from everyday life:

Imagine a car passing ... or a ball bouncing up and down ... notice the sensation that accompanies the image ... then let the eye muscles go negative and notice what happens to the images ...

Multiply 16 by 82 in your head ... when you have got the answer, notice how the eyes felt during the task ... then, rest the eyes and notice what happens to the figures ...

If the eyes are completely relaxed, the image disappears and the thought dies (Jacobson 1964). The individual, however, has made no effort to stop the thought process. He is asked only to release tension, 'letting other effects come as they may' (Jacobson 1976). Whether thought does in fact disappear in a totally relaxed body has not been scientifically established. Jacobson (1938) was, however, able to produce clinical evidence of the success of ocular relaxation in overcoming insomnia.

SPEECH MOVEMENTS

The speech muscles are also closely related to thought. Thinking with the use of words causes minute flickers of tension in the muscles of the tongue and jaw. Conversely, when these muscles

are relaxed, thinking with the use of words is no longer possible (Jacobson 1970).

The following script begins with tensing of the speech muscles and ends with sequences of counting using 'diminishing tensions'. As with the eye actions, it is customary today to present the whole group in one session. As a rough guide, 5–10 seconds can be allowed for each action and 30–40 seconds for 'going negative'. Each action is repeated once.

Close the jaws firmly, noticing the sensations you get from the action ... hold it ... and ... discontinue ... let your jaw drop ... feel the tension leaving you ... and continuing to leave you ... then repeat the sequence ...

Next, bare your teeth ... feel the tension in the cheeks ... hold it for a few seconds ... and cease the action ...

Make a tight 'O' with your lips ... hold it, while you register tension in the lips ... and ... go negative ...

Press your tongue against your teeth ... feel the pressure ... and discontinue ...

Now, pull the tongue back towards the throat. Feel the muscles drawing it back and note the sensations you get from this action ... and ... let it go negative ...

Tune in to the presence of residual tension in any of the muscles associated with speech and let that tension recede ... and go on receding ...

(Allow several minutes for the last phase.)

A counting sequence follows, using diminishing tensions.

Count aloud slowly from one to ten, picking up the sensations you get from the muscles in the mouth, throat, face and chest. Repeat it a few times ... then stop counting ... allow time for the full release of tension ...

Now, count again, half as loudly ... noticing the reduced amount of tension in the speech muscles ... discontinue ... next time, count softly ... notice the tension ... and let it go ... and now, under your breath ... still concentrating on the feelings you get in the mouth, jaw and throat ... rest a moment ... and now, simply imagine the counting ... here perhaps you can detect a flickering in the speech muscles ... finally, cease to count altogether ...

When the speech muscles ceased to be involved, Jacobson (1938, 1964, 1976) claimed that it was no longer possible to think in verbal terms. The notion that thought disappears in states of deep muscle relaxation is consistent with a theory which sees mental processes being influenced by the state of the skeletal musculature (Lehrer 1982).

FURTHER WORK OF JACOBSON

DIFFERENTIAL RELAXATION

Jacobson (1938) also investigated the degree of tension necessary for carrying out a particular activity. He drew a distinction between those muscles actually performing the activity and those muscles not involved in it. The first group needed the minimum level of tension consistent with performing the task; the second group could be totally relaxed or as relaxed as possible. This differential in the degree of tension required was studied by Jacobson for the purpose of reducing both the excessive effort often used by the first group and the unnecessary effort often used by the second. Differential relaxation is discussed in more detail in Chapter 12.

SELF–OPERATIONS CONTROL

In addition to progressive relaxation, Jacobson (1964) developed a method of instruction which he called 'self-operations control'. The principles of recognizing and eliminating tension are the same as those of progressive relaxation. The emphasis, however, is placed on self-direction: the individual controlling his muscle tension throughout the events of daily life, learning 'to go on and off … as different occasions may require' (Jacobson 1964). He learns to monitor all sensations of tension, simultaneously and automatically, and to release those tensions that are not desired, in a continuing process (McGuigan 1984). The result is a decreased consumption of energy, which effect extends to other body systems such as the autonomic nervous system, where sympathetic activity is reduced. Thought processes are also believed to benefit from the tension-decreasing effect (McGuigan 1981).

This method, however, takes as long to learn as Jacobson's original technique.

EVIDENCE OF EFFECTIVENESS

Jacobson used EMG, a technique which he invented, to measure muscle tension. By this means he showed that progressive relaxation had a direct effect on the release of tension in the skeletal musculature. The more practised the trainee, the greater the effect. He also showed that progressive relaxation had an indirect effect on anxiety levels, and that, via brain mediation, it promoted parasympathetic dominance (Jacobson 1938).

Jacobson, who was a pioneer in an unexplored area, carried out research which was meticulous by the standards of his day. However, despite careful attention to method, his work, by present day standards, suffers from certain shortcomings. One of these is the self-selection of participants, i.e. individuals volunteering to take part. Jacobson drew on his close associates and private patients for subjects, whereas modern standards would demand random selection.

A second methodological deficiency is the relative absence of statistical analysis. Jacobson seldom tested for significance, i.e. conducted analyses to estimate the probability that the results he obtained did not arise by chance (Lichstein 1988). It was not conventional to use probability statistics in his day (Lehrer 1982). In spite of this, however, his results often reached levels of statistical significance (Blanchard & Young 1973).

In her review of relaxation techniques Kerr (2000) cites studies which have shown reductions in both physiological and psychological indicators of stress following a course of PR. These results suggest that PR has the potential to promote relaxation (Kerr 2000). When PR has been compared with other stress-reducing approaches, PR often appears equally effective, as in Salt & Kerr's (1997) study where PR was compared with the Mitchell method in 24 normotensive participants. Whereas significant reductions in heart rate, respiratory rate and blood pressure were found in both methods, the study did not show any significant difference in effectiveness between the two interventions. Similarly, Crist & Rickard (1993) found no difference in outcome between muscular and imaginal relaxation in 100 healthy students, although both experimental conditions showed significant training effects.

Progressive relaxation, in one form or another, is widely used in the clinical field for reducing mental tension. Based on a substantial amount of evidence, it is believed that the mind becomes calmer as a result of relaxing the musculature. According to Jacobson (1938) this was best achieved by teaching minimal muscle contractions, as opposed to repeated strong contractions, a view which was supported in the findings of Lehrer (1982) and Lehrer et al (1988). Findings are not always consistent, however, and there are studies which show little or no correlation between anxiety level and muscle tension. It would seem that any influence exerted by the musculature on mental activity is part of an interactive process as yet not fully understood (Lichstein 1988, Kerr 2000).

The major disadvantage of Jacobson's original technique is its length, with accompanying problems of time and money. These problems have inevitably led to a plethora of modifications, one of which is described in the following chapter.

PITFALLS OF MUSCULAR RELAXATION

See Chapter 6 (pp 56–57).

Further reading

Jacobson E 1938 Progressive relaxation, 2nd edn. University of Chicago Press, Chicago

Jacobson E 1976 You must relax. Souvenir Press, London

McGuigan F J 1984 Progressive relaxation: origins, principles and clinical applications. In: Woolfolk R L, Lehrer P M (eds) Principles and practice of stress management. Guilford Press, New York

Chapter 5

Progressive relaxation training

HISTORY AND DESCRIPTION

Although Jacobson's method (Ch. 4) was found to reduce both pulse rate and blood pressure, it was time-consuming and unlikely to have wide appeal as it stood. Some form of abbreviation was needed. The first major attempt at shortening the format was made by Wolpe (1958), who reduced the training to six sessions and later reduced it further to one. Countless other modifications have followed, of which Bernstein & Borkovec's (1973) is one of the best known.

Named 'progressive relaxation training' (PRT) by its authors, the approach is defined as learning to relax specific muscle groups while paying attention to the feelings associated with both the tensed and relaxed states. Its aims are (Bernstein & Given 1984):

1. to achieve a state of deep relaxation in increasingly shorter periods
2. to control excess tension in stress-inducing situations.

The trainee works through the sequential tensing and releasing of 16 muscle groups. These are reduced to seven in the next stage and to four in a subsequent stage. The tension component is then withdrawn, in what is called 'relaxation through recall', and the final stage consists of a mental summary of the previously learned techniques. Proficiency at each level depends on the skill obtained in the previous stage. The tense–release element of PRT is described in this chapter (p. 45). Relaxation through recall is presented in

Chapter 7 (p. 60). Two additional components are described in later chapters: 'conditioned relaxation' in Chapter 8 (p. 71) and 'differential relaxation' in Chapter 12 (p. 101).

DIFFERENCES BETWEEN PROGRESSIVE RELAXATION AND PROGRESSIVE RELAXATION TRAINING

Although PRT is founded on Jacobson's principles of recognizing and eliminating tension, there are important differences between the two approaches (Table 5.1).

The contraction phase

One of these differences is the prominence given to the tensing component in the modified version. Bernstein & Borkovec (1973) describe an effect whereby the strength of the contraction determines the depth of the relaxation which follows it, in the manner of a pendulum which, when lifted high on one side, swings back to the same height on the other side. Thus, the stronger the initial contraction, the deeper the subsequent relaxation. Jacobson (1938, 1970) does not share this view. He sees the contraction phase simply as a means of cultivating the individual's sensitivity to the presence of muscle tension. He never intended it as a means of 'producing' relaxation (Lehrer et al 1988).

The strength of the contraction is not specified by Jacobson, except in such terms as 'Do not stiffen your arm to the point of extreme effort, but only in moderation' (Jacobson 1964); and the command to 'tense', even at greatest magnitude is taken to convey only a comfortable level, since the object is merely to enable the individual to identify the sensation of tension. To Jacobson, the lower the level of the contraction, the more useful it was. Bernstein & Borkovec, in contrast, use phrases such as 'tight fist' and refer to 'trembling neck muscles', suggesting a high level of tension. Wolpe & Lazarus (1966), similarly, in their version, urge clients to clench the fist 'tighter and tighter'.

Use of suggestion

Both Jacobson (1938) and Bernstein & Borkovec (1973) discuss suggestion. The argument in favour of using suggestion is that it increases cognitive awareness of the affective component which is believed to enhance the overall effect (Fig. 5.1) (M. E. Donaghy 1999, personal communication).

Addressing trainees who fear they might be put into a trance state, Bernstein & Borkovec point

Table 5.1 Differences between Jacobson's progressive relaxation method and Bernstein & Borkovec's progressive relaxation training

	Progressive relaxation	Progressive relaxation training
Position of relaxation	Lying or sitting	Reclining
Total number of muscle groups worked	40+	16
Number of new muscle groups worked in one session	1 or 2	All groups
Emphasis of technique	Releasing tension	'Producing' relaxation through tense–release cycles
Perceived value of the contraction	To alert the individual to the tension sensation	To deepen each relaxation component by providing a 'running start'; a strong contraction leads to a deep relaxation
Part played by suggestion	None: the technique is purely a muscular skill	Indirect suggestion is used to enhance the effect
Use of tapes	Not used	Advised against
Number of sessions needed	50+	8–12

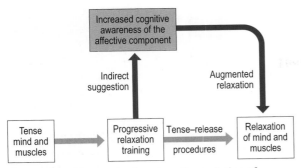

Figure 5.1 Diagram to show how the inclusion of suggestion might increase the effect of a muscular procedure. (M. E. Donaghy 1999, personal communication.)

out the difference between hypnosis and relaxation. In hypnosis, maximum use is made of direct suggestion, such as 'Now your arm is limp'. Direct suggestion, so crucial in hypnosis, is not appropriate in relaxation.

PRT does, however, use indirect suggestion, such as 'Notice how your muscles are feeling more and more relaxed' and 'Let a feeling of relaxation flow through your limbs', in order to deepen the sense of relaxation. Voice modulations to reinforce the distinction between tension and relaxation are also encouraged: crisp tones during the tensing component and soothing tones during the relaxation component.

To Jacobson, however, even indirect suggestion is unacceptable. He sees progressive relaxation exclusively as a muscular skill, the mastery of which is impeded by any kind of suggestion.

Relevant to this discussion is the work of Paul (1969) who has shown relaxation training to be more effective than hypnosis at reducing muscle tension.

RATIONALE

As with progressive relaxation, it is proposed that relaxing the musculature exerts a calming effect on the whole organism, including the mind. The contraction phase in PRT, however, is given greater prominence since it is believed that initial tensing actually produces relaxation.

THE PRT PROCEDURE

THE FIRST SESSION

In Bernstein & Borkovec's approach, training is governed by a fixed procedure.

1. The rationale of the technique is presented to the trainee, and the items involving the 16 muscle groups are then described and demonstrated. (See Introductory remarks section below.)
2. For the procedure itself the trainee is seated in a reclining chair. If this is not available, the trainee can sit in a chair with a high, sloping back and arms.
3. The procedure starts with the trainee being asked to focus attention on a given muscle group. (See Item one section below.)
4. A signal, such as the word 'Now', indicates that the muscle group is to be tensed.
5. The contraction is carried out all at once, not gradually.
6. Tension is maintained for 5–7 seconds during which the instructor asks the trainee to focus on the sensations of muscle contraction.
7. On a predetermined cue, such as the word 'Release', 'Relax' or 'Let go', the muscle group is relaxed (again, all at once).
8. As the muscle group relaxes, the trainee is asked to notice the feelings that accompany the relaxation while the trainer maintains a patter which is indirectly suggestive of relaxation.
9. This continues for the duration of the relaxation period which is 30–40 seconds.
10. All 16 muscle groups are worked in the first training session.

Introductory remarks to trainees

The method you are going to learn is called 'progressive relaxation training' and it consists of tensing and releasing muscle groups throughout the body. The object is to produce relaxation and this occurs after the tension is released. A firm contraction can lead to a deep relaxation, rather like a pendulum swinging high on both sides. You will be asked to concentrate on the feelings that accompany the tension and the relaxation; feelings that up to now, you may have taken for granted. There are 16 muscle groups to be tensed and released and it takes about 40 minutes to complete the whole schedule. First, I'll run through the items, demonstrating them and giving you a chance to try them out.

The trainer demonstrates the following items:

1. Making a fist with the dominant hand without involving the upper arm.
2. Pushing the elbow of the same arm down against the arm of the chair (activating the biceps), while keeping the hand relaxed.
3. } The non-dominant arm is worked
4. } separately.
5. Raising the eyebrows.
6. Screwing up the eyes and wrinkling the nose.
7. Clenching the teeth and pulling back the corners of the mouth.
8. Pulling the chin in and pressing the head back against a support, tensing the neck muscles.
9. Drawing the shoulders back.
10. Tightening the abdominal muscles (making the stomach hard).
11. Tensing the thigh of the dominant leg by attempting to contract the knee flexors and extensors together.
12. Pointing the dominant foot down (plantar-flexion).
13. Pulling the dominant foot up towards the face (dorsiflexion).
14. }
15. } The non-dominant leg is worked separately.
16. }

The trainer continues:

When we begin, I'll first describe each item but please do not tense the part until I give you the cue word 'Now'. Similarly, let it go only when I give you the cue word 'Relax'. Then let it go completely. Would you please close your eyes.

Item one

The first item involves the muscles of the right hand and forearm; the hand is drawn into a fist (Fig. 5.2):

We'll start with the right hand and forearm. I'm going to ask you to tense the muscles in the right hand and lower arm, by drawing up your hand into a tight fist ... Now ... clench the hand ... keep it

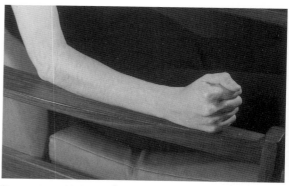

Figure 5.2   Making a fist.

tight ... feel the tension in the muscles as you pull hard ... and ... Relax ... let go immediately and as the fingers uncurl, notice the feelings you now have in the muscles of the hand ... focus on the sensations you are getting in the muscles of the forearm also, as they lose their tension ... feel relaxation flowing into the area as the muscles get more and more deeply relaxed ... completely relaxed ... notice the way your muscles feel at this moment, compared to how they felt when tensed.

All items are performed a second time, after which there is an extended relaxation phase lasting a full minute. Trainees can be asked to raise the little finger of the right hand to indicate that they are fully relaxed before the next item is introduced.

Item two and subsequent items

Item two involves the muscles of the right upper arm: the bent elbow is pressed down into the arm of the chair (Fig. 5.3). (A wooden arm rest can be softened with a cushion.)

Let the hand and forearm go on relaxing while you transfer your attention to the muscles in the right upper arm. I'd like you this time to press your elbow down against the arm of the chair. Do this without involving the muscles of the hand and forearm ... Now ... feel the tension in your upper arm as the elbow presses down ... and ... Relax ... let it go completely ... focus your attention on the relaxing muscles ... feel the tension flowing out ... enjoy the pleasant feelings of the muscles unwinding ... experience the feeling of deep relaxation and of

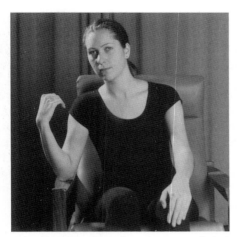

Figure 5.3   Pressing elbow down into arm of chair.

> comfort ... then notice if the upper arm feels as
> relaxed as the lower arm ... if it does, then signal
> with your little finger.

The above items give an idea of the nature of PRT, and in the first session the remaining 14 items are also worked through.

Ending the session

At the end, the trainer terminates.

> I am going to bring the session to an end by count-
> ing backwards from four to one ... four ... start to
> move your legs and feet ... three ... bend and stretch
> your arms and hands ... two ... move your head
> slowly ... and ... one ... open your eyes, noticing how
> peaceful and relaxed you feel ... as if you'd just
> woken from a short sleep.

PRACTICE

Two daily practice sessions of 15–20 minutes each are considered essential, the trainee picking moments when he is not under any pressure.

SUMMARIZED VERSIONS

When the trainee has learned the above procedure, it can be regrouped in a summarized form, enabling him to cover the process in a shorter time:

1. Right arm items combined.
2. Left arm items combined.

3. Face and head movements worked together.
4. Neck and shoulder region combined.
5. Torso items worked together.
6. Right leg items combined.
7. Left leg items combined.

A further summary cuts the process down to four items:

1. Both arms are worked together.
2. Face, head and neck items worked together.
3. Shoulder and torso movements combined.
4. Both legs are tensed together. (People who find this difficult should work the legs separately.)

RELAXATION THROUGH RECALL

PRT continues with relaxation through recall. This is described in Chapter 7 (p. 60).

EVIDENCE OF EFFECTIVENESS

PRT has produced favourable results in many conditions such as: anxiety (Rasid & Parish 1998), insomnia (Bootzin & Perlis 1992), asthma (Vazquez & Buceta 1993), hypertension (Yung et al 2001), epilepsy (Puskarich et al 1992), dyspnoea and anxiety in chronic obstructive pulmonary disease (Gift et al 1992) and rheumatic pain (Stenstrom et al 1996). The study of Stenstrom and colleagues compared the effects of dynamic muscle training with those of PRT in 54 patients with inflammatory rheumatic disease. Participants in both interventions trained for half an hour, 5 days a week for 3 months. At the end of that time the relaxation group exhibited marked improvements in muscle function which were significantly greater than those recorded in the dynamic exercise group. Comparison studies in general often show equal efficacy as in the study of Crist & Rickard (1993) where muscular relaxation was compared with imaginal relaxation in 100 healthy college students.

  Carlson & Hoyle (1993) reviewed studies featuring abbreviated progressive relaxation techniques such as PRT. The studies covered a wide range of conditions, but the largest effect sizes were found in tension headache. Other conditions such as cancer chemotherapy and hypertension showed smaller effect sizes. Overall, the intervention was found to be moderately effective.

Shortened and standardized versions of progressive relaxation such as Bernstein & Borkovec's are, in general, favoured by researchers and clinicians alike, although Lehrer (1982), re-evaluating Jacobson's work, argued for the superior benefit of the lengthy original. Lichstein (1988), reviewing studies comparing the two approaches, found the evidence inconclusive.

With regard to the 'pendulum effect', i.e. the stronger the initial contraction the deeper the relaxation which follows it, Lehrer et al (1988) found the evidence mixed. To these researchers it appeared unlikely that an automatic and immediate decrease in muscle tension to below base-line level would follow a strong muscle contraction.

The debate about the value of the initial contraction continues. While some authors, such as Bernstein & Borkovec, see the contraction as a means of promoting relaxation, others claim that it obstructs the process, and point to an increased muscle–nerve sympathetic activity resulting from the isometric contractions which feature in methods such as PRT (Farrell et al 1991).

Because of its various advantages, however, PRT is widely practised. With regard to the evidence, the picture is far from clear since some of the research suffers from methodological problems. In spite of this, Carlson & Hoyle (1993) conclude that the evidence is strong enough to support the continued use of such methods in the clinical setting.

PITFALLS OF PROGRESSIVE RELAXATION TRAINING

The pitfalls of muscular approaches are listed in Chapter 6 (pp 56–57).

Further reading

Bernstein D A, Borkovec T D 1973 Progressive relaxation training: a manual for the helping professions. Research Press, Champaign, Illinois

Bernstein D A, Given B A 1984 Progressive relaxation: abbreviated methods. In: Woolfolk R L, Lehrer P M (eds) Principles and practice of stress management. Guilford Press, New York

Chapter 6

A tense–release script

CHAPTER CONTENTS

The script set out below lies in the tradition of progressive relaxation. In procedure, however, it more closely resembles progressive relaxation training, except that reduced effort is put into the repeats in the manner of Jacobson's diminishing tensions. The exercises themselves are drawn from a variety of sources. Trainees may be lying or sitting in a high-backed chair to perform them, although, while the procedure is being introduced a sitting position is more suitable.

INTRODUCTION TO THE METHOD

I am going to lead you through some of the major muscle groups of the body, asking you to contract and relax them, one by one. Tensing and releasing muscles can help to induce a feeling of physical relaxation. You may also feel mentally relaxed. As you carry out the items, you'll experience sensations in the muscles. These sensations indicate tension which you will learn to identify and to release. This is a skill which enables you to relax yourself any time you want to and the more you practise it the easier it will become.

The following exercises should first be demonstrated by the trainer in order to familiarize participants with the procedure. Participants are then invited to try them out. It is worth spending time on the demonstration so that group members feel they know the exercises before the instruction begins.

THE EXERCISES

- Breathing (1).
- Arm: spider hand, rod-like arm.
- Leg: plantar and dorsiflexion (foot bending down and up), toe flexion (bending down) and extension (bending up).
- Breathing (2).
- Abdominal muscle tensing.
- Shoulder bracing.
- Shoulder hunching.
- Head pressing back.
- Upper face: brow raising, frowning, eye exercises.
- Lower face: jaw, lips, tongue.

Authors hold varying opinions as to the optimal duration of the tension and relaxation periods. Based on their collective judgements, the present author suggests 5 seconds for tensing, and 30–40 seconds for relaxing.

It is explained to participants that each tension phase is carried out on the command 'Now'. The signal for the release of tension is the word 'Relax'. When calling the items, the tone of voice can be varied from slightly crisp during the tension phase to soothing during the relaxation phase.

Participants may have their eyes open or closed. When they have taken up their chosen positions, the instructor begins.

BREATHING (1)

The section on hyperventilation in Chapter 15 (p. 134) is relevant to this exercise.

> Please make yourself as comfortable as you can. Let your breathing settle down and observe its natural rhythm. After a minute or two, follow a natural breath out, making it a little bit longer than usual ... then let the air in ... let it gently fill your lungs ... and ... breathe out slowly, releasing your tensions with the air ... and now let your breathing take care of itself ... do not immediately repeat this deep breath...
>
> You will recognize the exercises which follow. Please wait for the word 'Now' to perform the action.

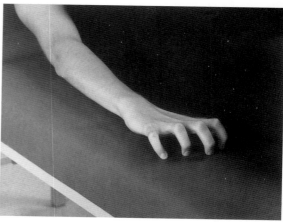

Figure 6.1   Spider hand.

ARM

Spider hand

This is adapted from Wallace (1980) (Fig. 6.1).

> I'd like you to focus attention on your right arm, whether it's lying alongside you or resting on the arm of your chair. With the hand placed palm downwards, slowly press the fingertips into the surface, drawing them towards your palm so that your hand gradually takes on the shape of a spider ... don't force the movement, just put a moderate amount of effort into it ... Now ... as you hold the position, notice the tensions in the hand and the underside of the forearm ... feel them build up ... then ... Relax ... let the tension go ... relax the muscles ... let the tension disappear and go on disappearing as you give the hand time to get more and more relaxed ... notice how it feels when it's fully relaxed...

The 'spider' exercise is repeated once using less effort.

Rod–like arm (Fig. 6.2)

> If you are seated, start with your right arm in your lap. Lying participants will have their right arm alongside them. I want you slowly to tense up all the muscles so that the arm becomes rigid. Begin with a little tension in the fingertips ... let it grow until the fingers are drawn into the palm making a fist shape. Then stretch out the arm, creating tension

Figure 6.2 Rod-like arm.

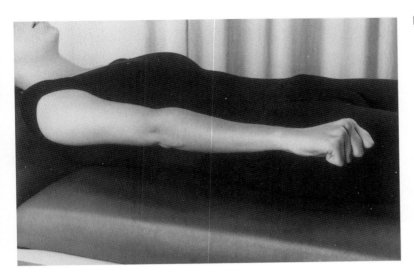

in the forearm and upper arm until the arm gets rigid like a rod ... Now ... feel the tension throughout the arm, but don't overdo it ... and ... Relax ... let it flop down ... feel the muscles going slack and the arm becoming limp ... notice the relief, the pleasant tingling and the sense of warmth ... let the arm go on relaxing ... and relaxing a bit more ... imagine the last remnant of tension flowing out through your fingertips ... notice how the arm muscles feel when they are fully relaxed.

The exercise is performed again, using less effort the second time.

'Spider' and 'rod' are then carried out with the left arm.

LEG

Next is a group of leg exercises. The first two are for those lying down and the second two are for those who are seated.

Feet pointing away from face

In this exercise the supine participant is asked to point his feet away from his face (Fig. 6.3).

Turning your attention to your legs which are lying flat on the ground, point your feet down, as if you were using them to indicate something. Don't overdo it especially if you are prone to develop cramp ... Now ... as you hold the position, study

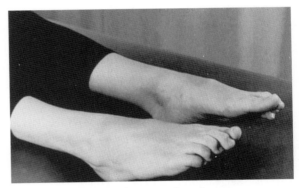

Figure 6.3 Feet pointing away from face.

the tensions in your calves ... and then ... Relax ... let go ... let all the tension dissolve ... feel comfort returning to your lower legs ... notice the sensations you get from relaxing the muscles ... continue letting go until you feel they won't relax any further...

Feet pointing towards face

The feet are now pointed towards the face (Fig. 6.4).

This time I'd like you to point your feet up towards your face, keeping the backs of your knees on the ground ... Now ... hold the position and notice the sensations you are getting in the working muscles around the shin bones ... and then ... Relax ... as you let go your leg muscles, feel the tension leaving them ... feel it draining out as your legs and feet become more and more relaxed...

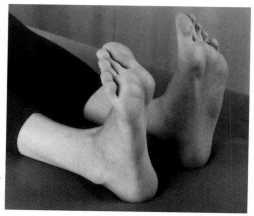

Figure 6.4   Feet pointing towards face.

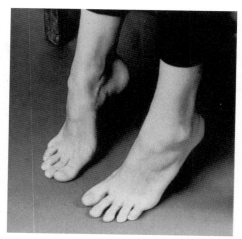

Figure 6.5   Heel raising.

These two exercises are repeated once with reduced tension.

The following two leg exercises are addressed to seated participants.

Heel raising

Here, the seated participant is asked to raise his heels off the ground (Fig. 6.5).

> Begin by making sure your feet are flat on the floor ... then, keeping your toes firmly in contact with the floor, raise your heels up in the air ... Now ... feel the tension in your calf muscles ... hold the action ... then ... Relax ... drop your heels to the ground ... notice the relief ... the comfort ... the warm, tingling sensation in your calves ... the enjoyable feeling of relaxing your feet ... go on letting those feelings continue until your feet and calves are completely relaxed ... then, a little bit further ...

Toe raising

In this exercise, the front part of the foot is raised off the ground (Fig. 6.6).

> This time, keep your heels on the ground, and raise the front part of your feet as if you were about to tap a rhythm ... Now ... keep your toes up in the air while you take notice of the tension sensation in the muscles around the shinbones ... and ... Relax ... let the feet fall down ... notice the relief in the shin area ... feel the tension leaving you ... draining out through your feet and toes ... and continuing to drain out a bit longer ...

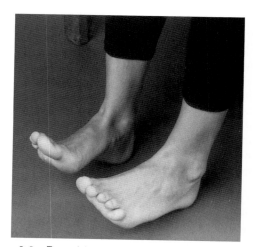

Figure 6.6   Toe raising.

These two exercises are repeated with diminished tension.

The next exercise is addressed to both lying and seated participants.

TOE FLEXION AND EXTENSION (Fig. 6.7)

> Let your attention focus on your toes. Whether you are lying or sitting, curl your toes down, restricting the action to the toes themselves. Some people can do it more easily than others, but just do what you can ... Now ... feel the tension in the sole of the foot and the calf of the leg ... then ... Relax ... let it go ... feel the muscles going slack ... feel them going

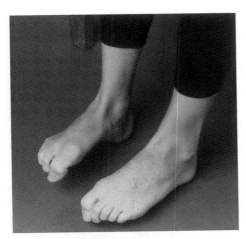

Figure 6.7   Toe flexion.

slacker still as the tension disappears ... notice how the muscles feel when they are relaxed.

The exercise is repeated once using less tension.

It is followed by a similar exercise in which the toes are bent upwards. Here, muscle tension is felt along the top part of the foot and the shin.

BREATHING (2)

At least a minute can be allotted to this item.

Turn your attention to your breathing again ... notice its rhythm ... place one hand over your upper abdomen and notice the gentle swell and recoil of the area underneath it ... avoid any inclination to alter the rhythm ... just let the breathing take care of itself...

ABDOMINAL MUSCLE TENSING

Focus next on the abdominal muscles ... make the area over your internal organs go flat and hard as you pull the muscles in ... Now ... feel the tension under your ribs, over your organs and around the back of your pelvis ... then ... Relax ... let go ... allow your muscles to spread themselves ... feel a sense of deep relaxation ... and let that relaxation become deeper as the moments pass...

One repeat is carried out using less tension.

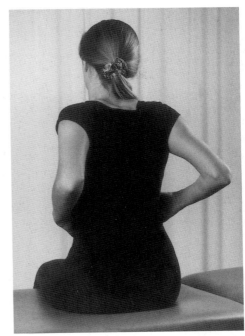

Figure 6.8   Shoulder bracing.

SHOULDER BRACING (Fig. 6.8)

Moving to the region of the back, bring your attention to the blade-bones behind your shoulders. Draw them back so that they get nearer to each other (without putting too much effort into it) ... Now ... feel them being gently squeezed together ... notice also, how your chest is lifted away from the supporting surface ... and then ... Relax ... release the tension ... let the muscles soften ... feel your back lying once again in contact with the supporting surface ... notice the feeling of relaxation and let that feeling continue on and on...

The exercise is repeated once with less tension.

SHOULDER HUNCHING (Fig. 6.9)

Moving to the neck region, I'd like you to lift your shoulders ... hunch them up as if to touch your ears ... Now ... feel the tension in the lower neck ... register the sensation ... and ... Relax ... let the shoulders drop ... and go on dropping ... further and further as the tension ebbs away ... feel your shoulders completely relaxed...

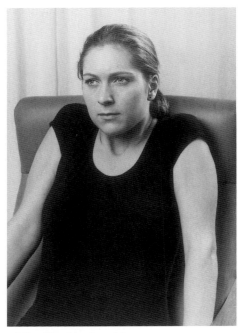

Figure 6.9 Shoulder hunching.

The exercise is performed once more using diminished tension.

HEAD BACK

And the head: keeping your chin in, press your head back against the support (against the floor or back of the chair) ... press it back, making double chins in the front ... stop short of discomfort ... Now ... notice the feelings you get from the working muscles ... tension in the back of the neck ... and ... Relax ... let go ... feel the area relax ... notice the sense of ease that floods into the area ... allow the relaxation to deepen until all the tension has left your neck ...

One repeat is carried out using less tension.

UPPER FACE

Eyebrow raising (Fig. 6.10)

Moving to the face, to the many muscles which control your facial expressions: would you now raise your eyebrows ... raise them high, creating horizontal furrows ... Now ... feel the tension in the muscle that stretches across the brow ... and ...

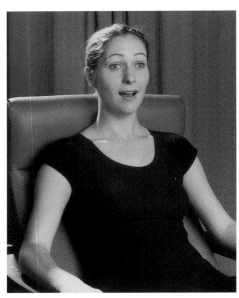

Figure 6.10 Eyebrow raising.

Relax ... let the tension flow out ... feel the furrows being smoothed ... continue until there is no tension left in your brow ... then a little bit further ...

The repeat is carried out using less tension.

Frowning (Fig. 6.11)

Focus on your frowning muscle ... bring the eyebrows closer together, buckling the skin between them into a deep frown ... Now ... hold it a few moments, taking note of the sensation you get from the action ... then ... Relax ... release the tension ... feel the eyebrows spread sideways ... imagine the space between them getting wider and continuing to get wider ... notice the comfortable feeling that accompanies this idea ... continue until all the tension dies away ...

The exercise is repeated once using diminished tension.

Eyes

We come to the eyes. First, I'd like you to screw them up and notice the sensation you get from the action ... Now ... spend a moment registering it ... then ... Relax ... let go ... let the muscles loosen ... notice the feeling you get from loosening them ... feel the skin smoothing out ...

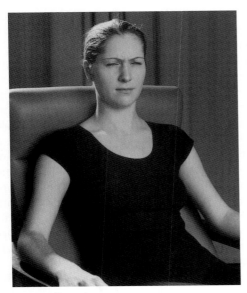

Figure 6.11   Frowning.

The exercise is performed once more using diminished tension. For the following exercise, the trainee's eyes should be closed. The format is slightly different in that, because there are so many eye movements, the relaxation is postponed until the end.

Next, without moving your head, turn your eyes upwards behind your closed lids ... Now ... hold your gaze up for a few moments ... notice the tension in the muscles ... and ... bring your eyes back to a central position ... and, look down, as if towards your feet ... Now ... hold it a few moments ... then return to the centre ... look to the right ... Now ... keep a steady hold ... and return to the front ... and, to the left ... Now ... hold it ... then bring your eyes back to the front ... and ... as they rest in a middle position, notice how they feel ... compare this with how they felt when they were working ... let them go on relaxing ... continue relaxing for a full minute...

Finally, roll your eyes in a clockwise circle ... Now ... notice the sensations of tension ... pause ... roll them in an anticlockwise direction ... Now ... notice the feelings ... and ... Relax ... let them fully relax ... let them go on relaxing until all the tension has left them...

One repeat may be carried out using less tension. A further exercise consists of focusing at different distances behind closed lids: first on a faraway object, then on an object placed close to the eyes (adapted from Madders 1981).

With your eyes still closed, imagine you are looking at an object on the distant horizon. You can't see it clearly but you are trying to make it out ... Now ... notice how it feels as you strain to identify it ... then, releasing the tension, bring your eyes to focus on a piece of writing held very close ... Now ... notice the sensations as you make the effort to read the words ... and, Relax ... let your eyes settle on the middle distance ... feel the relief as you let go the tension in the muscles which control the focusing ... enjoy the feeling of releasing that tension...

After a short rest, repeat the action with reduced tension.

LOWER FACE

Jaw

Bring your back teeth together ... do it firmly but without actually clenching them ... Now ... feel a sensation in your jaw as if you'd been chewing tough meat ... hold it ... and ... Relax ... release the jaw muscles ... feel the tension fading ... continuing to fade ... and then further still...

The exercise is repeated with diminished tension.

Lips

Press your lips tightly together as if you were rejecting some unpleasant medicine ... Now ... hold your lips pursed ... then ... Relax ... let them go ... and as they relax, notice feelings such as the warmth of the blood flowing back into your lips ... tune in to the feelings of relaxation...

One repeat is carried out using less tension.

Tongue

Finally the tongue: press your tongue against the roof of your mouth and hold it there ... Now ... feel the tension in the tongue ... and ... Relax ... notice how it feels when your relax it ... and press it against the inside of your right cheek ... Now ... hold ... and Relax ... and against your left cheek ... Now ... hold ... and Relax ... and pull it back

> towards your throat (not too strongly) ... Now ...
> hold ... and Relax ... and then let your tongue
> settle in the middle of your mouth, just touching
> the backs of your front teeth ... feel it releasing
> tension ... let it go on relaxing ... enjoy the feeling
> of relaxation ... let that feeling spread throughout
> your mouth and over your face, making them
> feel warm, glowing and relaxed ... then, let it spread
> to cover your neck and shoulders ... your arms ...
> back ... abdomen ... and legs, so that your entire
> body experiences a feeling of complete
> relaxation ... continue relaxing for several
> minutes...

TERMINATION

> And so, I'm going to bring this session to an end ...
> gradually I'd like you to return to normal activity,
> but first I'll count from one to three to help you
> make the adjustment ... when I get to three, I'd like
> you to open your eyes, feeling fresh and alert and
> ready to carry on with your day ... one ... two ...
> three ... before getting up, give a few gentle
> stretches to your arms and legs.

PITFALLS OF MUSCULAR APPROACHES

It would seem that progressive relaxation is appropriate in any circumstances where rest is prescribed (McGuigan 1984). The method is unlikely to create negative effects and Jacobson did not refer to any.

Some points, however, need to be considered:

1. Training in relaxation should never be viewed as a substitute for medical treatment; wherever a disorder is present or suspected, medical help should be sought.

2. Relaxation training is not generally recommended for people suffering from hallucinations, delusion or other psychotic symptoms, as the exercises can lead to out-of-body sensations. It is traditionally held that imagery is never appropriate, but benefit has been derived from a tense–release and physical exercise approach during a non-active period of psychotic illness (Bloom & Gonzales 1981). Keable (1997) has emphasized the value of this finding for individuals who experience stress in

addition to their psychosis. Discussion with the attending psychiatrist or psychologist would first be necessary.

3. Variations in the blood pressure may occur in the course of relaxation training: it can rise when limbs are being tensed and fall during deep relaxation. The first can be counteracted by allowing a rest between the tensings, and the second by asking trainees, when the session is over, to bend and stretch their limbs a few times before resuming active life. The fall in blood pressure which accompanies deep relaxation is only that which occurs under any resting conditions. It is, however, important to allow time for the individual to adjust to active life following a session of relaxation. Suddenly jumping up from a relaxed lying position can induce faintness.

For people whose blood pressure is already high, a release-only method (Ch. 7) is preferable to one which consists of muscle tensings.

4. Tension-based exercises can induce heart arrhythmias in cardiac patients (McArdle et al 1986) and are therefore considered unsuitable for patients following myocardial infarction. An alternative relaxation method is suggested for people suffering from heart conditions.

5. Antenatal and labouring mothers are no longer given tense–release exercises because of the possibility of interference with uterine contractions (Ch. 25). Release-only forms (i.e. passive relaxation) would, however, be appropriate.

6. Tense–release procedures performed with excessive tightening may lead to cramp. In order to avoid this, trainees can be advised to stop short of discomfort. Recurrent cramp would indicate the unsuitability of the technique for that individual. Overtensing the spine and the neck should also be avoided since it can lead to spinal damage.

7. Some researchers have reported a fear of relaxing in certain individuals (Lehrer 1979), and others report that relaxation occasionally induces anxiety (Borkovec & Heide 1980). This can be recognized by excessive perspiration, trembling, rapid breathing or general restlessness. The training (for that individual) should immediately be stopped. These symptoms may, however, be the result of a fear that letting-go might lead to loss of control. To individuals who harbour such fears, the wording can be changed to 'as relaxed as you

want to be'. It is worth mentioning that the researchers who studied the reaction (Borkovec & Heide 1980) were not using Jacobson's original method, but one of its modifications.

Disturbing feelings may rise to the surface during any kind of relaxation: in the process of releasing tension, psychological defences can be weakened (Hough 1991).

8. Abromowitz & Wieselberg (1978) reported that a few individuals undergoing relaxation training became angry when asked to relax. It was unclear what had caused the anger but one reason suggested was that they had found difficulty in mastering the technique.

9. Progressive relaxation training has been found effective for many people suffering organic pain. It provides a physical approach to a physical disorder (Davidson & Schwartz 1976). Some individuals, however, find that focusing on the body intensifies their perception of pain (Snyder 1985), and for them, muscular approaches may be less useful than cognitive ones such as imagery or meditation.

10. Trainees who, because of disability or disorder, are in doubt as to the suitability of any exercise, should begin by performing it very gently. This applies, for example, to individuals with back or neck problems.

11. As attention to breathing is a feature of most muscular approaches, the hazards of hyperventilation should be borne in mind (p. 134).

12. Some tense–release scripts make use of imagery. They will therefore, in addition, be subject to the pitfalls listed in Chapter 18 (p. 170).

Chapter 7

Passive muscular relaxation

INTRODUCTION AND RATIONALE

Muscular relaxation is a process by which contractile tension in voluntary muscles is reduced. The methods described in the previous three chapters are examples of the tense–release technique. Because of the contraction component, this is essentially an active procedure. When the contraction component is withdrawn, however, relaxation becomes a passive procedure. Jacobson's work covers both tense–release and passive relaxation.

Passive muscular relaxation consists of a systematic review of the skeletal muscle groups in the body. As attention is focused on each one in turn, the individual spots any tension and then releases it. Passive relaxation has certain practical advantages over active methods in that:

1. The sequences can be carried out without drawing attention to the individual performing them. They are thus potentially useful in the workplace or other public locations where stress arises.
2. Passive routines take less time to work through than tense–release ones.
3. The method is available to those with physical disabilities, the nature of which might preclude some of the tension routines.

Passive muscular relaxation, on the whole, requires previous knowledge of the tense–release approach. It is through tense–release that the individual learns to become aware of the sensations associated with muscle state; sensations that help him identify and release the tension.

Evidence of the value of passive relaxation comes from Lucic et al (1991), whose work supports the view that muscles relax more fully when the process is not preceded by a strong contraction. In other words, the tensing of muscle groups prior to relaxation may actually hinder their capacity to relax. These findings are thus in line with the view of Jacobson, whose work was essentially passive (though he did not use that word to describe it). Although his method has already been described in Chapter 4, reference must be made here to the position he holds as the pre-eminent exponent of the passive muscular approach. It is true that he used tensing procedures, but the central idea of his work lay in the release of tension.

The authors whose work is described here are:

- Bernstein & Borkovec (1973)
- Everly & Rosenfeld (1981)
- Madders (1981), and
- Kermani (1990).

These authors have been included primarily because of the precise form of their presentations. Bernstein & Borkovec (1973) describe a release-only routine which they call 'relaxation through recall' in which muscle groups are relaxed by recalling the sensations associated with the release of tension.

Everly & Rosenfeld (1981) have developed a release-only approach which they call 'passive neuromuscular relaxation', defining it as a focusing of sensory awareness on particular muscle groups followed by their relaxation. These researchers see passive neuromuscular relaxation as a form of mental imagery which, together with its overtones of suggestion, departs from the strictly physical nature of Jacobson's progressive relaxation. On this account, the pitfalls of visualization (Ch. 18, p. 170) as well as those for muscular relaxation (Ch. 6, p. 56) should be read when adopting this approach.

The authors mentioned above are psychologists. Madders, a physiotherapist, includes passive relaxation in her book *Stress and Relaxation* (1981), while Kermani (1990), an autogenic training therapist, presents a scanning procedure.

RELAXATION THROUGH RECALL

While giving prominence to tense–release sequences in progressive relaxation training (Ch. 5), Bernstein & Borkovec (1973) also offer a release-only technique. 'Relaxation through recall' is the name given to this technique which is described here in an adapted form. It requires the trainee to have first learned the active form of progressive relaxation training, since the passive form is based on the memory of those routines.

The muscle groups involved are the final summarized groupings of arms, head and neck, trunk, and legs (p. 47). Two steps are involved.

1. The individual focuses on one of the groups, noticing any tension.
2. He recalls the sensation associated with releasing tension, and spends 30–45 seconds relaxing any tension that he finds.

Trainees are prepared by a short introduction (adapted from Lichstein 1988):

> Tensing and relaxing has made you highly sensitive to the feelings which accompany changes in the muscles, and now that you know the technique, I want to lead you to a more advanced version of it. I would like you to cast your mind back to the four-group tense–release procedure, but this time, to drop the tensing part. As we travel through these four groups, I'm going to ask you simply to look for any tension, and then, by recalling the sensations associated with its release, to let it go.

The trainee sits in a reclining chair or something that resembles it and the following script is presented:

> Would you close your eyes please. I'd like you first to concentrate on the muscles of your hands and arms. See if you can identify any feeling of tension in them. If so, notice where it is ... notice how it feels ... and relax it away, remembering previous feelings of releasing tension in these muscles ... go on releasing tension as you recall those sensations ... go on until the muscles become more and more deeply relaxed ... until you feel relaxation flowing through all the muscles of your arms ... until they are totally free of tension ... signal with a lifted finger when the arms feel fully relaxed.

The trainer continues in this way for 30–45 seconds.

> Next, bring your mind to focus on the muscles of your face and neck. Is there any tension there? If so, notice where it is and what it feels like ... then, recalling the feeling of letting the tension go, relax it ... feel the tension leaving the muscles ... note the pleasant feeling of relaxation ... allow the relaxation to deepen and go on deepening as you concentrate on the peaceful state of those muscles...
>
> Next, concentrate on the muscles of the trunk. Pick up any sensation of tension you may find ... notice where it is and what it feels like ... remember what it felt like when you previously relaxed tension in those muscles ... and relax them now ... relax any tension you find ... continue letting the tension go until your muscles feel quite loose. Go on relaxing them ... feel them getting looser and looser.
>
> Finally, give your attention to your legs ... do you notice any tension there? ... notice exactly where it is ... notice how it feels ... and release it ... recalling the sensation of releasing it ... remembering that feeling ... letting all the tension dissolve ... further ... then further still ... until the muscles feel entirely relaxed...

By practising relaxation through recall the trainee will be able to reduce the time it takes to relax each muscle group from 45 to perhaps 15 seconds.

RELAXATION THROUGH RECALL WITH COUNTING

When the trainee feels skilled at relaxing through recall, the procedure can be still further shortened by introducing counting. Here, recited numbers correspond to the groups in the recall procedure as follows:

> I'm going to count slowly from one to ten. As I count, I'd like you to focus on the same muscle groups as in the recall procedure, relaxing them as you did then.
>
> One ... two, focusing on the arms and hands as they become more relaxed ... three ... four, relaxing the face and neck muscles ... five ... six, focusing on the muscles of the chest, back, shoulders and abdomen, feeling them becoming more and more relaxed ... seven ... eight, allowing relaxation to flow through the muscles of the legs and feet ... nine ... ten, relaxed all over...

It is suggested that the counting be done at a pace which corresponds with the trainee's respirations. Once mastered, this technique can be used by the trainee when faced with challenging situations.

PASSIVE NEUROMUSCULAR RELAXATION

The technique described here is the work of Everly & Rosenfeld (1981). This method owes much to autogenic training (Ch. 19) in its use of suggestion and its images of warmth and heaviness. It is, however, considered by its authors to be a muscular method and so belongs in this chapter.

Trainees are introduced to the approach with a short explanation on the following lines:

> Tension in the muscles is associated with tension in the mind. If tension is eliminated from the muscles, then the subjective feeling of stress is reduced. In this method you will be asked to focus attention on one muscle group at a time, releasing any tension that exists. No activity is involved; the method is a passive one. It has been found that by concentrating on the muscles in this way, deep levels of relaxation can be achieved. Of course, the more you practise, the more effective it becomes.

The necessary conditions include a warm, quiet room where interruptions are unlikely to occur, and a comfortable chair to sit in or flat surface to lie on. The following script is adapted from Everly & Rosenfeld (1981).

> Settle into the chair you're in or the surface you are lying on, letting your body weight sink into it. Close your eyes. To start with, I'd like you to turn your attention to your breathing ... follow the next breath out ... then, let the air in ... feel it gently filling your lungs ... pause for a moment ... and breathe out slowly ... then allow your breathing to follow its natural rhythm: gentle and slow ... getting gentler and slower...
>
> Now bring your attention to the muscles of your head. Begin to feel a slow warm wave of relaxation gathering at the top of your head and beginning to descend towards your forehead ... focusing on the muscles above your eyes ... feel those muscles becoming heavy and relaxed ... concentrate on the heavy feeling you are getting from them ... now

shift your attention to the muscles of your eyes and cheeks and feel them also becoming heavy and relaxed ... now, focus on the muscles of your mouth and jaw ... allow them to grow heavy and relaxed...

Pause for 10 seconds.

As your head and face continue to relax, let the wave of relaxation slowly descend into your neck ... focus your attention on the neck muscles and feel them becoming slacker and more relaxed with every moment that passes...

Pause for 10 seconds.

The wave of relaxation continues to roll down, this time spreading warmth over your shoulder muscles ... focus on this area ... allow it to become heavy and relaxed as you concentrate your attention on it.

Pause for 10 seconds.

The head, neck and shoulders remain relaxed while you focus on your arms ... letting the wave of relaxation bring heaviness and warmth to them ... concentrate on the feelings in the arms...

Pause for 10 seconds.

Now feel the wave of relaxation descending into your hands as you focus on them ... feel the muscles of your palms and fingers relaxing ... feel warmth flowing into them as they become more relaxed...

Pause for 10 seconds.

Now, as the upper part of your body remains in deep relaxation, switch your attention to your abdomen and the wall of muscle covering your internal organs ... let those muscles loosen and spread ... then feel the wave of relaxation beginning to descend into your thigh muscles ... and as you concentrate on them, feel your thighs becoming heavy ... heavy as lead...

Pause for 10 seconds.

The wave of relaxation continues to descend into your lower legs ... focus on your calf muscles ... feel the sense of heaviness and relaxation in your calves...

Pause for 10 seconds.

Now, as the rest of your body remains relaxed, turn your attention to your feet ... feel the warm wave of relaxation descending into your foot muscles ... feel them becoming warm, heavy and relaxed...

Pause for 10 seconds.

Then, as you feel all your muscles to be in a state of relaxation, start to recite the phrase, 'I am relaxed'; repeat it every time you breathe out.

After a 5-minute pause:

I'd like you now to bring your attention back to the room in which you are lying. I am going to count from one to five, and as I count, begin to feel more and more awake, more and more refreshed, with a clear head. When I reach five, I'd like you to open your eyes. One, begin to feel alert ... two ... three, more alert still ... four ... five ... open your eyes and gently stretch your arms and legs...

THE RELAXATION 'RIPPLE'

Closely related to the above method is the relaxation 'ripple'. Adapted from Priest & Schott (1991), the technique consists of one continuous wave of relaxation which begins at the crown of the head and progresses down through the body to the toes. As the wave descends, the individual briefly scans the muscle groups, releasing tension. If he is lying down, all tension can be released; if he is standing, excess tension can be released. The effectiveness of the exercise is increased if it is timed to coincide with the outbreath. However, the participant should be discouraged from extending the outbreath too long.

The exercise can be better understood if the first relaxation ripple is preceded by a tensing of the whole body (Schott & Priest 2002). Thereafter, it can be performed in a passive manner.

A PASSIVE RELAXATION APPROACH

The script presented here is adapted from Madders (1981). It is addressed to trainees who are lying down. A supplementary section enables the instructor to adapt it for the seated participant.

INTRODUCTORY REMARKS TO TRAINEES

This is a method which helps to relax your muscles and your thoughts. It consists of focusing on different parts of the body in turn and releasing any tension you find. There are no physical actions involved; relaxation occurs by virtue of a thought process. In spite of its length, the method is one which you can easily use to induce relaxation on your own.

PROCEDURE FOR TRAINEES WHO ARE LYING DOWN

A firm support with a soft surface is needed, e.g. a length of foam spread out on the floor. The script could begin with the passage called 'Sinking' in Chapter 2 (p. 17), and continue as follows:

With your eyes closed, notice how slow and regular your breathing is becoming ... easy, calm and even ... leaving you more relaxed than you were before...

I'm going to ask you to take a trip round the body, checking that all the muscle groups are as relaxed as possible and letting go any tension that might still remain. If outside thoughts creep in, hold them in a bubble and let them float away. I'll begin with the feet.

Bring your attention to your toes ... are they lying still? If they are curled or stretched out or in some way not entirely comfortable, waggle them gently. As they come to rest, feel the tension ebbing away ... feel the tension leaving them as they lie motionless...

Let your feet roll out at the ankles. This is the most relaxed position for them. Let all the tension flow out of them ... enjoy the sensation of just letting them go.

Moving on to the lower legs: feel the tension leaving the calf muscles and the shins. As the tension goes, so they feel heavier ... so they feel warm and pleasantly tingling.

The thighs next: to be fully relaxed they need to be slightly rolling outwards ... feel the relaxing effect of this position ... make sure you have released all tension, and feel your thighs resting heavily on the floor.

Focus for a moment on the sensation of sagging heaviness throughout your legs ... let the muscles shed their last remaining hint of tension and settle into a deep relaxation.

And now, think of your hips. Let them settle into the surface you are lying on ... recognize any tension that lingers in the muscles ... then relax it

away ... let it go on relaxing a bit further than you thought possible.

Settle your spine into the rug or mattress ... become aware of how it is resting on the floor. Let it sink down, making contact wherever it wants to ... all tension draining out of it.

Let your abdominal muscles lose their tension. Let them go soft and loose. Feel them spreading as they give up their last vestige of tension ... notice how your relaxed abdomen rises and falls with your breathing ... rises as the air is drawn in and falls as the air is expelled ... abdominal breathing is relaxed breathing.

Moving up to your shoulders, to muscles which are prone to carry tension ... feel them letting go ... feel them spreading ... feel them easing into the floor, limp and heavy ... feel them dropping down towards your feet ... imagine them shedding their burdens ... and as the space between your shoulders and your neck opens out, imagine your neck a bit longer than it was before.

Now, direct your thoughts to the muscles of your left arm. Check that it lies limply on the ground. Notice the feeling of relaxation and allow this feeling to sweep down to your wrist and hand. Think of the fingers, are they curved and still? ... neither drawn up nor stretched out ... in a hand that is neither open nor closed, but gently resting ... totally relaxed. As you breathe out, let the arm relax a little bit more ... let it lie heavy and loose ... so heavy and loose that if someone were to pick it up, then let go, it would flop down again like the arm of a rag doll.

Repeat the last paragraph with the muscles of the right arm.

Your neck muscles have no need to work with your head supported, so let them go ... enjoy the feeling of 'letting go' in muscles which work so hard the rest of the time to keep your head upright. If you find any tension in the neck, release it and let this process of releasing continue, even below the surface ... feel how pleasant it is when you let go the tension in these muscles.

Bring your attention now to your face, to the many small muscles whose job it is to manage your expressions. At the moment there's no need to have any expression at all on your face, so allow your muscles to feel relaxed ... imagine how your face is when you are asleep ... calm and motionless...

Now, think about the jaw ... and as you do, allow it to drop slightly so that your teeth are separated ... feel it relaxing with your lips gently touching. Check that your tongue is still, and lying in the middle of your mouth, soft and shapeless. Relax your throat so that all tension leaves it and the muscles feel smooth and resting.

With no expression on your face, your cheeks are relaxed and soft. If you think of your nose, let it be just to register the passage of cool air travelling up your nostrils while warmer air passes down ... breathe tension out with the warm air ... breathe stillness in with the cool air.

Check that your forehead is smooth ... not furrowed in any direction ... and as you release its remaining tension, imagine it being a little higher and a little wider that it was before ... let this feeling of relaxation extend through your scalp muscles, over the crown of your head and down behind your ears ... feel a sense of calm as you do this.

Let your attention focus on your eyes as they lie behind gently closed lids. Think of them resting in their sockets, floating rather than fixed ... and as they come to rest, so do your thoughts also.

Spend a few minutes continuing to relax, deepening the effect of the above sequences...

You have now relaxed all the major muscle groups in your body. Think about them now as a whole ... a totally relaxed whole ... soothed by your gentle breathing rhythm, feel the peacefulness of this idea...

Images may drift in and out of your mind ... see them as thoughts passing through. Feel yourself letting go of them. Say to yourself: 'I am feeling calm, I am feeling peaceful'. Let your mind conjure up a scene of contentment.

Trainees can relax quietly for a few minutes, before the session is brought to an end.

TERMINATION

I am going to ask you to bring yourself slowly back to the room you are lying in. Gradually become aware of it. Gently move your arms and legs ... wriggle your spine, and in your own time, allow your eyes to open. Slowly sit up and take in your surroundings. Give your body plenty of time to adjust from the relaxed to the alert state.

Before the meeting breaks up, the value of practice should be emphasized. If carried out on a daily basis, the technique will help the trainee to relax himself more effectively.

ADAPTED PROCEDURE FOR SEATED TRAINEES

The trainee picks the chair he finds most comfortable, although in a public building the choice may be limited. For deep relaxation the body needs to be well supported. The procedure begins in the following way:

Settle into your chair, sitting well back into the seat, your feet flat on the floor and your hands in your lap. Close your eyes. Become aware of the parts of your body that touch the chair and the floor. Feel the weight of your body passing through those points: hips, thighs, feet, back and arms, some of them carrying more weight than others. If the back of the chair is high enough, use it to support your head. If not, your head may be dropping forwards which is all right if you find it comfortable, but it tends to put a strain on the neck muscles if held for a long time. Try raising your head and seeing it as a weight supported by a pole. If you can balance it in this way, on your spine, you will be giving your neck muscles a rest.

The same script as for the lying position may be used, substituting the word 'sitting' for 'lying', and 'chair' for 'floor'. The paragraph about the neck muscles can be deleted, and also the one referring to the feet.

KERMANI'S SCANNING TECHNIQUE

To 'scan' in this sense, is to run the attention over all the voluntary muscles.

Scanning may be used for at least two purposes: on the one hand, as a means of checking to see if tension exists, and on the other, as a device to enable the individual to feel in touch with his body as a whole. Both purposes are relevant in the context of relaxation, and the method forms a quick and simple version of the passive relaxation approach.

Here is an example adapted from Kermani (1990).

> I'll ask you to spend a moment getting in touch with the different parts of your body, acknowledging them as part of you and checking that they feel relaxed and comfortable. Begin by bringing your attention to your feet. First the toes ... working up through the ankles ... to the calves and shins ... over the knees ... along the thighs ... the abdomen ... then the chest. Think now of your shoulders ... of travelling down to the elbows ... through the forearms ... and into the wrists ... hands and fingers. Become aware even of your fingertips.
>
> Next, move across to the lower spine and the pelvis. Give your attention to the lumbar region ... rising to the back of the chest and the blade bones ... continuing up into the neck and scalp ... to the crown of the head ... then slowly begin to descend to the forehead ... ending with the jaw ... feel that every part of your body is relaxed...
>
> You might like to think of a giant paint brush sweeping over your body, following the same route.

RELEASE–ONLY

A release-only method is described in Chapter 8 (p. 70) as one component of Öst's applied relaxation.

PITFALLS OF PASSIVE RELAXATION

Passive relaxation is subject to the pitfalls of other muscular approaches (Ch. 6, p. 56). Because passive methods often include imagery and suggestion, the pitfalls relating to visualizations should also be taken into account (Ch. 18, p. 170).

Further reading

Bernstein D A, Borkovec T D 1973 Progressive relaxation training: a manual for the helping professions. Research Press, Champaign, Illinois

Everly G S, Rosenfeld R 1981 The nature and treatment of the stress response. Plenum Press, New York

Jacobson E 1976 You must relax. Souvenir Press, London

Kermani K S 1990 Autogenic training. Souvenir Press, London

Madders J 1981 Stress and relaxation: self-help ways to cope with stress and relieve nervous tension, ulcers, insomnia, migraine and high blood pressure, 3rd edn. Martin Dunitz, London

Chapter 8

Applied relaxation

HISTORY

The methods described in previous chapters have, on the whole, been concerned with the induction of deep relaxation. Their purpose is to equip the individual with routines to be performed in the privacy of his own home. As such, these methods are useful for unwinding after a stressful day, but may not, however, provide strategies for coping with stress as it occurs. For this, some kind of shortened version that can be linked into life activities is required. Jacobson's (1938) differential relaxation (p. 40) and Wolpe's (1958) systematic desensitization represent early attempts at applied formats. However, it was Goldfried (1971) who, recognizing the extent of the gulf between relaxation in the therapeutic environment and relaxation in the stressful situation, focused expressly on the issue of the application of the skills. He emphasized the need for a portable and shortened form of progressive relaxation; a form which could be used to defuse anxiety as it occurred, and one which the individual could use as a general coping skill in everyday life. In so doing, he gave the individual a new role, defining him as an active agent in his treatment rather than a passive client. The approach was called 'training in self-control' because it implied active mastery of anxiety by the individual himself.

DESCRIPTION

Öst's (1987) applied relaxation method is a recent version of Goldfried's approach. Using progressive relaxation as a core technique, the method teaches the individual to relax in successively shorter periods and to transfer these relaxation effects to everyday situations. Thus the individual is equipped with a strategy to control his reactions to stressful events as they occur.

The method consists of six components, in each of which a particular aspect of relaxation is taught:

- tense–release technique
- release-only technique
- cue-controlled (conditioned) relaxation
- differential relaxation
- rapid relaxation
- application training.

It is estimated that by using the tense–release method taught here (Wolpe & Lazarus 1966), the trained individual can achieve a relaxed state in 15–20 minutes; by using the release-only technique he can achieve it in 5–7 minutes; using the cue-controlled, in 2–3 minutes; the differential technique, in 60–90 seconds and using rapid relaxation, in 20–30 seconds. The final goal is to be able to apply relaxation skills to the experience of everyday stressful events.

The components must be taught in a precise order since progression to each depends largely on mastery of the preceding one. A total of 8–12 sessions of tuition is required, backed up by home practice which should be carried out twice a day, and is itself an important part of the programme.

RATIONALE

As with all versions of progressive relaxation, applied relaxation is said to calm the thoughts as a result of relaxing the musculature. Thus, it can be used for coping with day-to-day stress. Öst's method, however, was designed principally for use with people who suffer from panic and other kinds of anxiety. In this context, an understanding of anxiety as a state is crucial to the success of the training and an explanation should be given to the participant at the outset.

Anxiety may be seen as having three aspects: the physiological, the cognitive and the behavioural. The physiological aspect is represented by such phenomena as raised heart rate and blood

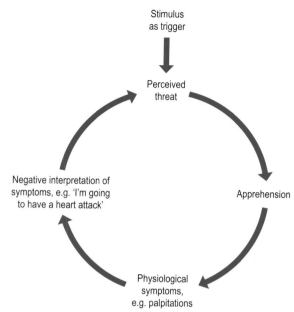

Figure 8.1 A cognitive model of panic attacks. (Adapted from Clark 1986.)

pressure, sweating and increased muscle tension; the cognitive aspect by negative thoughts such as 'This is too much for me to cope with' or 'I'm going to have a heart attack', and the behavioural aspect by tense posture and different kinds of unrelaxed activity. These effects can escalate with one inflaming the other. In particular, the physiological and cognitive aspects can create a vicious circle with negative thoughts leading to sympathetic changes which are themselves interpreted in a negative way. The result can be a spiralling of anxiety (Clark 1986) (Fig. 8.1).

One way of breaking the circle would be to reinterpret the bodily changes in a more positive light, i.e. instead of thinking he is about to collapse with a heart attack, the individual could reassure himself that everyone gets palpitations sometimes. This constitutes a cognitive approach. Another way of breaking the circle would be to neutralize the anxiety with the use of a relaxation technique such as progressive relaxation. This draws on physiological theory. A third way would be to introduce graded exposure to the feared item which represents a behavioural approach. All three are incorporated in Öst's applied relaxation which can

Date	Situation	Reaction, i.e. anxiety signals	Intensity (0–10)	Action taken

Figure 8.2 A form for recording self-observed early anxiety signals. (Adapted from Öst 1987.)

thus be seen as a cognitive behavioural method (Heimberg 2002).

Because anxiety is easier to relieve when it is mild, it should be addressed before it reaches a peak. Early signals or signs of rising anxiety levels such as a pounding heart, sweating, fast breathing or tense muscles can be used as cues to employ the technique. Experiences of anxiety-provoking events can be recorded by means of 'self-monitoring', where the individual notes on a printed form the situations, the intensity of his anxiety and the remedial action taken by him (Fig. 8.2). This form, over time, reflects his progress in coping with such events.

PROCEDURE

It is suggested that participants sit for the exercises since daily stress frequently occurs in this posture rather than in a lying one. The chair should be comfortable and have arm rests.

INTRODUCTORY REMARKS TO PARTICIPANTS

Before beginning the programme of relaxation, the rationale of the treatment is presented to participants:

As its name suggests, this method will show you how to apply relaxation skills in everyday life. This means the techniques have to be quick-acting and unobtrusive. The ultimate aim is to be able to relax in 20–30 seconds and to transfer this skill to situations of stress.

When people experience anxiety they tend to react in three different ways: a physiological way in which their blood pressure rises and they become breathless with a pounding heart and a cold sweat; a psychological way in which distressing thoughts go through their head; and a behavioural way whereby they find themselves trying to escape.

If the physiological symptoms are viewed as threatening, the body will respond by intensifying those symptoms, which in turn will make the thoughts more negative. This is the way a panic attack develops.

However, this vicious circle can be broken and one way of doing this is by learning not to react so strongly. This will reduce your feeling of distress and your symptoms will tend to subside.

I am going to lead you through a well-tested method which will help you to achieve this. You'll be learning a skill, so it's important to practise it, but once you've mastered it, you'll find it useful in nearly all situations.

The approach starts by introducing you to progressive relaxation which consists of tensing and releasing the muscles throughout the body. When that is learned and practised daily, the tensing part of the exercise is dropped.

Next, you'll be asked to repeat the word 'relax' to yourself when you are in a state of relaxation. Attaching the word to the state has the effect of turning the word into a cue; a cue to invoke a state of relaxation. This only happens, of course, after repeated associations.

Learning how to use reduced amounts of muscle tension when carrying out specific tasks is the next procedure, followed by a rapid-acting technique for maintaining low levels of stress throughout the day. Finally, these skills are applied to particular situations of stress.

These exercises enable you to achieve relaxation in progressively shorter periods of time. Success depends on practice.

TENSE–RELEASE

Two sessions of tuition are devoted to learning this version of progressive relaxation. The procedures are first demonstrated by the trainer and carried out by the trainee to ensure that they have been understood. The trainee then closes his eyes while the instructor runs through the programme. At the end, the trainee rates the degree of relaxation gained on a 0–100 scale.

First session

This is spent working on the hands, arms, face, neck and shoulders. Each muscle group is taken through one tense–release cycle in which 5 seconds are allotted for the tension and 10–15 seconds for the release, as follows:

Begin by clenching the right hand ... make a fist ... make it tight ... notice the sensation of tension in the hand and forearm while you hold it for 5 seconds ... then let it go ... feel the hand and forearm becoming relaxed and comfortable ... warm and relaxed ... relaxed and heavy ...

The other actions featuring in session one are:

- clenching the left hand
- bending the right elbow
- straightening the right elbow by pressing the wrist down on the arm of the chair
- bending the left elbow
- straightening the left elbow
- raising the eyebrows and wrinkling the forehead
- bringing the eyebrows together and frowning
- screwing the eyes up tight
- biting the teeth together
- pressing the tongue against the roof of the mouth
- pressing the lips together

- pressing the head against the back of the chair
- pressing the chin down on to the chest
- hunching the shoulders up to the ears
- bracing the shoulders back to bring the blades together.

Termination. When the above exercises have been worked through, the session is brought to an end.

The relaxation session is over now, and to help you return to activity, I'm going to count from one to five, and when I get to five, I want you to open your eyes, feeling calm and relaxed ... one, feeling calm ... two, feeling relaxed ... three, very calm ... four, very relaxed ... five ... open your eyes, feeling ready to carry on with your everyday life.

A debriefing session follows. Participants are instructed to practise for 15 minutes twice daily. They are asked to record the level of relaxation achieved, using a 0–100 scale where 0 = total relaxation, 100 = maximum tension, and 50 represents normal. They are also asked to keep a note of the length of practice time taken to reach the level achieved. The form shown in Figure 8.3 serves to motivate the individual to practise as well as to record the details of the homework session.

Second session

Session two starts with a review of the work done in the first session followed by tense–release exercises for the chest, stomach, back, legs and feet. These are:

- tensing the muscles which pull the stomach in
- arching the back so that the spine leaves the back of the chair
- tensing the buttock muscles by pressing the feet down into the floor
- raising the heels with the toes remaining on the ground
- raising the front part of the foot keeping the heels on the ground.

The second session is terminated in the same way as the first and trainees are reminded to practise.

RELEASE–ONLY

In this phase of instruction, the 'tension' part of the sequence is eliminated, leaving just the 'release'

0 = totally relaxed
100 = maximum tension

Date	Time	Component	Degree of relaxation (0–100)		Time taken to achieve it
			Before	After	

Figure 8.3   Form for recording relaxation training homework. (Adapted from Öst 1987.)

part. As a result, the relaxed state can be achieved in less time than when working with the full sequence; 5–7 minutes are suggested instead of the 15 of the tense–release session.

The training session begins with breathing instructions, followed by a scanning of all the voluntary muscles starting with the head and working down to the toes. The following instructions are adapted from Öst (1987):

In a moment I'm going to ask you to focus your attention on your breathing and, in particular, on the movement of your upper abdomen ... notice how it swells slightly as you breathe in, and sinks back as you breathe out ... do not change it in any way ... just tune in to its rhythmic pattern ... feel yourself relaxing more with each breath ... feel your muscles letting go from the top of your head ... your forehead ... eyebrows ... eyelids ... cheeks ... temples ... jaws ... throat ... tongue ... lips ... feel your entire face relaxed ... now ... your neck ... shoulders ... arms ... and down to the tips of your fingers ... and while you are doing this, let your breathing continue at its own pace, expanding the stomach region in particular ... Now, relax your back ... now, the lower part of your body ... hips ... thighs ... knees ... calves ... shins ... feet ... toes ... still breathing gently and noticing the relaxing effect of each breath ... feel yourself relaxing more and more ...

The sequence is terminated in the same way as for the first component.

Again, the homework assignment is a twice-daily practice, the trainee being asked to record afterwards the level of relaxation achieved and how long it took to reach it.

CUE–CONTROLLED OR CONDITIONED RELAXATION

This component of the training focuses on the breathing. It begins by asking the trainee to relax himself by employing the release-only method of progressive relaxation. Once relaxed, he is asked to begin silently to recite the word 'relax'; he recites it once each time he breathes out. Following many repetitions, an association is built up between the word and the relaxed state whereby the word alone becomes capable of inducing a measure of relaxation. The word has thus become a cue. The stronger the association, the greater the power of the cue word. Expressed in other terms, a conditioning process has been set up, as a result of which the trainee feels himself relaxed whenever he thinks the word 'relax'.

The trainer introduces the exercise in the following manner:

> Spend a few moments with your eyes closed ... relax yourself by running through the release-only routine ... signal to me by raising your right index finger when you feel fully relaxed ... if you are ready, turn your attention now to your breathing ... tune in to its rhythm ... let it adopt its own pace ... do not be tempted to alter it ... and just before you breathe in, think the word 'inhale' ... just before you breathe out, think the word 'relax'...

Leading with the instructions of 'inhale' and 'relax' for five breaths, the trainer then asks the participant to continue on his own for a further five breaths. After a few minutes' rest, the full sequence is repeated.

If there is more than one participant, the trainer will not attempt to synchronize their respirations but will let them conduct their own exercise. As proficiency increases, the command 'inhale' can be dropped, and the word 'relax' used on its own.

Homework consists of 20 pairings a day of the word 'relax' with the state of relaxation. Participants should be warned against overbreathing, i.e. allowing the breathing to become deeper or more rapid (p. 134). The trainee keeps a record of the level of relaxation achieved and the time taken to reach it.

Once learned, it takes only 2 or 3 minutes to get fully relaxed by this method.

DIFFERENTIAL RELAXATION

So far, the sessions have been concerned with teaching basic techniques. The application of those skills now begins. Differential relaxation focuses on controlling the levels of muscle tension while the individual is engaged in some activity. Although

some tension is needed in order to carry out the task, the level is often greater than is necessary and may need to be reduced. Also there may be unnecessary tension in the muscles not directly engaged in the task. Different levels of tension (or relaxation) are required for each.

Since an ability to recognize muscle tension at its varying levels is essential for developing this skill, differential relaxation is presented after the individual has been trained in progressive relaxation.

Two sessions of tuition are indicated, one dealing with sitting and the other with standing activities. Both sessions begin with a revision of cue-controlled relaxation.

The first session: sitting

In the first, the trainee, seated in an armchair, is instructed to make certain movements while maintaining a relaxed state in the rest of the body.

> Please make yourself as comfortable as possible. Settle into the chair with your feet flat on the floor. With your eyes closed relax yourself using your cue word with breathing ... when you are ready, would you raise your right index finger ... I'd like you now to open your eyes and look around the room without moving your head ... notice the tension in the eye muscles but keep the body relaxed...
>
> Next, look around the room allowing your head to move in order to increase your range of vision. Keep a minimum of tension in the neck muscles while you do this, and check that the rest of your body is free from tension...
>
> Would you now lift one arm, and as you do, remember to keep the other parts of your body relaxed ... and, lower the arm. Continue to scan your body for signs of unnecessary tension.
>
> Now, lift one leg off the ground, keeping the rest of your body as relaxed as possible ... and, let it down.
>
> If you had any difficulty with this exercise, perhaps we could discuss it before moving on.

The routine is then carried out on the other arm and leg, after which the trainee is moved from his armchair to an upright chair. He relaxes himself in this new sitting position before being led through the same procedure of eye, head and limb movements.

Next, he is seated at a table and asked to write something short such as his name and address, using the minimum of muscle tension needed to accomplish the task. As an alternative, in practice sessions, he could make a short telephone call, adopting the same relaxed state.

The second session: standing

In the second session of differential relaxation, the trainee stands. His position should be near a wall or some form of support, in case he feels unsteady, but he should not be leaning on it. The session begins with cue-controlled relaxation, after which the same schedule of head, arm and leg movements is worked through.

Lastly, the trainee is asked to practise relaxation while walking. Emphasis is placed on finding an easy way of moving, and on relaxing the muscles not used, such as those of the face and hands. Any initial awkwardness will disappear as the individual discovers more relaxed ways of holding his body.

With the skills he has learned and practised, the individual will be able to achieve a state of relaxation consistent with effective task performance within 60–90 seconds. Differential relaxation is expanded in Chapter 12.

RAPID RELAXATION

As its name implies, this component is designed to reduce still further the time it takes to become relaxed; it also gives the trainee opportunity to practise in everyday situations. First, the trainee's environment is arranged so that a regularly used appliance acts as a cue to relax; for example, the wristwatch or the telephone are marked with a coloured dot which reminds the individual to relax whenever he sees it. Every time he looks at his watch or makes a telephone call he is reminded to release tension. This means that stress is in general held at low levels in the everyday setting. Rapid relaxation consists of the following routine performed each time the individual sees the coloured dot:

Take a slow breath ... think 'relax' ... then exhale. Repeat this twice ... scan the body for unnecessary tensions ... and release them.

Regular practice of this short sequence (15–20 times a day) makes the technique more effective and results in the trainee being able to relax in a still shorter space of time. It has been found that after 1 or 2 weeks' practice, he can relax himself by this method in as little as 20–30 seconds.

APPLICATION TRAINING

Applying relaxation skills to situations of potential stress is the subject of this phase. The trainee is provided with a wide range of opportunities in which to use the techniques he has learned. Anxiety-provoking situations should, however, be presented at a level of challenge which the trainee can cope with.

Take yourself to a situation that you know is likely to provoke stress for you. Relax yourself before entering the scene. Observe your reactions. If you feel anxiety levels beginning to rise, bring out your cue word 'relax'. Continue to apply it until you feel your anxiety levels falling.

It may not work the first time because, like any skill, practice is necessary to achieve success, but gradually you will find you are gaining more control over your anxiety levels.

As a preliminary, the individual could visualize himself successfully coping in the stress-provoking situation before exposing himself to the same event in real life (see Ch. 18).

MAINTENANCE PROGRAMME

However successful the treatment, Öst suggests keeping up the habit of scanning the body for unnecessary tension and using rapid relaxation to release it.

EVIDENCE OF EFFECTIVENESS

Öst addresses three modes of anxiety with the applied relaxation approach: the physiological, the cognitive and the behavioural. The physiological aspect is addressed through muscle relaxation; the cognitive through the cue word; and the behavioural through differential relaxation and exposure to the stressor. A multivariate approach such as this has advantages in a condition, such as anxiety, where changes occur in different modes.

Applied relaxation has been tested in the treatment of a large number of conditions including phobia, panic disorder, headache, epilepsy and tinnitus. In a review of 18 controlled studies, it was found to be significantly more effective than no treatment or placebo conditions. Follow-up, at varying times from 5 to 19 months, showed that the effects were maintained and in some cases augmented (Öst 1987).

A study which compared applied relaxation with progressive relaxation training showed applied relaxation to be more effective on most measures immediately following treatment. At follow-up 19 months later, however, applied relaxation was shown to be more effective on all measures (Öst 1988). Thus the method seems to provide long-term benefit.

More recently, Spence and colleagues (1995) tested the effect of applied relaxation on chronic upper extremity pain caused by cumulative trauma. Forty-eight patients were randomly allocated to four groups: applied relaxation, electromyographic feedback, a combination of both and a waiting list control. After treatment twice weekly for 4 weeks significant reductions in pain, depression, distress and anxiety were found in all the relaxation groups, while minimal change occurred in the waiting list control. The greatest benefit, in the short term at least, was reported in the group who received applied relaxation.

Studies comparing applied relaxation with other psychological methods often find very little difference in effectiveness. For example, in a study comparing the method with cognitive therapy on a population of 33 people experiencing generalized anxiety, it was not possible to declare one method superior to the other. Both however, were found to be effective (Öst & Breitholtz 2000).

PITFALLS OF APPLIED RELAXATION

Since applied relaxation is based on progressive relaxation, it is subject to the same pitfalls. They may be found in Chapter 6 (p. 56).

Further reading

Hawton K, Salkovskis P M, Kirk J, Clark D M 1996 Cognitive behaviour therapy for psychiatric problems. Oxford University Press, Oxford

Öst L-G 1987 Applied relaxation: description of a coping technique and review of controlled studies. Behaviour Research and Therapy 25: 397–407

Chapter 9

Behavioural relaxation training

HISTORY AND RATIONALE

A person who is tense adopts a characteristic pattern of muscular activity in the form of frowning, clenching and general body tenseness. The muscles of a relaxed person, by contrast, are free from excessive muscle tension. As a result, people who are tense look different from people who are relaxed. Their feelings are associated with a different posture in each case. Don Schilling, a psychologist working in the early 1980s, found the converse also occurred, that is, people adopting a relaxed posture reported feeling more relaxed.

Schilling, who was teaching progressive relaxation to adolescent boys, noticed they were better at tensing than relaxing; in fact, they found it difficult to respond to the request to relax. He suggested to his pupils that instead of trying to *become* relaxed, they should adopt the more concrete objective of trying to *look* relaxed: to take up postures they would expect to see in people who *were* relaxed. The result was that the pupils not only succeeded in looking relaxed but reported actually feeling more relaxed. Thus, by adopting postures characteristic of relaxation, they had induced a subjective feeling of relaxation.

The idea is reminiscent of the facial and postural feedback hypotheses which state that feedback from facial expression and posture induces feelings that match those expressions and postures. In other words, people feel the emotions that correspond with their poses. This theory is referred to again in Chapter 24 (p. 215).

Based on these ideas, Schilling & Poppen (1983) set up a method of relaxation which they called behavioural relaxation training (BRT). Liberal comment from the trainer provided reinforcement or corrective adjustment. The method is thus underpinned by behaviourist principles.

DESCRIPTION

BRT is a method in which tense postures are replaced by relaxed ones. The trainee is required to take up specified relaxed postures based on the way people look when they are relaxed. He then registers the feeling of adopting that posture.

PROTOCOL FOR BEHAVIOURAL RELAXATION TRAINING

SETTING

The ideal setting is a warm, quiet room with dimmed lighting. A padded recliner is the chair of choice but, since this may not be available, any flat surface will serve. Pillows may be used under the knees, forearms and head, as required. Women will find it convenient to wear trousers.

INTRODUCTION OF METHOD TO PARTICIPANTS

Participants are introduced to the method in the following way:

We can all recognize signs of tension: tightly drawn face muscles, clenching of teeth and fingers. These are typical postures that people adopt when under stress. When people are relaxed, muscle tensions are released and a new posture results. The central idea of behavioural relaxation training is that by adopting the posture of a relaxed person, we can make ourselves feel more relaxed.

In this method you will be asked to make different parts of your body look as relaxed as possible and then to notice the effect the new position has on you; to notice how the new position feels. I'll describe and demonstrate each item before we begin. Please try out the items on yourself.

The postures, as described in Table 9.1, are then demonstrated and the trainee asked to copy them.

Table 9.1   Relaxed and unrelaxed behaviours (Adapted from Lichstein © 1988 Clinical relaxation strategies, p. 137, with permission from John Wiley and Sons Inc, New York)

Item	Relaxed	Unrelaxed
Breathing	Breaths regular and fewer in number than recorded on the baseline	Breaths irregular and greater in number than recorded on the baseline
Quiet	No audible sounds such as sighs, words or movements	Talking, whispering, sighing, coughing, snoring or other audible sounds
Body	Symmetrical and fully resting on supporting surface	Holding any part tense or twisted
Head	Motionless and supported with nose in midline	Head-turning or other movements; head unsupported or tilted; nose outside midline
Eyes	Lids lightly closed with eyes still	Eyes open; or if closed, darting about under tense and fluttering lids
Mouth	Lips parted at centre of mouth with teeth separated	Lips firmly closed with teeth held together; or mouth uncomfortably open
Thoat	No activity	Swallowing, twitching or preparing to speak
Shoulders	Dropped, and level with each other; resting against support	Both hunched or one higher than the other; not resting on support
Hands	Both resting at sides, on armrests or on lap; palms down, fingers gently curled	Clasped, clenched tight or gripping the armrest
Feet	Comfortably rolled out so that the toes point away from each other	Pointing vertically, crossed or excessively rolled out

The unrelaxed postures are also demonstrated to emphasize the point. Feedback is provided by the trainer in the form of praise or corrective instructions. The trainee is asked particularly to take note of the proprioceptive events, i.e. the joint and muscle feelings which convey the sense of body position as each new posture is adopted.

Following the demonstration, the trainee rests quietly with his eyes closed. After a few minutes, the instructor may make an initial assessment (see the section on the Behavioural Relaxation Scale, p. 79).

TRAINING PROCEDURE

The training procedure is then presented in its entirety. Below is a slightly paraphrased version of the protocol laid out in Poppen (1988), where it is suggested that each relaxed posture be held for 30–60 seconds. Trainees are asked to close their eyes.

Feet

Starting with the feet: these are relaxed when you feel they are flopping, with the toes slightly pointing away from each other. No effort is involved; it is the posture of rest. If you are putting any effort into it, then your muscles will be working and your feet will be tensed. Notice how your feet feel in the relaxed position.

Body

The next item is called 'body'. Your body is relaxed when your hips and shoulders are in line with each other and resting on the supporting surface. If you are lying in a crooked fashion, your body is not relaxed. If there is any movement you are not relaxed. Make a note of the sensation of having a relaxed body.

Hands

This posture is called 'hands'. Your hands are relaxed when they are resting on a surface with the fingers gently curled, that is to say, neither clenched nor stretched out. Notice the sensations in your hands as you relax them.

Shoulders

And now the shoulders: these are relaxed when they are level and dropped. If you feel one is twisted or higher than the other, then they are not relaxed. Register the feeling of having relaxed shoulders.

Head

The next posture is called 'head'. Make sure your head is resting on its cushion and facing forwards. Feel it being supported. Any attempt to turn or twist it will cause your neck muscles to work. Notice the feelings you get as you relax your neck muscles.

Mouth

The next posture is called 'mouth'. Your mouth will be relaxed if your teeth are parted and your lips gently touching. If you are smiling, grimacing, licking your lips or pressing them together, your mouth is not relaxed. Take note of the feelings you get as you relax your mouth.

Throat

Now the area called 'throat': this is relaxed when you can feel no movement there. If you are swallowing or if your tongue is twitching, then your throat is not relaxed. However, if you need to swallow, do so, then return to your relaxed state. Notice the sensations in your throat as you relax it.

Breathing

The next item is called 'breathing'. Relaxed breathing is slow and gentle. Unrelaxed breathing is rapid, jerky and may be interrupted by coughing, sighing and yawning. Register the effect of your relaxed breathing.

Quiet

And now we come to an item called 'quiet'. This means that you are not making any sounds such as sniffing, umm-ing, or talking. If you feel you have to clear your throat, that's all right, but return to your state of quiet afterwards, noticing the sensation of stillness.

Eyes

> The last relaxed area is called 'eyes'. These are relaxed when the lids rest over them in a lightly closed position and when the eye movements are brought to rest. Eyes are unrelaxed when they dart about and when the lids are twitching. Notice the feelings you are getting from your eyes as you relax them.

The order is not important, but it is suggested that the eyes are left until the end, since the trainee needs to use them mentally to observe the other behaviours (Poppen 1988).

A training session will last about 15–20 minutes, after which the trainee is instructed to continue relaxing as he silently reviews the items for a further 10–15 minutes. At the end of this period, the trainer may carry out a post-treatment assessment (see p. 79).

AROUSAL

Arousal takes place in the following manner:

> Very slowly, I would like you to prepare to end the session. To help you transfer from your deeply relaxed state, I am going to count slowly from one to five: one ... two ... three, open your eyes ... four ... five ... begin to move your limbs ... and in your own time, sit up.

Practice. Since behavioural relaxation training is a skill, practice is necessary. Trainees are urged to spend 20 minutes a day practising. Poppen suggests that benefit can be derived from combining BRT with cognitive relaxation methods, such as autogenics or meditation. In this way, the one can augment the effects of the other.

VARIATIONS OF THE PROTOCOL

Variations of the above protocol exist for different situations: first, where the only available chair is an upright chair and second, where the need for relaxation occurs in the middle of a task (termed 'mini-relaxation' by Poppen 1988).

SCRIPT FOR TRAINEE SITTING IN AN UPRIGHT CHAIR

Where the trainee is seated in an upright chair, the following four areas of legs, back, arms and head

should be substituted for feet, body, hands and head in the protocol given above.

Legs

> This area is called 'legs', and these are relaxed when you have both feet flat on the floor with a right angle at the knees. Allow the knees to fall outwards into a comfortable position. The legs are unrelaxed when crossed, extended or tucked under the chair. Notice the sensations in your legs when they are in the relaxed position.

Back

> The next area is called 'back'. It is relaxed when your shoulder blades and hips touch the chair symmetrically. It is unrelaxed when you are bending forwards, arching backwards or leaning to one side. Register the feelings you get from the relaxed posture.

Arms

> Next is the area called 'arms'. These are relaxed when the wrists are resting on the thighs; they are unrelaxed when hanging down, when crossed or when being leant on. Notice the sensations as you relax your arms.

Head

> Now we come to the area called 'head', and this is relaxed when it is held upright and is looking forwards. The head is unrelaxed when it is tilted or turned in any direction. Notice the feelings you get from holding your head in the relaxed position.

'MINI-RELAXATION'

Tension can arise in the course of any task or situation. For example, while talking, the individual might develop tension in the hands; while typing, in the shoulders, and while focusing on a difficult job, in the mouth and throat. Breaking off to release these tensions is what Poppen means by mini-relaxation. He suggests that a person, when engaged in any task, should take mini-relaxation breaks periodically. Thus, mini-relaxation can be seen as a form of differential relaxation (Ch. 12).

Mini-relaxation can be practised throughout the day and reminders to do so provided by placing coloured dots on the telephone, watch, steering wheel, typewriter, kettle-handle or any other frequently used appliance.

PITFALLS OF BEHAVIOURAL RELAXATION TRAINING

As with any relaxation approach, possible pitfalls should be considered before taking it up. Chapter 6 (p. 56) contains a discussion of hazards relating to muscular approaches.

THE BEHAVIOURAL RELAXATION SCALE

There are no universally accepted procedures of assessment in relaxation; a reliable and valid measuring device has yet to be found. Schilling & Poppen's (1983) Behavioural Relaxation Scale (BRS) is an attempt to fill one aspect of this gap. It was designed as an easy method for measuring the motor element of relaxation, i.e. that relating to the voluntary muscles. Although it specifically measures the behaviours taught in BRT, it may be used to assess the motor aspect of any relaxation procedure.

The scale is based on the assumption that a person who feels relaxed also looks relaxed. As a result, some kind of judgement of the degree to which a person is relaxed can be made by an onlooker. Using the same items that feature in BRT, the scale allows an objective assessment to be made, without the need for expensive equipment such as electromyographic instruments. Each posture is checked for its degree of relaxation with reference to the table of relaxed and unrelaxed postures (see Table 9.1). The order of the items in Table 9.1 is seen by Poppen (1988) as being the most convenient for assessment purposes.

USING THE BEHAVIOURAL RELAXATION SCALE

Establishing the baseline breathing rate

The first measure concerns the breathing rate. This is counted over a 30-second interval (each count representing a complete cycle of inhalation and exhalation). The process is repeated 15 times and the total sum of the respirations divided by 15 to give the mean or average number of respirations in 30 seconds. The mean is then entered in the box marked 'breathing baseline' on the score sheet (Fig. 9.1).

Name .... Date .... Time .... Session no. ....

Breathing baseline ☐

+ relaxed
− unrelaxed

INTERVALS

	1		2		3		4		5		Total
Breathing	−	+	−	+	−	+	−	+	−	+	
Quiet	−	+	−	+	−	+	−	+	−	+	
Body	−	+	−	+	−	+	−	+	−	+	
Head	−	+	−	+	−	+	−	+	−	+	
Eyes	−	+	−	+	−	+	−	+	−	+	
Mouth	−	+	−	+	−	+	−	+	−	+	
Throat	−	+	−	+	−	+	−	+	−	+	
Shoulders	−	+	−	+	−	+	−	+	−	+	
Hands	−	+	−	+	−	+	−	+	−	+	
Feet	−	+	−	+	−	+	−	+	−	+	Score

Self-ratings 1 2 3 4 5 6 7

Figure 9.1 Behavioural Relaxation Scale score sheet. (Adapted from Poppen R. Behavioral relaxation training and assessment, p. 123, © 1988 by Pergamon Press. Reprinted by permission of Sage Publications, Inc., Thousand Oaks, CA, USA.)

A diaphragmatic form of breathing is recommended (Ch. 15, p. 132).

General assessment

A general assessment covers five 1-minute periods in which the individual is observed for outward signs of relaxation. Each minute begins with a further count of the breathing rate lasting 30 seconds; it is entered in the empty box in the column marked '1' in Figure 9.1. If the answer is less than the baseline rate, then the adjacent plus sign is ringed; if it is more, the minus sign is ringed. The following 15 seconds are spent scanning the trainee's key postures, picking out any unrelaxed ones and repeating the appropriate word label, for example 'shoulders' for a hunched arm. The succeeding 15 seconds are spent ringing the items; plus for relaxed postures, minus for any that continue to be unrelaxed.

After the first minute, the procedure is repeated and the answers recorded under the figure '2', and so on until five columns have been completed. The ringed plus signs are added up and entered under 'total'.

Working out the score

Scoring is expressed as a percentage arrived at in the following way: the total number of ringed 'plus' signs is counted and the sum divided by the total number of observations (i.e. the 10 behaviours multiplied by the five testings). The resulting figure is then multiplied by 100. For example: if there were a total of 40 ringed plus signs, they would be divided by the 50 observations. After multiplying the resulting fraction by 100, a figure of 80% would be obtained.

The pre-treatment baseline

At the beginning of the course one pre-treatment assessment is carried out. It acts as a baseline against which to measure progress, but should itself be carried out after a short period of rest to avoid confusing the effects of training with those which occur naturally whenever a person enters a restful environment (Lichstein et al 1981). Thereafter, assessment follows each training session to monitor progress.

RELIABILITY AND VALIDITY OF THE BEHAVIOURAL RELAXATION SCALE

The reliability of the scale, i.e. its ability to produce the same scores when used on different occasions, has been tested. It was found that higher levels of reliability were obtained with trained observers than with untrained ones. Thus the training of observers is important.

Two forms of validity have been demonstrated: one, procedural, where participants receiving other accepted forms of relaxation training showed statistically significant changes in relaxation scores on the BRS, while controls did not (Schilling & Poppen 1983) and the other, concurrent. Here, significant correlations were found between electromyographic measures of frontalis muscle and BRS scores, i.e. low EMG readings were associated with scores which reflect relaxed postures as described in the BRS, while high readings were associated with scores which reflect unrelaxed postures (Poppen & Maurer 1982). Further work has tended to strengthen confidence in these results (Norton et al 1997) but more research is needed.

OTHER METHODS OF ASSESSMENT OF BEHAVIOURAL RELAXATION TRAINING

Because relaxation involves responses in subjective, physiological and behavioural spheres, a full assessment would take account of all three modalities. Poppen indicates the need to view behavioural assessment as part of a broader system of measurement. One of its components is self-report.

SELF-REPORT

As relaxation and anxiety are subjective states, it is appropriate and customary to include a self-rating measure when assessing their levels. Self-report can take the form of free description, but since this is difficult to quantify, pre-set descriptive phrases with associated numbered ratings are often used. The individual rings the number corresponding with the phrase that most accurately reflects his state.

A behavioural relaxation self-rating scale, adapted from Poppen (1988), is shown below.

Behavioural Relaxation Self-rating Scale

1. Feeling extremely tense and upset throughout my body.
2. Feeling generally tense throughout my body.
3. Feeling some tension in some parts of my body.
4. Feeling relaxed as in my normal resting state.
5. Feeling more relaxed than usual.
6. Feeling completely relaxed throughout my entire body.
7. Feeling more deeply and completely relaxed than I ever have.

Discrepancy between self-report and objective testing

There are often wide discrepancies between self-reports and objective measurements. One of the reasons is that self-report may be coloured by factors of social desirability, for instance where the trainee gives the answer he thinks is expected of him. These matters are discussed further in Chapter 26 (p. 225).

EVIDENCE OF EFFECTIVENESS

Behavioural relaxation training offers both therapy and a scale of assessment. As a therapy it provides a form of body scanning in which relaxed postures are adopted and feelings of relaxation experienced. As an assessment tool it provides a numerical measure of the level of relaxation present in the musculature.

The approach does not ask participants to recognize subtle degrees of arousal or to be conscious of different levels of relaxation; moreover, the method is easily learned and readily applied. These attributes make it a convenient technique for reducing anxiety in people with learning disabilities. In this context, Lindsay and colleagues have carried out a series of studies charting its effect on cognitive performance. Results showed that where the disability was severe, short-term memory and learning significantly improved following 12 sessions of BRT, compared with quiet reading where no significant differences were reported (Lindsay & Morrison 1996).

In a later study, Lindsay et al (1997) tested concentration and responsiveness in eight participants, this time with profound learning disabilities. Several different procedures were compared: snoezelen, aromatherapy massage, BRT and active therapy. Following each therapy participants were set simple concentration tasks. The treatments which led to the most successful outcomes were snoezelen and BRT, where significant effects were recorded. There was no improvement in the aromatherapy group and the active group even showed a deterioration.

Brain injury is another area where the approach has been applied. Guercio et al (2001) taught BRT skills to one adult with an ataxic tremor resulting from an acquired brain injury. Having learned the skills, the participant was then connected to a biofeedback facility. Results demonstrated a significant reduction in the severity of the tremor.

The benefits of BRT can be seen after very little teaching: Schilling & Poppen (1983) observed benefit within as few as two training sessions. They also reported that effects were retained at follow-up 4–6 weeks later.

Further reading

Poppen R 1988 Behavioural relaxation training and assessment. Pergamon Press, Oxford

Schilling D J, Poppen R 1983 Behavioural relaxation training and assessment. Journal of Behaviour Therapy and Experimental Psychiatry 14: 99–107

Chapter 10

The Mitchell method

CHAPTER CONTENTS

HISTORY AND RATIONALE

In 1963 a new method of relaxation was introduced. Its originator was Laura Mitchell, a physiotherapist with a wide experience of teaching and practice in the field of obstetrics. She argued that it was useless to ask a person to notice tension in his muscles since there are no nerve endings in muscle tissue capable of conveying such information to the conscious brain. The sensory apparatus in the muscle connects only with the lower brain and spinal cord. Consequently, exhortations to become aware of the presence or absence of muscle tension are inappropriate. However, proprioceptive structures in the joints, and skin pressure receptors, do have links with the conscious brain. The first tell us where our limbs are in space, and the second tell us where the skin is being stretched or compressed. It is only, she claims, by moving the joints and stretching the skin that information about muscle state is relayed to the higher centres. Thus, the joints and the skin are the organs on which we need to focus attention.

Mitchell's approach is based on the physiological principle of reciprocal inhibition, i.e. when one group of muscles acting on a joint is working, the opposing group is obliged to relax. As the fibres of one group contract, the fibres of the opposing group become slack. It is a built-in mechanism to allow the smooth performance of movement.

Mitchell exploits this principle and makes it the nub of her approach. Stress-related posture, or what she calls 'the punching position', is studied, the working muscle groups are identified, and then relaxed by activating the opposing groups. The resulting changes of position of the joints, and the accompanying skin sensations, are then mentally registered as the part settles into the posture of ease. Thus, her approach consists in moving the body out of the posture of defence or stress, and training the mind to recognize the posture of ease or relaxation.

The aim of the procedure is to reduce stress and relax the mind. Mitchell proposes that the relaxation induced by her method spreads throughout the organism to include the mind.

DESCRIPTION

Mitchell's method is composed of 13 items, referred to as joint changes (although they do not all involve joint activity). These changes reverse different aspects of the punching position, which is described below:

- shoulders hunched
- arms held close to sides
- fingers curled into the palms
- legs crossed
- feet dorsiflexed (drawn up towards face)
- torso bent forwards
- head held forwards
- breathing rapid with noticeable movement in the upper chest
- jaw clenched
- lips pursed
- tongue pressed into upper palate
- brow furrowed into a frown.

Mitchell does not suggest that the punching position is actually adopted under stress; rather, that the muscles responsible for it are contracting to a slight extent.

PROCEDURE

STARTING POSITIONS

Three starting positions are described:

1. Supine lying with a pillow under the head (Fig. 10.1). A pillow under the thighs is optional.

2. Forward-lean sitting, i.e. leaning forwards with head and arms resting on a table (Fig. 10.2).
3. Sitting in a high-backed chair with arm rests on which the hands are supported, palms downwards (Fig. 10.3).

Varying the starting position is useful in order to extend the range of application of the method. The eyes may be open or closed.

INSTRUCTIONS

The instructor begins by giving an order to direct a part of the body away from its posture of tension. The order is followed by the word 'Stop'. This means that the part is no longer being actively moved; it also means that the muscles responsible for the movement are no longer contracting. The part then falls naturally into the position of ease. This position is then mentally registered. Below is a list of the items to be worked:

ITEMS OF THE MITCHELL METHOD OF RELAXATION

1. Pull your shoulders towards your feet.
2. Slide your elbows away from your body.
3. Stretch your fingers and thumbs.
4. Turn your hips outwards.
5. Move your knees until they are comfortable.
6. Push your feet away from your face.
7. Breathing.
8. Push your body into the support.
9. Push your head into the support.
10. Drag your jaw downwards.
11. Press your tongue downwards in your mouth.
12. Close your eyes.
13. Think of a smoothing action which begins above your eyebrows, rises into your hairline, continues over the top of your head and down into the back of your neck.

Each item is modelled by the instructor who asks the trainee to copy it.

INTRODUCTORY REMARKS TO PARTICIPANTS

Trainees are introduced to the method by a short description of the rationale and procedure.

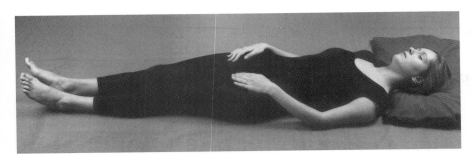

Figure 10.1   Starting position: supine.

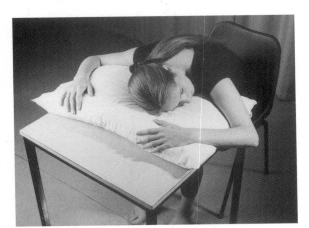

Figure 10.2   Starting position: forward-lean sitting.

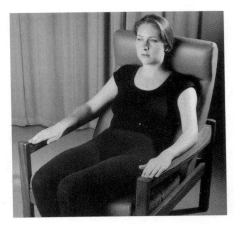

Figure 10.3   Starting position: sitting.

I just want to say something about the Mitchell method before we begin. When people are under stress, there is a position which they tend to adopt. We could call this 'the punching position'. Although people don't actually present themselves in a punching posture, the muscles which create it are tensing to a minute degree. This happens instinctively and helps to promote a feeling of being ready for anything.

If we move the body into the opposite of the punching position, we will be taking it into a position of ease or relaxation.

You might ask: 'How do we get the punching muscles to relax?'. This is where the physiological principle comes in: when one group of muscles acting on a joint is tensed, the opposing group automatically relaxes.

The trainer demonstrates.

When I bend my wrist forwards, the bending-back muscles relax, and vice versa. It's a reciprocal mechanism without which smooth action could not take place.

The method itself consists of a succession of changes of position. Each change moves a body part out of its position of defence and into its position of ease. As the part settles into the position of ease, you'll be asked to notice how it feels. The aim is to learn to recognize the relaxed position so that you can reproduce it more easily. I'll first demonstrate the items.

WORKING THROUGH THE SCHEDULE

The schedule is then worked through in its entirety. It is presented here with the orders expressed in inverted commas:

1. Shoulders

'Pull your shoulders towards your feet.' Do this gently, but go on until you can't pull them down any more. Feel the space between your shoulders and your ears getting greater. 'Stop pulling.' Notice the feel of the new position. Take plenty of time to register the sensations you are getting from it.

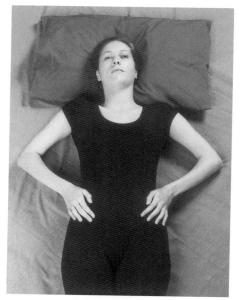

Figure 10.4 'Elbows out and open' in supine position.

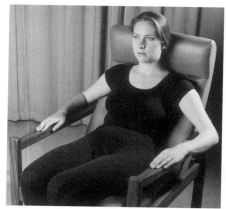

Figure 10.6 'Elbows out and open' in sitting position.

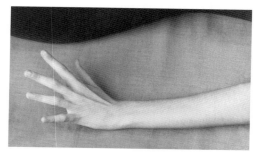

Figure 10.7 'Fingers and thumbs long.'

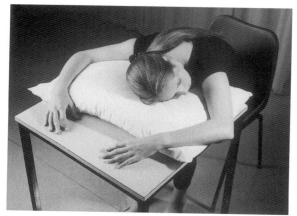

Figure 10.5 'Elbows out and open' in forward-lean sitting position.

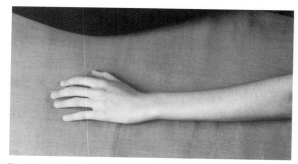

Figure 10.8 Fingers recoiling.

2. Elbows (Figs 10.4, 10.5 and 10.6)

'Elbows out and open.' For participants lying supine or sitting in a high-backed chair: slide your elbows sideways, carrying your arms away from your body until you reach a comfortable point (Figs 10.4, 10.6). For participants in forward-lean sitting: slide your arms away from your body, opening your arms at the elbow joint (Fig. 10.5). 'Stop moving.' Check that your arms are resting on the supporting surface

and notice how it feels to have a space between your arms and your body. Feel this position.

3. Hands (Figs 10.7 and 10.8)

'Fingers and thumbs long.' Stretch and separate your fingers and thumbs while the heels of both hands remain in contact with the floor, the table or the arm of the chair. While the fingers and thumbs

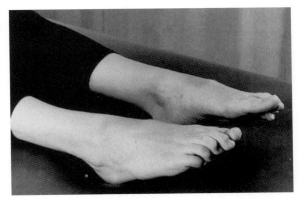

Figure 10.10   'Push your feet away from your face' in supine position.

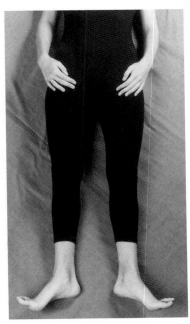

Figure 10.9   'Turn your hips outwards'.

spread (Fig. 10.7), feel the palms getting taut. 'Stop.' As you stop, the fingers recoil and fall on to the supporting surface where they lie with the hand gently open, fingertips touching the surface underneath (Fig. 10.8). Notice how the hand feels; notice also, without disturbing your fingers, the texture of the surface under your fingertips. Spend a moment or two taking in these sensations.

Extra time should be spent on the hand because of its disproportionately large sensory area in the brain.

4. Hips (Fig. 10.9)

'Turn your hips outwards.' If you are lying, this means rolling your thighs outwards (Fig. 10.9). If you are sitting, it means swinging your knees apart. 'Stop!' Let your legs settle comfortably, noting how they feel in this position.

5. Knees

'Move your knees until they are comfortable.' This simply means adjusting their position in whatever way enhances their comfort. 'Stop' and register that sense of ease.

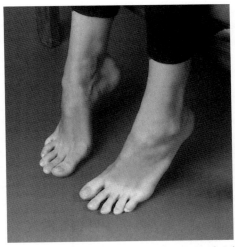

Figure 10.11   'Push your feet away from your face' in sitting position.

6. Feet and ankles (Figs 10.10 and 10.11)

'Push your feet away from your face.' If you are lying, point your feet and toes down, being careful not to induce cramp. If you are sitting with your feet on the floor, keep your toes in contact with it and raise your heels. You are working the calf muscles and reciprocally relaxing the muscles around the shin. 'Stop.' As you stop, your calf muscles stop working too. (If you are sitting, your heels drop down.) Take note of the feelings you are now getting from your feet and ankles. Spend a few minutes enjoying the sensation of ease in your legs.

7. Breathing

There are no orders for this item because people have their own breathing rates. I'll describe the action first, then you can perform it in your own time.

I'd like you to think of the soft triangle between the front edge of your ribs and your waist. As you breathe in you can feel it swelling slightly; at the same time you can feel your ribs spreading outwards. As you breathe out, that soft area sinks back and your ribs recoil.

Allow your breathing to take place slowly and comfortably, without putting any effort into it and without attempting to alter its rhythm.

8. Torso

'Push your body into the support.' Press against the support whether it is underneath you or behind you. 'Stop.' Feel your body slumped into the floor, table or chair. Feel its weight being supported. Notice the points where your body touches the support.

9. Head

'Push your head into the support.' This will be the floor for those lying down, the table for those leaning forwards and the back of the chair for those seated. 'Stop.' As you stop pushing, notice that the support carries the weight of your head. Feel your head being supported.

10. Jaw

'Drag your jaw downwards.' Let your teeth come apart and your jaw hang down inside your mouth. 'Stop.' Feel the new position. Notice also the contact between your gently touching lips.

Spend a bit longer on this item because the lips, in common with the fingertips, are richly supplied with sensory nerve endings.

11. Tongue

'Press your tongue downwards in your mouth.' Draw it away from the upper palate. 'Stop.' Feel your tongue lying loosely behind your teeth. Notice also your throat slackening.

12. Eyes

'Close your eyes' (if they are not already closed). Simply lower your eyelids and gently keep them down. Let your eyes be as still as they can be. Feel the peace of the darkness.

13.   Forehead and scalp

'Think of a smoothing action which begins above your eyebrows, rises up into your hairline, continues over the crown of your head, and down to the back of your neck.' Savour the effect.

The above 13 items may be repeated.

Mind

Mitchell ends with a sequence for the thoughts.

Let your mind focus on a topic you find pleasant. Pick one that flows, like a poem or a walk in the country, and let it hold your attention as it develops. Continue for a few minutes.

Termination

When you are ready, I'd like you to begin to make a gradual return to normal activity. Give your arms and legs a good stretch. Sit up slowly, giving your body plenty of time to adjust to an active state.

PRACTICE

The Mitchell method of physiological relaxation is a skill which can be learned; the more it is practised, the greater will be the benefit gained from it. It is through practice that the individual can cultivate his awareness of the relaxed posture, thus enabling him to reproduce it at will.

FURTHER ASPECTS OF THE MITCHELL METHOD

'KEYS' AND 'TRIGGERS'

The items in Mitchell's schedule cover the whole body. Many individuals, however, have characteristic ways of displaying tension. This means that they will be likely to benefit more from some joint changes than from others. The joint change that an individual finds most effective in reducing tension is referred to by Mitchell as the 'key change', because it is instrumental in releasing tension in other parts of the body. The key change can be identified by asking the individual how he tends to react when experiencing anger, pain, anxiety or conflict. If he tends to make fists, his key change will be finger-lengthening; if he tends to clench his teeth, it will be jaw-dropping. Key changes, by their generalizing effects, can promote a sense of ease throughout the whole body.

Mitchell applies her technique to everyday activities, using the concept of 'triggers of tension', i.e. events which tend to provoke feelings of stress, such as waiting at traffic lights or being interrupted by bells and alarms. She suggests sticking coloured tabs on potentially stressful appliances, such as the steering wheel and the telephone, as reminders to adopt the key change. Thus, to become more relaxed in daily life, there is first a need to recognize the triggers, and second, a need to diminish their effect by using the key change to move the body into the ease position.

Benefit can also be gained from a partial use of the schedule. Mitchell suggests that selected joint changes be used during specific activities; for example, the face items can be carried out while driving, or the leg items while reading. The idea is not far removed from the concept of differential relaxation (Ch. 12).

THE 'THREE-POINT PULL'

This is a variation of the shoulder item where, in addition to pulling the shoulders down, the head gently reaches upwards. (It should be done without tilting the head backwards.) The action is useful for stretching the joints in the neck, and may be practised in public situations without attracting attention.

APPLICATION OF THE METHOD TO SPECIFIC CONDITIONS

The Mitchell method lends itself to a range of conditions including insomnia, psychiatric disorders, dyspnoea, osteoarthritis and cardiac rehabilitation, as well as to everyday stress. It is widely used in the field of obstetrics where its advantage lies in its avoidance of tensing procedures (Ch. 25). The required relaxation is achieved by simply moving the body part.

Mitchell's insistence that breathing should be slow and easy and never include breath-holding, is another reason for the method being favoured by those working in the obstetric field (Mantle et al 2004). For the same reasons the method is often adopted by those who work in the field of respiratory medicine (Hough 2001).

COMPARISON WITH OTHER APPROACHES

Both Jacobson (Ch. 4) and Mitchell see their approach as a skill to be learned. Neither favours the use of tone of voice to influence the message. Instead, the participant is required simply to respond to the basic order. Again, like Jacobson, Mitchell avoids using the order 'Relax'. Her reason is that she finds it 'vague, generalized and ambiguous'. Jacobson avoided using it because he felt it provoked the trainee into making an effort which was superfluous, when 'going negative' was the effect he wanted. On other points they are, of course, fundamentally opposed: Mitchell placing the highest value on joint and skin sensations and rejecting the idea of information coming from the muscles, while Jacobson is only interested in muscle feelings, dismissing any value that joint sensations might have.

Greater resemblance may be found between Mitchell and Alexander (Ch. 11) in the value they both place on proprioceptive stimuli and awareness of posture. There is little difference between the three-point pull of Mitchell and the 'neck lengthen' injunction of Alexander.

EVIDENCE OF EFFECTIVENESS

Mitchell's method promotes awareness of relaxed postures. The method is simple and quick and many of the 'changes' can be carried out unobtrusively. It is widely practised as a stress-relieving strategy, and clinical findings testify to its effectiveness. Scientific evaluation of the method, however, has only just begun. Jackson (1991) studied four rheumatoid arthritis sufferers trained in the Mitchell method, comparing them with controls who simply rested. Using electromyography to measure activity in the frontalis muscle (a sensitive indicator of general muscle state), she found a marked reduction of tension in the study group and very little change in the control group. No statistical analysis was reported.

An interesting comparison between the methods of Mitchell and Jacobson was made by Salt & Kerr (1997). With a sample of 14 men and 10 women, these authors measured the effects of both approaches on the cardiovascular and respiratory systems. The study was designed with a control condition of supine lying. Participants were randomly assigned to three groups in which they received the two trainings and the control condition, presented in different sequences to avoid order effects. Heart rate, systolic blood pressure, diastolic blood pressure and respiratory rate were recorded before and after every treatment.

Results showed significant reductions after treatment on all measures for both methods, with no significant differences between them. The control condition itself showed significant reductions in heart rate and respiratory rate; however, when compared to the control, both treatment methods were found to be significantly superior on measures of systolic blood pressure. On a subjective level, there was some evidence of participants finding the Mitchell method easier to follow and less demanding in concentration than progressive relaxation.

Thus, while each approach demonstrated greater effectiveness than supine lying on certain counts, the study has been unable to demonstrate a substantial difference in the separate capacities of the two approaches to induce physiological relaxation. This is the first study to investigate the Mitchell method using statistically analysed data. A later study compared the Mitchell method with diaphragmatic breathing (Bell & Saltikov 2000) and also found a lack of significant difference between the two. The study is reported in greater detail in Chapter 15, page 134.

PITFALLS OF MITCHELL'S METHOD

These are similar to the pitfalls of other muscular approaches (Ch. 6, p. 56).

Further reading

Mitchell L 1987 Simple relaxation: the Mitchell method for easing tension, 2nd edn. John Murray, London

Acknowledgement

The author acknowledges the permission granted by the publisher, John Murray Publishers, to reproduce the phrases from Simple Relaxation 1987 by L. Mitchell.

Chapter 11

The Alexander technique

HISTORY AND RATIONALE

Posture refers to the way an individual habitually holds himself against the forces of gravity and is one of his recognizable features. A look round our acquaintances tells us that they all have characteristic ways of holding themselves; each one stands differently, walks differently and sits differently. Although a person's posture may be largely of genetic origin and thus beyond his control, we are inclined to think that it is also governed by the way he looks at and reacts to life.

Teachers of the Alexander technique point to the way young children use their bodies, describing the effect as 'poise'. They also indicate how this natural poise can become distorted by emotional and physical influences as the child grows towards maturity, resulting in the development of tension habits which interfere with healthy functioning.

This notion had earlier captured the attention of Matthias Alexander, at a time when he was experiencing a problem with his voice. An actor by profession, he noticed that he was developing hoarseness and a painful throat whenever he began to perform. Intuitively, he felt that posture lay at the root of it. Mirrors revealed that he was pulling his head back and tightening his neck muscles to the extent that he could not breathe properly. By freeing his neck and lengthening his spine he discovered he could regain control of his voice, and the manner in which he accomplished this forms the basis of the Alexander technique.

PRINCIPLES OF THE ALEXANDER TECHNIQUE

The Alexander technique is not underpinned by any established theory but it is based on principles of body positioning:

- primary control
- use and misuse
- faulty sensory perception
- inhibition
- 'end-gaining' and the 'means whereby'
- integration of mind and body.

PRIMARY CONTROL

Alexander believed that the primary control of human posture lay in the relationships of the head to the neck and of the neck to the rest of the spine. So convinced was he of their crucial nature, that an almost magical significance was attached to these relationships in his day. This status has, however, been modified over the years, and the Alexander teacher of today sees primary control less as an inviolable principle than as a useful starting point.

Primary control has three components:

- a neck that is free and whose muscles contain only enough tension to keep the head upright
- a head moving forward and up (Fig. 11.1), not back and down to crumple the spine (Fig. 11.2)
- a spine that feels lengthened, thus counteracting any tendency towards sagging.

USE AND MISUSE

'Use' refers to the characteristic way we have of holding our bodies. It is a neutral term. When there is harmony between the tension necessary to support the body and the relaxation necessary to allow it to move, the use is said to be 'balanced'. When, however, this is upset by too much or too little tension, a state of misuse is said to prevail (Barlow 2001). Examples of misuse are hunching of the shoulders, head sinking into the spine, chin thrusting out.

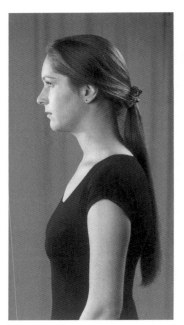

Figure 11.1   Head held forward and up.

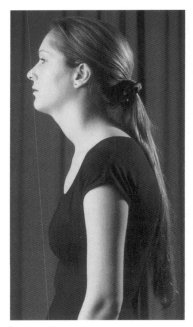

Figure 11.2   Head held back and down.

The regaining of 'balanced use' means the recovery of natural movement patterns, which can only occur if we review the messages we are getting about the position of the body in space.

FAULTY SENSORY PERCEPTIONS

All movement in the healthy organism is accompanied by sensory feedback in the form of proprioceptive impulses from the moving part. This gives us information about the position of body parts in space. In the young child these messages lead to responses which are natural, economic (in terms of energy consumption) and uncontaminated by emotional factors, while those in the adult may be distorted by trauma (mental or physical).

Responses carried out repeatedly, turn into habits which are then interpreted by the higher centres as normal, i.e. the way we habitually use our bodies will feel normal to us simply because we are used to it. Alexander's experience with the mirror showed him he was still pulling his head back even after he felt he had corrected it. This could only be because his body had got used to the 'bad' posture and had internalized it as normal, so that even the smallest degree of correction was interpreted by his conscious mind as overcorrection.

The phrase 'faulty sensory perception' refers to the way messages are interpreted in a misused body.

INHIBITION

Many of our movements are automatic. If they show patterns of misuse which we want to change, it will be necessary to intercept them, i.e. to examine them before they are automatically executed. A pause is required. This act of pausing constitutes what Alexander called 'inhibition'. It allows the individual to question the validity of his response. It gives him the chance to reconsider his action and to redirect his movement.

Inhibition, not to be confused with the Freudian meaning, is what happens when the individual ceases to react automatically to stimuli, thereby leaving him free to respond appropriately; to do nothing for a moment while the maladaptive, automatic response pattern is broken. 'When you stop doing the wrong thing, the right thing does itself' (Alexander 1932).

'END-GAINING' AND THE 'MEANS WHEREBY'

Inhibition provides the opportunity to focus on the means whereby we achieve a certain end. It draws attention away from 'end-gaining', where action is performed too quickly and too energetically for one to give any thought as to the manner in which the end is gained. Alexander would say that if you pay attention to the means, the end will take care of itself (Maisel 1969).

INTEGRATION OF MIND AND BODY

Central to the teachings of Alexander is a belief that the mind and the body are interdependent. Not only does the body posture reflect the individual's thoughts, but his mind responds to the way he uses his body. Such notions introduce a new dimension to the concept of body movement, and can be said to lie at the heart of the statement that 'we *are* our posture' (Barlow 2001).

THE TECHNIQUE

The technique itself re-educates the body to perform in a balanced and energy-economical way (Gray 1990). Habits of misuse are identified and replaced by more appropriate ways of using the body. Assessment and correction are carried out in positions of lying, sitting, standing and walking. Gently using her hands, the teacher guides the pupil's body both in motion and at rest while the pupil mentally focuses on the message he is getting from the teacher's hands. For example, a supine pupil might be told to think of the words: 'Shoulder release and widen', as the teacher is repositioning one of his shoulders. Thus, without actively performing the movement, the pupil directs his body to cooperate.

Some of the principal orders or directions are listed below, beginning with the three elements of primary control:

1. 'neck free'
2. 'head forward and up'
3. 'back lengthen'.

Other directions include:

4. 'keeping length'
5. 'back widen'
6. 'shoulder release and widen'.

THE THREE ELEMENTS OF PRIMARY CONTROL

1. 'Neck free'

This means that the head is carried in such a way that no undue strain is put on the neck muscles. The image of the nodding dog in the back of the car may help to convey the feeling of a free neck.

2. 'Head forward and up'

The phrase applies to pupils who are sitting or standing. 'Head forward and out' is the phrase for those who are lying. It means that the head is held with the chin pointing to the toes, not poking out. It also means that the head is lifted up or out of the vertebral column. The result is that the individual feels taller or longer, having 'grown' from a point at the back of the crown of the head. It is the opposite of a head that sinks into the shoulders with the chin thrust out. At the same time no excessive effort should be made to extend the body. The effect described can often be achieved simply by 'thinking up'. Figures 11.1 and 11.2 illustrate the correct and incorrect ways of carrying the head.

3. 'Back lengthen'

An erect spine anteroposteriorly displays a succession of natural curves: concavities in the cervical and lumbar regions, convexity in the dorsal region. In urging 'back lengthen', it is not implied that efforts should be made to obliterate these natural curves, but rather that the curves should not be allowed to become overemphasized, since that would result in shortening or crumpling of the spine. Actions which particularly shorten the spine are:

1. overextension of the cervical vertebrae (thrusting out the chin)
2. overextension of the lumbar vertebrae (exaggerated lumbar concavity) (Fig. 11.3).

Similarly, slumping is to be avoided. Slumping occurs when the whole spine is rounded into a long C-shaped curve, with the neck hyperextended in order to allow the eyes to look forwards. Slumping also creates shortening of the spine (Fig. 11.4).

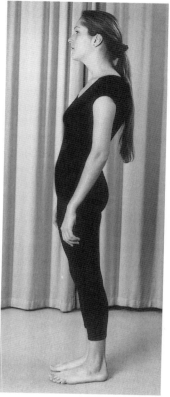

Figure 11.3   Standing with exaggerated cervical and lumbar curves.

'Back lengthen' indicates that the spine should be allowed to reach its full length (or height) as opposed to being either crumpled (where spinal curves are exaggerated) or slumped (where the back is too rounded). An image that evokes the idea of lengthening the back is that of a jet of water springing up in the spine and lifting it gently. The head should feel lightly balanced on top.

Alexander's view of a balanced standing posture is one in which the body weight passes through the front of the heel, the knees are unbraced, and the pelvis is in midposition, with the 'tail' neither thrown out, nor forcibly tucked under. The direction to 'think up' helps to convey the idea of standing straight but without making any forced effort to do so. Some teachers introduce the image of a helium-filled balloon lifting the head (Gray 1990). Figure 11.5 illustrates the correct standing position.

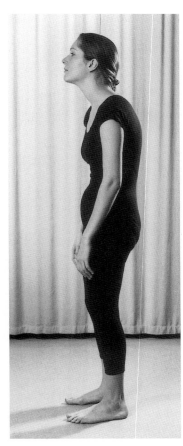

Figure 11.4   Standing with spine slumped into a long C-shaped curve.

'Neck free', 'head forward and up' and 'back lengthen' are fundamental to the technique.

OTHER DIRECTIONS

4. 'Keeping length'

The order 'keeping length' is related to 'back lengthen'. Alexander applies it to the action of sitting down where he sees particular benefit to be gained from the avoidance of crumpling. His method of lowering the body is illustrated in the following passage (Leibowitz & Connington 1990):

Place your feet slightly apart and positioned so that the backs of your legs are lightly in contact with the chair seat. Let your arms hang loosely by your sides. Before lowering yourself, let your mind focus

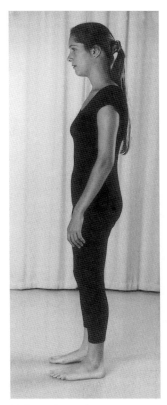

Figure 11.5   Balanced standing posture.

on the idea of 'keeping length', i.e. not crumpling the spine. Keep the head and neck in the same relation as they were in the standing position and as you lower yourself, flatten the lumbar curve. Although you are looking at the floor as you go down, make a point of thinking 'UP' to prevent any tendency of the spine to crumple.

Figure 11.6 demonstrates the correct way of lowering the body into a chair.

The wrong way of sitting down, according to Alexander, is to overextend both the neck and lumbar regions, i.e. to thrust the chin out and exaggerate the lumbar concavity. Their combined effect crumples and shortens the spine (Gray 1990). Figure 11.7 shows an incorrect way of lowering the body into a chair.

On rising from the chair, the head should start the movement and lead the body forwards. From that point the motions of sitting down are put into reverse.

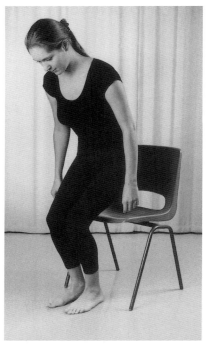

Figure 11.6 Sitting down with the spine 'keeping length'.

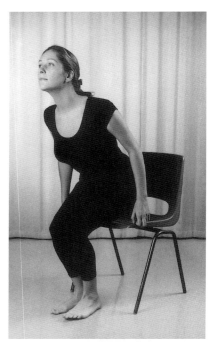

Figure 11.7 Sitting down with a 'crumpled' spine.

What Alexander is saying is that the lumbar spine should be slightly flexed and the cervical spine prevented from extending itself in the actions of sitting down and rising. He urges applying the same ideas to other activities which carry the centre of gravity forwards, such as leaning over a basin to clean the teeth.

Alexander compared the action of toothbrushing in humans to the peeling of fruit by erect primates in the wild. Both actions take place anterior to the body itself. On noticing that primates adopted a particular stance to carry out their task, he concluded that mechanical advantage was being gained from it. The stance itself is characterized by bent knees, and slightly flexed (flattened) lumbar and cervical spines; a posture which is referred to as the 'monkey stance' (Fig. 11.8).

The effect of the monkey stance is to keep the centre of gravity as close to the spine as possible, thereby relieving the strain on the lumbosacral junction. Where the monkey stance is not adopted for comparable tasks, a position of mechanical disadvantage is created. Figure 11.9 illustrates this idea: the arms and head reach forwards, pulling the centre of gravity with them, while the cervical and lumbar spines retain their concavities.

Common to both the monkey stance and the act of sitting (as recommended by Alexander) is a slight flexion of the lumbar spine. Alexander's insistence on the value of this posture has been supported by research (Adams & Hutton 1985, Adams et al 1994) which is discussed later in this chapter.

5. 'Back widen'

This phrase applies to the posterior part of the thorax which should be allowed to feel wide in order to permit full expansion of the ribs. To convey the idea of 'back widen' Gray (1990) promotes the image of the rib cage filling out into the back as the air enters the lungs.

6. 'Shoulder release and widen'

This is aimed at relaxing the muscles of the shoulder girdle which are often held more tensely than they need to be.

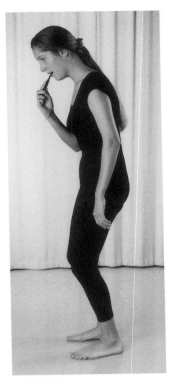

Figure 11.8 Task performance in a position of mechanical advantage (monkey stance).

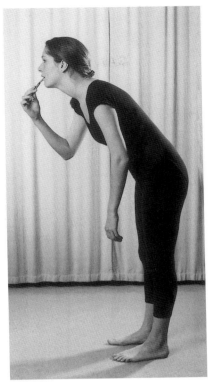

Figure 11.9 Task performance in a position of mechanical disadvantage.

RECOGNIZING AND CORRECTING MISUSE

Test for body alignment

As mentioned in the section on faulty sensory perception, an habitual posture, whether balanced or not, will feel 'right' to its owner. This makes it difficult for him to recognize misuse in himself. A procedure to solve this matter has been worked out by Barlow (2001):

Stand with your heels 5 centimetres (2 inches) from a wall, with your feet 46 centimetres (18 inches) apart. Let your body sway back until it touches the wall.

Figure 11.10 shows this position.

If your shoulders and hips touch simultaneously with each side level, your alignment is correct. However, you may find that one side touches the wall before the other or that your shoulders touch before your hips. Do what you can to realign yourself. Next, bend your knees slightly and notice that

this action will tend to bring the lumbar vertebrae into contact with the wall (lumbar curve flattened).

Figure 11.11 demonstrates this effect.

If you can hold this position with relative comfort, then your body is not in a misused state. If you find it unduly tiring, then practice will make it easier and help to restore alignment.

Changing posture

Alexander sees misuse as resulting, largely, from stress and the demands of contemporary life; in its turn, misuse can be the cause of physical stress leading to muscle and joint problems.

A person wishing to change his posture needs to consider three points. He should:

- be aware of the particular habit-governed movement that he wants to alter

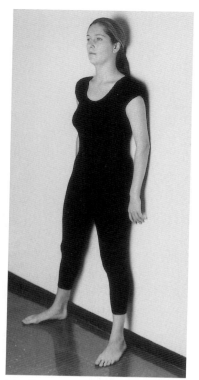

Figure 11.10 Testing for body alignment 1: leaning against wall.

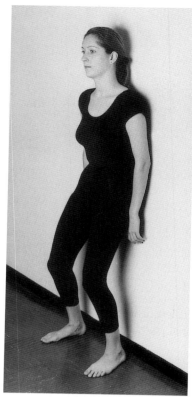

Figure 11.11 Testing for body alignment 2: flattening the lumbar concavity as the body is lowered.

- refuse to react automatically. This implies pausing to reassess the 'means whereby', i.e. being ready to say 'no' to the old method
- redirect his muscles by a thought process. In the early stages of re-education this signifies *thinking* about the corrected movement rather than driving the muscles to perform it. Such an approach allows the neuromuscular system to re-structure its response. 'The mind gives the instruction, and little by little, the body absorbs the message' (Fontana 1992) until the corrected form of the movement becomes automatic.

Regularly practising new responses will result in a gradual weakening of the old ones and turn a pattern of misuse into one of more balanced use. There are no defined stages of progress nor specified goals of perfection. Individual problems call for individual remedies. Common to all remedies, however, is the cultivation of a sensitive approach to the movement of one's own body (Barlow 2001).

RELAXATION EFFECTS

Although proponents speak of 'balanced use' rather than relaxation, the technique can nonetheless be seen as a method for promoting relaxation. Balanced use results in the elimination of excess muscular activity and in the establishing of minimum levels of muscle tension. These are concepts that are found in Jacobson's differential relaxation. For Alexander, however, they form the basis of his technique, whereas for Jacobson they are subsidiary to his main concern, which is the release of residual tension.

Alexander suggests a daily 15-minute session of rest, to be carried out in a crook lying position (knees bent up, feet flat on the ground) with a book under the head (where the height of the book is determined by the shape of the spine). The object is to allow the body to regain its natural symmetry; the procedure is also, however, a relaxing one (Fig. 11.12).

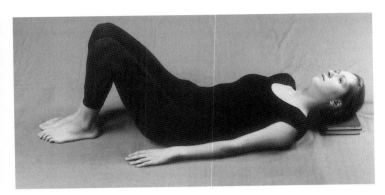

Figure 11.12   Promoting body symmetry in a relaxed position.

TEACHING THE ALEXANDER TECHNIQUE

The purpose in writing this chapter is to give a general idea of the principles underlying the Alexander technique, rather than to show how to teach it; such training involves a 3-year course. The principles, however, may be woven into other approaches, particularly where posture is a key item.

Trained teachers of the Alexander method often work in the field of the performing arts in the belief that the approach can identify unwanted movement patterns which interfere with performance (Batson 1996). The technique, however, has universal relevance.

EVIDENCE OF EFFECTIVENESS

Alexander's method is among the few approaches to focus systematically on relaxation of the body while it is in motion (Woolfolk & Lehrer 1984). As such, it is a form of kinesthetic re-education. The technique is based on the assumption that the way we use our bodies affects our general functioning. However, there is no ideal; it is for each to explore his or her possibilities and find better ways of using the body. For this, and other reasons, the technique does not readily lend itself to systematic investigation and has not until recently begun to receive scientifically rigorous assessment.

One of the few controlled trials is that of Austin & Ausubel (1992). They studied the effects of the technique on respiratory strength and endurance in performing artists. Results demonstrated a significant association between the Alexander instruction and increased respiratory resources, a finding which has implications for individuals who develop muscular tensions related to anxiety and fatigue which interfere with their performance.

In contrast to the above physiological study is the work of Valentine (1993), whose investigation looked at psychological as well as physiological dimensions of performance anxiety. The participants in her controlled study were 27 music students: 6 singers and 21 instrumentalists. Following a programme of 15 lessons she found some evidence that anxiety was reduced in low stress situations such as the classroom, but little evidence that this effect transferred to the highly stressful recital situation. Thus, conclusions drawn from this study would suggest that anxiety-reducing benefit from the Alexander technique in the context of musical performance is slight.

Wide use is made of the Alexander technique in the field of motor problems. Stallibrass et al (2002) tested its efficacy in people experiencing symptoms of Parkinson's disease. Ninety-three participants were randomly divided into three groups: one received 24 lessons in the Alexander technique, one received 24 sessions of massage and there was a control group which received no treatment. Results showed that, from pre- to post-intervention, motor symptoms in the Alexander group improved significantly compared to the no-treatment group and this improvement was maintained at 6-month follow-up. These benefits were not demonstrated in the massage group. Both intervention groups, however, recorded positive changes on the Beck Depression Inventory whereas the control group registered no such changes.

In her critical review of relaxation techniques, Kerr (2000) finds that the available research suggests that the Alexander technique may offer benefit in states of stress; it may also have positive effects in conditions such as anxiety and depression.

The work of the anatomist Adams (Adams & Hutton 1985, Adams et al 1994) is relevant with regard to some of the postural claims made by Alexander. Adams has studied the effect of actions which impose physical stress on the lumbar spine. He has found that a moderate degree of flexion (i.e. flattening of the lumbar curve) is mechanically advantageous, which supports Alexander's views about the action of sitting down and the value of the monkey stance.

There is, however, a need for more research, both psychological and physiological, into the effectiveness of the Alexander technique. Until that has been carried out and conclusions drawn, the technique must, in Barlow's words, continue to be regarded as a hypothesis (Barlow 2001).

Further reading

Alexander F M 1932 The use of the self. Dutton, New York

Barlow W 2001 The Alexander principle. Orion, London

MacDonald G 2002 The Alexander technique: a practical programme for health, poise and fitness. Element, London

Park G 2002 The art of changing: exploring the Alexander technique and its relationship to the human energy body. Ashgrove, London

Chapter 12

Differential relaxation

DEFINITION AND RATIONALE

Differential relaxation, a phrase introduced by Jacobson (1938), means, in his own words: 'the minimum of tensions in the muscles requisite for an act, along with the relaxation of other muscles' (Jacobson 1976). This is to say that the muscles engaged in performing any activity, for instance typing, should exhibit a minimum level of tension consistent with task efficiency, while those not directly engaged in the task are relaxed. This leaves the body as relaxed as it can be while achieving the objective, i.e. typing the page. Thus, differential relaxation is progressive relaxation applied to everyday tasks.

We need muscle tension in order to live our lives. It is essential for carrying out purposeful activity, of the type that Jacobson calls 'primary'. Purposeful activity, however, may be accompanied by tension in muscles whose action does nothing to promote the outcome, such as grimacing while writing. This is referred to by Jacobson as 'secondary activity'. Differential relaxation calls for the recognition and elimination of all secondary activity and of any excessive tension in the muscles performing or helping to perform the primary activity.

The approach is underpinned by the same theoretical principles as progressive relaxation (Ch. 4). A thorough knowledge of progressive relaxation provides the skills to carry out differential relaxation.

DESCRIPTION

JACOBSON'S METHOD

Jacobson has described a method in which he isolates the task, reduces muscle tension to below the level at which the task can be performed then, gradually, reintroduces tension to the minimum level where the task can be carried out efficiently. He gives an example (Jacobson 1976):

> Sit holding an open book on your lap. Reduce the tension in your posture so that the book nearly falls off your lap. Relax your eye and speech muscles so that you are unable to follow the words. Then little by little, increase the tension until the book is secure on your lap and you can see the words ... then, gradually increase the tension enough to take in their meaning.

A similar routine can be applied to writing:

> Take up a pen with the intention of writing your name, but using too little energy to make a mark on the paper. Repeat the action, this time putting a little more force into it. Continue putting slightly more force into it until you reach a point where you are able to write in a way which you recognize as your style. Keep it relaxed. You are now combining effective outcome with economy of effort.

A good time to test for the presence of secondary tensions is when opening the morning mail. The anticipation and apprehension of what it might reveal can raise tension levels far beyond what is necessary for the simple task of opening envelopes.

BERNSTEIN & BORKOVEC'S METHOD

In their manual on progressive relaxation training, Bernstein & Borkovec (1973) develop the idea of differential relaxation. They single out three aspects of complexity; position of the body, level of activity and the situation in which the activity takes place. Variations of each are worked into an 8-step schedule starting with 'sitting, doing nothing in a quiet room', and ending with 'standing, performing some activity in a busy environment'. Four of the items occur in the sitting position while the level of activity and the situation are varied; the other four occur in the standing position. During the performance of these exercises the pupil is asked to monitor his tension levels, using 'recall' (p. 60) to relax the appropriate muscle groups.

ÖST'S METHOD

This approach is described in Chapter 8.

EXAMPLES OF THE USE OF DIFFERENTIAL RELAXATION

SEATED AT A DESK TYPING

> Using just enough power in the hands to control the keys, type a few sentences. Then break off to check your body for tension. If you find any, relax it away using 'recall' (p. 60) or cue-controlled breathing (p. 71). Resume typing, checking again for tension. Make a telephone call, maintaining a relaxed posture, using only enough tension to hold the receiver.

DRIVING TO THE SUPERMARKET

> As you settle yourself into the driving seat, spend a minute checking all your muscle groups for tension. Identify the muscles you need for driving. If you notice excess tension in any of these muscles, relax it. Check that the muscles you don't need, such as the face muscles, are relaxed. Maintain relaxation while steering and changing gear until you arrive at the store. Park the car and walk towards the entrance, relaxing any tension in your face and shoulders. Pick a trolley and as you push it around, continue to check your body, relaxing those muscles you do not need and putting the minimum of tension into the ones you need for the task. Pause regularly to scan your body for unnecessary tension.

DIGGING THE GARDEN

> As you pick up the spade, feel the weight of it in your hand, fleetingly judging the degree of muscle work required to use it. Remind yourself that you can put

too much effort into tasks of this nature. Relax your face muscles while you carry out the digging.

STRESSFUL SITUATIONS

Differential relaxation is relatively easy to achieve in activities which do not pose any threat, but is more difficult in situations of stress, e.g. delivering a speech. In such cases additional strategies may need to be employed, such as mental rehearsal of the event and positive self-talk, to help reduce excessive tension (see Ch. 18, p. 163).

STANDING AND WALKING

The principles of differential relaxation can also be applied to the postures of standing and walking, where certain muscle groups, such as those of the back and the legs, hold the body vertical and propel it along while uninvolved groups, such as those of the face, can be relaxed.

The following two examples illustrate these ideas.

Standing

Have your eyes open. Stand with shoes off, feet parallel and 5–7.5 centimetres (two or three inches) apart. Release excess tension with cue-controlled breathing. Unlock your knees, slightly bending and stretching them a few times to feel the weight falling evenly down through them to your feet. Rock forwards and backwards over them until you find a comfortable position for your hips. Feel your spine rising above your hips ... feel it supporting your head, and let your head reach up as high as it wants to go. Nod it gently to find its best position. Relax your face muscles. Let your arms hang down by your sides with your shoulders dropped. Feel your body relaxed and resilient. Enjoy being inside it. There should be no effort involved. When the posture feels as comfortable as possible, notice what makes it feel like that.

Walking

One way of finding your own energy-economical way of walking is to experiment with different kinds of walking. Marching, sailor's roll and tiptoeing are, of course, artificial ways of walking; however, by exploring different styles, you may find it easier to distinguish between unnatural and natural forms, and be helped to find your own natural way of walking. This will be the one that gives you most comfort and ease. Practise it, enjoy it. Feel your whole body relaxing into the rhythm of your walking. Feel that the muscles responsible for carrying you along are no more tense than they need to be ... and that your face and shoulder muscles are relaxed.

PREREQUISITES

Differential relaxation is thus concerned with minimum tension levels during activity and task performance. There are two prerequisites: knowing which muscle groups are needed for each activity and which are not; and possessing the skill of muscle relaxation.

COMPARISON WITH OTHER METHODS

The Alexander technique, with its concept of 'balanced use' (p. 92), is grounded in the principle of differential relaxation. Here, the crucial elements are the relationships of head, neck and spine which, when correct, allow the body to adopt balanced and relaxed postures while engaged in activity. Alexander's procedures for the actions of sitting down and rising are essentially techniques of differential relaxation.

Mitchell (1987) is advocating differential relaxation when she urges the partial use of her schedule during task performance; for example, practising 'joint changes' for the shoulders and the jaw while driving or typing. Her 'key changes' can also be seen as a differential technique, in that they are directed at switching off unnecessary global tension while allowing specific movements to take place (p. 88).

Poppen's (1988) mini-relaxation is another differential form. Here, relaxed-looking postures are adopted in the muscle groups not engaged in the task; for example, the legs can be relaxed while writing a letter (p. 78).

Further reading

Bernstein D A, Borkovec T D 1973 Progressive relaxation training: a manual for the helping professions. Research Press, Champaign, Illinois

Jacobson E 1976 You must relax. Souvenir Press, London

Öst L-G 1987 Applied relaxation: description of a coping technique and review of controlled studies. Behaviour Research and Therapy 25: 397–407

Chapter 13

Stretchings

INTRODUCTION AND RATIONALE

Flexibility is one of the properties of muscle tissue which mild stretching helps to maintain. Gentle stretchings also help to promote the mobility of the joints and stimulate the flow of synovial fluid. This fluid lubricates the joint and creates a smooth action.

In the case of the spinal joints, stretchings help the discs to recover after activity which changes their shape. The intervertebral discs are soft structures whose shape is altered when the spine is moved. Bending in any direction transforms the discs into wedge-shaped bodies with their fluid content squeezed towards the thick end of the wedge. When a body position such as leaning over a desk, for example, is held for long periods and under load, even the load of the body's own weight, this effect becomes more pronounced (Twomey 1993). It is known as 'creep' and is defined as the progressive deformation of a structure under constant load by forces which are not large enough to cause permanent damage (Kazarian 1975). The condition rights itself as the body resumes its normal position, but it takes time. Stretchings in the opposite direction can aid the recovery and may help to reduce the risk of injury, since the spine is vulnerable during the interval.

For this reason, motorists who have driven long distances, creating conditions in which creep occurs, should avoid lifting heavy loads immediately afterwards and should perform stretchings, not only at the end of the journey, but at regular intervals throughout its course (Twomey & Taylor

1987). Stretchings will not guarantee protection from injury, but they may make it less likely to occur. (See the sections on Back arching and Crouching/squatting.)

Many jobs require work postures which throw strain on body structures. Stretches help to relieve this strain. The stretch exercise is designed to carry the body or body part in the opposite direction from the posture determined by the work; for example, a seated worker could stand and stretch upwards, whereas a standing operator might arch himself backwards or crouch down on his haunches. Activities which involve precision movements with flexed arms and fingers would call for wide arm stretches.

Stretching is something we do unconsciously after being in one position for a long time. The body seems to ask for it. We stretch after sleeping, after working at a desk, after bending down to weed a flower bed. All three trigger the need or the desire to stretch the body. Subjectively, stretches result in a feeling of comfort, pleasure and relief.

Stretching is essentially a physical action. The process of stretching links in with physiological principles in that the stretched group is responding in a reciprocal way to the action of the prime mover. Charles Carlson, a psychologist at the University of Kentucky, has looked at the effects of stretching and suggests mechanisms by which it might help to promote relaxation (Carlson et al 1990):

1. It has been found that a greater contrast can be obtained between stretching and releasing than between tensing and releasing, because more length-sensitive receptors in the muscle are activated during stretching than during tensing (Anderson 1983). This more pronounced contrast effect might make it easier for individuals to release body tensions.

2. Stretch-based exercises have been found to lower the excitability of the motorneurone pool (Scholz & Campbell 1980), a finding which suggests a resulting decrease in levels of muscle tension, pain and ischaemia.

DESCRIPTION

Carlson and colleagues have devised a procedure consisting of muscle stretchings on the lines of progressive relaxation training, i.e. the tensing routines in the abbreviated version of Bernstein & Borkovec's protocol are replaced by stretch-based actions. Each stretch lasts 10 seconds and is followed by a relaxation period of 60 seconds (Carlson et al 1990). The purpose is to induce an overall sense of relaxation.

Stretchings presented here consist of a range of large body movements and are similar to those in Carlson's schedule. Each stretch is carried out slowly, held for 5–10 seconds, then released quickly. An interval of approximately 30 seconds can be allowed between each stretch (Heptinstall 1995). Participants are asked to notice the feelings in the relevant body part and to compare the sensations during and after the action.

INTRODUCTORY TALK TO PARTICIPANTS

The method you are about to learn consists of a series of stretches. It is believed that stretching a muscle helps to relax it and there is evidence to support this idea. The exercises are arranged so that each stretch lasts about 5 seconds after which there is a rest period of 30 seconds. Please don't overdo the actions – they should be comfortable, even pleasant. Let the stretch build up slowly and take note of the sensations that accompany it. Then, when you release it, register the feelings of relaxation and notice how they contrast with the feelings of the stretch. I'd like you to settle into a comfortable position before we start.

PROCEDURE

The exercises are arranged according to their starting positions:

LYING

The floor or ground provides the best surface, softened by a mat or a carpet. Grass or firm sand also give the degree of hardness required. A bed is too soft.

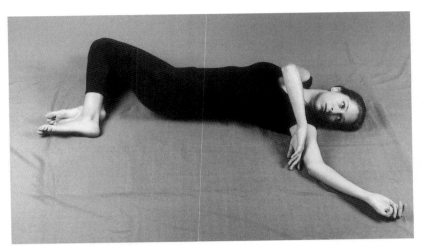

Figure 13.1   Body rotations.

Body rotations (Fig. 13.1)

Lie flat on your back. Bend both knees and place the feet flat on the ground. Now roll your bent knees to one side; roll them as far as they will easily go. At the same time, carry both your arms and your head to the other side. You are now twisting your body and stretching one set of oblique trunk muscles. Make it a comfortable stretch. Hold the position for a few seconds. Then bring your knees back to midline, resting your feet on the ground and your arms by your sides. Repeat the exercise in the other direction.

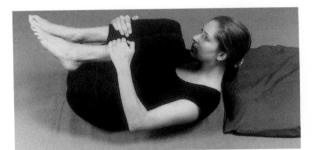

Figure 13.2   Curling into a ball.

Curling into a ball (Fig. 13.2)

Lie flat on your back. Draw your knees up. Gather them in your hands and gently pull them towards your face. Still holding your knees, release the pull. Repeat the pull a few times.

Here the soft structures on the posterior aspect of the spine are being stretched. Some lower back conditions respond favourably to this exercise and the previous one, Body rotations.

Hip joint stretches (Fig. 13.3)

Sit on the ground (cushion optional) and draw your legs into a bent position with your knees pointing sideways. Have the soles of your feet facing each other and in contact. Place your hands around your ankles and rest your elbows on your thighs. Apply

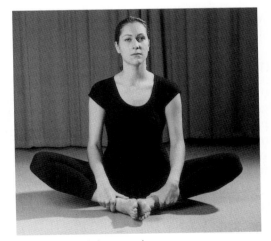

Figure 13.3   Hip joint stretches.

pressure to your thighs, gently and slowly. You should feel a comfortable stretching in the hip area. However, the range of movement in hip joints varies greatly, so do not compare yourself with other

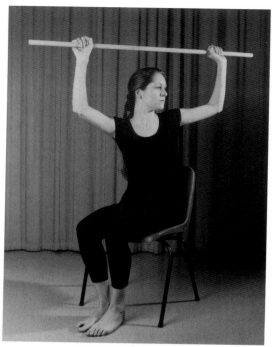

Figure 13.4   Body turning.

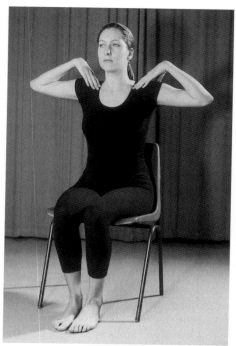

Figure 13.5   Shoulder circling.

people. Perform the exercise just to the point where you feel it is giving you a comfortable stretching sensation and no further. Then take a rest. Reapply the pressure.

SITTING

An upright chair or stool is used for this group of stretchings. For the first item, a long stick such as a broom handle is needed, in an exercise which stretches the trunk and shoulder muscles. Other exercises in this group stretch the shoulder area in different ways.

Body turning (Fig. 13.4)

Sit with your feet flat on the ground. Grasp the broom handle with your hands 90 cm (3 ft) apart and raise your arms so that the stick just clears your head (your elbows are bent). Turn the upper part of your body to the left. This moves the stick through about 90°. Just go as far as you need to in order to get a comfortable stretch. Do not

overstretch or bounce. Then return to the starting position. Repeat in the other direction.

Shoulder circling (Fig. 13.5)

Bend your elbows and place your fingertips on your shoulders. With your elbows, draw slow circles in the air. After two or three circles, break off and repeat in the opposite direction.

Arms stretching above head (Fig. 13.6)

Bend your elbows and lift your arms above your head. Feel yourself pushing the air above you with your open hands. When your elbows are straight, spread your arms sideways and lower them to your sides. Let them rest limply. Repeat once or twice.

Head pressing backwards (Fig. 13.7)

Clasp your hands behind your head and, resting your head in them, arch backwards. Take care not to lean back too far if you are in a lightweight chair. Return your body to a vertical position.

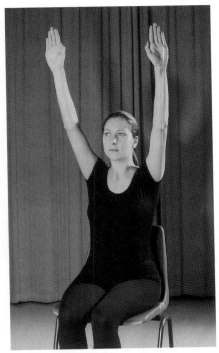

Figure 13.6   Arms stretching above head.

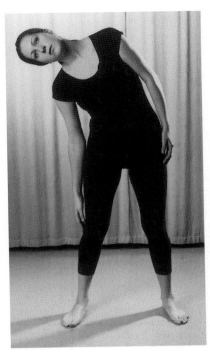

Figure 13.8   Trunk bending sideways.

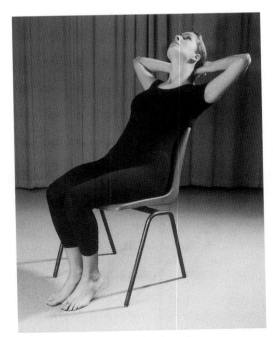

Figure 13.7   Head pressing backwards.

STANDING

Trunk bending sideways (Fig. 13.8)

Stand with your feet apart and your hands by your sides. Bend your body sideways, giving it a good stretch. Return to the upright position and repeat on the other side.

Arm and trunk bending sideways (Fig. 13.9)

This exercise resembles the previous one except that the sideways bend is performed with one hand over your head. Maintain an easy stretch in each direction.

Arms stretching back (Fig. 13.10)

Clasp both hands behind your back and straighten your elbows, drawing your shoulders back at the same time. Feel a stretch in the shoulder area, but do not overdo it. Then relax your arms and repeat the exercise.

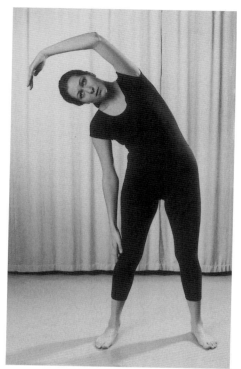

Figure 13.9   Arm and trunk bending sideways.

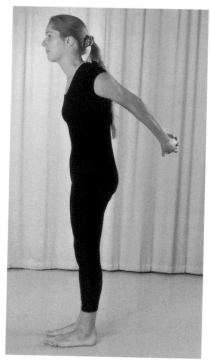

Figure 13.10   Arms stretching back.

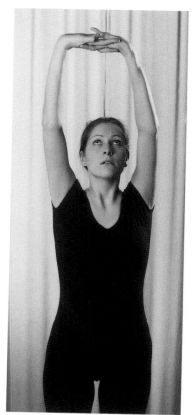

Figure 13.11   Arms reaching upwards.

Arms reaching upwards (Fig. 13.11)

Stand with your feet slightly apart. Clasp your hands, then raise your arms above your head, turning the palms towards the ceiling as you straighten your elbows. Hold them there a few seconds, then lower them.

Arms stretching sideways (Figs 13.12 and 13.13)

Stand with your feet apart, and your arms bent at the elbow and raised to shoulder level. Gently swing one arm sideways and as you do so, allow your elbow to straighten. Return your arm to the bent position. Repeat with the other arm.

The previous five exercises are particularly useful for people who are leaning over a desk or a workbench. The last two can also be performed in a sitting position.

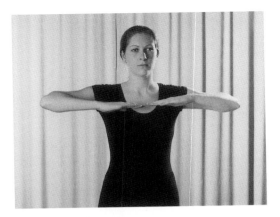

Figure 13.12   Arms stretching sideways: 1.

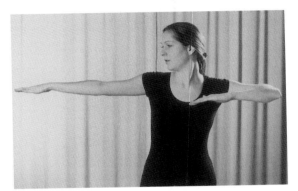

Figure 13.13   Arms stretching sideways: 2.

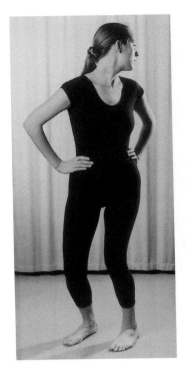

Figure 13.14   Trunk twisting.

Trunk twisting (Fig. 13.14)

Stand with your hands on your hips. Slightly bend your knees and twist the upper part of your body to the left. Feel a comfortable stretch, then return to the starting position. Repeat on the other side.

Back arching (Fig. 13.15)

Place the palms of your hands over the bones that run sideways from your lumbar spine. Using that point as a fulcrum, bend over backwards. Go as far as is comfortable. No further! Then return to an upright position. Repeat. If the exercise makes you feel dizzy, keep your head and eyes looking forwards as you perform it.

Benefit can be gained from this exercise when driving long distances, brushing paths, vacuuming carpets or leaning over a table to sort papers.

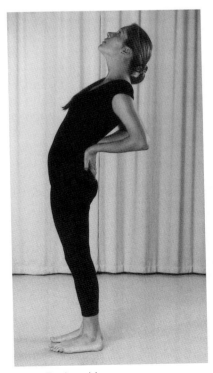

Figure 13.15   Back arching.

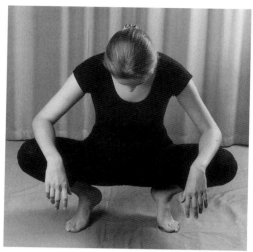

Figure 13.16   Crouching.

Crouching/squatting (Fig. 13.16)

Get into a crouching or squatting position with your head down. Hold the position for 5–10 seconds. If you can, lay your feet flat on the ground; otherwise, perch on your toes. That is all that most people can do.

This is another exercise which may be found to ease the lumbar spine during long-distance drives. Its somewhat bizarre appearance will escape attention if the driver pretends to be examining the tyres of his vehicle. The squat position seems to be beneficial for back health in general since it has been found that in populations where it is habitually adopted, lumbar disc degeneration is rare (Fahrni & Trueman 1965). For people with painful knees, however, it is not advisable.

Calf stretching (Fig. 13.17, Read 1984)

Take your shoes off and stand facing a wall with your toes about 30 cm (12 in) away from it. Have your feet parallel and 10 cm (4 in) apart. Raise your arms and lean your forearms vertically on the wall. Rest your body weight on your forearms. With your heels on the ground and your knees straight, let your hips sink forwards.

You will feel a stretching in the calf muscles. Let it be a comfortable stretch, not a punishment. If you do not feel any stretching, take your feet further back until you do. As you stretch the calf

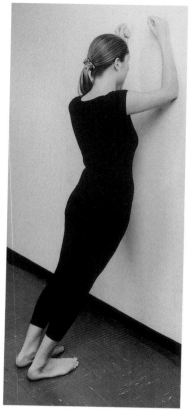

Figure 13.17   Calf stretching.

muscles, hold the position for 5 seconds, then release it. Repeat a few times.

Inner thigh stretching (adductor stretching) (Fig. 13.18)

Stand with your feet about 50 cm (20 in) apart, hands on your hips. Swing your weight over the left knee, bending it as you do so. This puts a stretch on the inside of the right thigh. Hold the position for about 5 seconds, then release the stretch. Repeat. Then swing your weight over the other leg.

EVIDENCE OF EFFECTIVENESS

In a controlled study on volunteers who rated themselves as moderately tense, Carlson et al (1990) compared the effects of stretching exercises with those of tensing routines. Their results, based on both subjective and objective measures, suggest

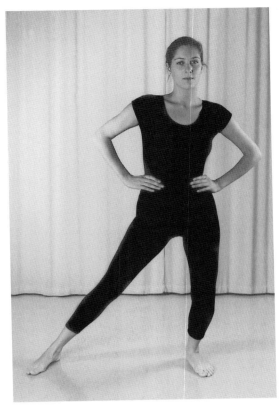

Figure 13.18   Inner thigh stretching.

that stretch-based exercises could be a useful way of promoting relaxation, and particularly in conditions where muscle contractions give rise to pain.

A further study, which investigated the effect of muscle stretching in the treatment of chronic neck tension, supported the earlier findings (Kay & Carlson 1992). In this study 60 individuals with muscle tension in the neck were randomly assigned to three groups: stretch-based, tense–release and a resting control group. After exposure to a mental stressor they performed the relaxation procedure allotted to them, with the result that significantly greater reductions in muscle tension were found in the stretch-based group than in either the tense–release group or the resting control. Thus, in this study, stretch-based relaxation appeared superior to tense–release methods. An additional finding, that skin temperature increased significantly in the stretch-based group, suggested that this method might contribute to a reduction in autonomic activation, whereas the tense–release group, which showed no increase in skin temperature, appeared to offer no such advantage. In conclusion, the authors proposed that stretch-based procedures be viewed as an effective alternative to tense–release ones.

A review of the literature (Carlson and Curran 1994) indicated that a number of conditions including generalized anxiety and excess muscle tension responded favourably to stretch-based procedures. However, although the method offers benefit, it should be seen as only one component of a much wider treatment plan in the management of anxiety and musculoskeletal disorders.

PITFALLS OF STRETCHING EXERCISES

1. A participant may be undergoing medical treatment which contraindicates a particular stretching exercise. Priority should always be given to any medical instructions he has received.

2. The stretching must be done slowly to avoid causing microscopic tearing of the connective tissue (Anderson 1983). It should also be done without straining. At no time should any exercise feel uncomfortable. If it does, it should be stopped. Reasons for possible discomfort are that:
    a. the trainee is overdoing it
    b. he has innate restriction of joint movement
    c. he has an incipient disorder.

3. The number of repetitions carried out is a matter for the individual to decide. Only he knows if he is still benefiting from the exercise.

4. When working in a group of people there is often a temptation to do better than, or at least as well as, the others. Minor injuries can occur when participants feel challenged by neighbours (perhaps older than they) who outshine them. People often feel they have a duty to prove themselves. This of course is mistaken thinking. The only 'duty' imposed on the individual in this context is to make his body feel as comfortable as possible.

Chapter 14

Physical exercise

There is now solid evidence that exercise contributes to the well-being and consequent peace of mind of the individual. So convincing is this evidence that a book like this would be seriously deficient without some reference to it. However, as small group work does not usually provide opportunities for exercise of the type recommended below, the many ways of taking exercise will not be described. Nevertheless, the topic may be discussed within a group, along with plans for the introduction of exercise into the lives of hitherto inactive participants. Individuals can be encouraged to take up a form of exercise of their choice, since enjoyment adds to any resulting sense of well-being.

In this chapter, the effects of exercise on some areas of health are examined. Three areas are included:

- the heart and blood vessels
- the bones
- psychological well-being.

The first two are discussed only briefly since they are not central to the main burden of this work. The third area, psychological well-being, is considered in greater detail and includes sections devoted to depression, anxiety, schizophrenia, mood states, self-esteem, alcohol misuse, sleep and women's health. The chapter continues with a reference to tools which measure exercise intensity and it ends with a list of some of the pitfalls associated with physical activity.

THE CARDIOVASCULAR SYSTEM

RATIONALE

Inactivity can lead to coronary disease. It appears to be so powerful a factor that some researchers suggest it doubles the risk of the disease developing (Powell et al 1987). Dynamic (aerobic) exercise, on the other hand, when carried out regularly, results in a decreased heart rate for any given level of activity (Box 14.1). The demand for myocardial oxygen is thus reduced and exercise tolerance is increased (Royal College of Physicians 1991).

In a well-exercised body, changes occur in the peripheral vascular system which enable the voluntary muscles to function with a lower blood-flow than they had hitherto needed. As a result, blood is not diverted from the viscera until a higher level of activity is reached. Thus, the circulatory system undergoes less disturbance during exertion than previously occurred (Royal College of Physicians 1991).

The value of exercise is underlined in the findings of the National Fitness Survey (Allied Dunbar National Fitness Survey 1992). In women over 54 years of age who had never carried out recreational activity, 15% of the sample suffered from heart disease, angina or breathlessness, compared with only 3% who had exercised for three-quarters of their adult lives. In men these percentages were 21% and 14% respectively. Further evidence of the value of exercise can be found in a study of over 9000 English civil servants (Morris et al 1990). The participants who regularly took part in vigorous exercise (Box 14.2) experienced less than half the coronary heart disease of their sedentary counterparts.

Box 14.1 Aerobic, non–aerobic and anaerobic exercise

Aerobic exercise
Aerobic exercise is sustained rhythmic activity such as distance running, swimming, walking, jogging, dancing and cycling. Dynamic activity of this kind raises the heart rate and increases the oxygen consumption. As defined by the Royal College of Physicians (1991), it is exercise which 'involves repetitive contractions of large muscle groups at levels of energy expenditure less than about 60% of maximum capacity ... performed for prolonged periods on the available oxygen supply'. It results in cardiovascular fitness and the improved endurance of muscles.

Non–aerobic exercise
This term covers activity where the principal aim is to increase strength, flexibility, balance or coordination. The enhancement of cardiovascular fitness is not the primary purpose.

Anaerobic exercise
This consists of high intensity work. The muscle contracts so strongly it compresses the arteries within it, thus reducing the blood and oxygen supply (Royal College of Physicians 1991). This creates the need for a metabolism which does not rely on oxygen and is therefore anaerobic. Examples are weight-lifting, press-ups, isometric work and strong resisted actions. Exercise of this nature causes a temporary rise in blood pressure.

Box 14.2 Grades of exercise intensity. Adapted from Allied Dunbar Fitness Survey (1992)

Vigorous
Activity in which the individual exerts himself to the point of getting out of breath and sweating. It includes squash, football, tennis, strong sustained swimming, long-distance running, cycling over difficult terrain, and energetic aerobics.

Moderate
The same activities (except squash) are carried out but the individual stops short of getting out of breath and sweating. Less demanding activities such as golf, social dancing, table tennis, garden digging, long brisk walks, climbing stairs or gentle uphill gradients are included, performed at an intensity which causes breathing to be somewhat harder than normal and sweating to occur for some of the time.

Light
A few of the above activities such as golf, social dancing and table tennis are performed in a light manner; also included are fishing, darts, snooker, bowls, weeding, planting, light DIY and long walks at an average pace.

HYPERTENSION

Hypertensive individuals also benefit from exercise programmes. This condition, which is a prominent risk factor in the development of heart disease, stroke and congestive heart failure, responds favourably to physical activity, and significant decreases in blood pressure have been recorded following exercise programmes. Arroll and Beaglehole (1992) reviewed 13 controlled trials and found an average lowering of 6–7 mmHg in both systolic and diastolic pressures.

Just how intensive the exercise should be has not been determined, although it seems that lower levels can provide as much if not more benefit than high ones (Box 14.2). Hagberg and Brown (1995) reviewed studies which looked at the resting blood pressures of hypertensive people who carried out exercise of specified intensities. They found that the lower intensity exercisers, i.e. those who trained at levels <70% $\dot{V}O_2$max (maximum oxygen uptake) decreased their systolic blood pressure to a greater extent than those who exercised at higher levels of intensity.

By contrast, some authors consider that the more vigorous the exercise, the greater the benefit. Against this must be weighed the increasing risk of musculoskeletal injury and, in the case of coronary patients, further infarction. Setting these factors together, most authors consider the best approach is to adopt a programme of moderate intensity exercise as being suitable in the majority of cases (Hardman 1996).

With regard to duration, it has been found that half-hourly sessions give the best result; however, a few studies have shown that benefit can still be gained when the exercise period is broken into three 10-minute sessions, suggesting that the intensity of training may be less important than the total energy expended (Hardman 1996). Breaking the sessions into short bouts has also been found to increase adherence rates: people seem to find it easier to structure the day around repeated short sessions than one continuous long one (Jakicic et al 1995).

Guidelines come from the American College of Sports Medicine (ACSM) who recommend that healthy adults should accumulate 30 minutes or more of moderate-intensity physical activity over the course of most (preferably all) days of the week (Pate et al 1995). The emphasis has moved away from high intensity exercise performed three times a week to lower intensity work performed more frequently.

It is agreed that previous regular exercise, if not maintained into middle age, provides no protection from coronary disease (Hardman 1996). However, once training is reintroduced, beneficial effects may occur quite soon, with measurable falls in blood pressure after as little as one week (ACSM 1993).

CORONARY HEART DISEASE

Exercise has been found useful in the rehabilitation following myocardial infarction: meta-analysis shows a reduction in mortality of 20% in the post-infarction period among individuals who carry out exercise, compared with those who do not (Finlayson 1997). Angina also seems to respond favourably to exercise. Bethell & Mullee (1990) reported a decrease of 10% in its occurrence following a training period of 3 months. The non-exercising group, with whom participants were compared, experienced a 60% increase.

Exercise has been shown also to reduce the anxiety and depression associated with heart attack. Kugler and colleagues (1994) conducted a meta-analysis, involving 15 studies, from which they concluded that exercise can have psychological as well as physiological advantages in coronary disease, although exercise should not be relied on as the only treatment in cases of emotional distress.

It should, however, be stressed that any fitness training programme for a heart that does not have a normal blood supply should be constructed under the guidance of a relevant health professional, or at least with his or her cooperation. While the aim of training is to improve the individual's physical capacity, the training must be carried out within the restrictions of the disorder.

THE BONES

Bone mineral density in both men and women undergoes a progressive decline from its peak in the early thirties. In women there is a sharp decline

Box 14.3   Osteoporosis

Osteoporosis is a disease characterized by low bone mass and deterioration of the microarchitecture of the bone tissue. The bones become fragile and are liable to fracture (Cooper & Dennison 1997). The World Health Organization classifies bone density in three categories measured relative to the mean in a population of young adults:

- normal, where values lie within 1 standard deviation (SD) below the mean
- osteopenic, where values lie between 1 and 2.5 SDs below the mean
- osteoporotic, where values are more than 2.5 SDs below the mean (World Health Organization 1994).

Box 14.4   Risk factors of osteoporosis

Risk factors include:

- being female
  - having passed the menopause
  - having had an early menopause
  - having experienced amenorrhoea and consequent oestrogen deficiency
- physical inactivity
- low calcium intake
- inherited tendencies
  - familial
  - ethnic: being of North European extraction
- thin body build
- oral corticosteroid treatment
- excess consumption of tobacco and alcohol.

in the first five years following the menopause, as a result of diminishing oestrogens, and the decline continues, although less sharply, into old age. This can result in osteoporosis (Box 14.3).

The mineral density of bone is determined by the concentration of calcium salts per unit volume (Law et al 1991). It is subject to two influences: the peak mineral content achieved during early life, and the rate of loss sustained during middle and old age. Recent data suggest that environmental influences are responsible for as much as half the variation in peak bone mass among women (Krall & Dawson-Hughes 1993). This implies that factors such as exercise and nutrition play a role in establishing bone mass in the female child and young adult (Snow-Harter et al 1992). It has been suggested that these factors are also important in controlling the loss in later years (Box 14.4).

PREVENTIVE MEASURES

Recent guidelines have advised post-menopausal women to take 1 g of calcium a day in the belief that it helps to reduce bone loss (Cooper & Dennison 1997). Testing this assumption, McMurdo et al (1997) compared the effects of a calcium-only regimen with a calcium-plus-exercise regimen on bone mineral content in 118 volunteers aged between 60 and 73 who were not taking hormone replacement therapy. The calcium dose was 1 g a day; the exercise consisted of 45-minute sessions of weight-bearing exercise (activity which applies longitudinal pressure to the long bones) three times a week. After 2 years a modest significant increase in bone mineral content occurred in the calcium-plus-exercise group, compared with the calcium-only group where there was a decline. The only two fractures reported were in the calcium-only group. A number of the participants had falls but these occurred more in the calcium-only group than in the calcium-plus-exercise group, and as the study moved into its second year the difference became significant. Such findings question the value of calcium supplementation and highlight the value of exercise.

Thus, a policy which addresses bone mineral content alone might not be focusing on the most productive area. Instead, it is suggested that since fractures occur as a result of falls, attention be given to exercises designed to reduce the possibility of falls, i.e. exercises which improve balance, flexibility and strength (McMurdo et al 1997). Current advice to women looking for ways of protecting themselves from osteoporotic fractures is to adopt a combined policy of exercise with a dietary supplementation of calcium and vitamin D (Collier 2002).

These approaches are non-pharmacological. It is widely held, however, that hormone replacement therapy is the most effective way of controlling bone loss in the later life of women. This is difficult to refute, although some authors report that appropriate weight-bearing activity can provide a comparable level of benefit. Mutrie (1997) cites trials in which exercise had resulted in a bone density gain of 4%.

Exercise at an intensity of 60–70% of HRmax (maximum heart rate) has been shown to enhance the psychological as well as the physical health of osteopenic women. In a programme of mixed activity (brisk walking, stepping on and off benches, aerobic dancing and flexibility exercises) for 1 hour three times a week over 12 months, the women experienced an increase in well-being and self-perceived health. This was in addition to the physical benefit gained whereby bone mineral density in the spine was found to stabilize (Bravo et al 1996).

Exercise offers some degree of protection against bone loss throughout life: the bone density of women who exercise at least three times a week is higher than the bone density of sedentary women in their age group, whether they are 20 or 80 years of age (Talmage et al 1986).

TYPES OF EXERCISE

Weight-bearing (often referred to as load-bearing) activity is considered necessary for maintaining bone density. No bone response occurs unless the area is stressed, which means the load must be specific to the site targeted (Smith 1995). For improving the bone mineral density of the spine, for example, aerobic weight-bearing exercise seems to be the most effective activity; this means that swimming and cycling are less effective than walking, jogging and dancing. For improving the bone density of the forearm and wrist, resisted localized strengthening work has been found the most effective exercise. This is illustrated in the finding that the dominant arm of tennis players shows a greater density of bone than the non-dominant arm (Smith 1995).

A few studies have suggested that high impact exercise, e.g. jogging, may be more effective than low impact exercise, e.g. walking, for gaining bone response. When the former is performed three times a week for 18 months it can lead to significant increases in bone mineral density of the femoral neck (Heinonen et al 1996). Lower impact exercise

is also found useful, however, and a meta-analysis of six trials, which included both forms, demonstrated that the incidence of fracture at this site may be reduced by 50% following activity programmes (O'Brien 1996).

Although results of research on this topic are not consistent, a pattern does emerge which indicates the benefits of regular, moderate, dynamic, weight-bearing exercise. It must, of course, be appropriate to the age group and take account of the presence of other restricting factors.

PSYCHOLOGICAL WELL-BEING

RATIONALE

Exercise seems to be closely linked to mental health. There is evidence of the link in healthy populations, but in clinical populations it is even stronger (North et al 1990, Scully et al 1998). Psychological assessment suggests that a sense of well-being is derived from regular exercise, with participants reporting less tension, fatigue, aggression, depression and insomnia (Royal College of Physicians 1991). The psychological benefits of exercise include distraction from worries, release of frustrations, a sense of achievement, a feeling of improved physical appearance and enjoyment in the company of other individuals in the pleasant surroundings of the exercise activity. In addition to the above benefits, exercise is inexpensive, non-invasive and has few side effects.

As a therapy, exercise is not underpinned by any particular theory. However, rather than being conceptualized as an atheoretical approach, Mutrie & Faulkner (2003) suggest it should be viewed as a process through which therapeutic goals can be reached.

What is the mechanism?

Many hypotheses are put forward in an attempt to explain the mechanism underlying the association between exercise and mental well-being. Some of these are physiological, such as an increase in brain oxygenation which might result from aerobic exercise (Donaghy & Mutrie 1999). Others pose questions about biochemical changes. For example, to what extent are the catecholamines involved? It has been suggested that exercise can help to maintain a healthy balance in the neurochemistry of the body (Chaouloff 1989). Or again, how do the beta-endorphins fit into the picture? We know that exercise is accompanied by raised levels of endogenous morphines, but not how those raised levels might influence the mental state. De Coverley Veale (1987) has indicated that for a few hours following a period of activity, the mood of a person who regularly takes exercise can become altered: a depressed person becomes less depressed, an anxious person less anxious and an angry person less angry; and Sher (1996) reports that intravenous administration of beta-endorphin reduces both anxiety and depression. This creates a persuasive picture but leaves open the question of how such changes are brought about.

Moving away from biochemical concerns to psychosocial ones, we can ask other questions in an attempt to discover the mechanism. For example, does the sense of physical well-being transfer to the psychological sphere, making the thoughts more positive? Does the active coping strategy engender a feeling of mastery? Mutrie (1997) refers to the association of regular exercise with raised self-esteem, but it is not known whether this is brought about by virtue of weight reduction, improved physical health, or sense of achievement.

Then again, is there some connection with people's expectations? Do people feel positive mood changes following a bout of exercise because they expect to? Does distraction play a part?

La Forge (1995) has reviewed all the possible mechanisms. He sees them as integrated mechanisms rather than separate ones. His model shows the mechanisms to overlap, sharing the same neural pathways. In this light, an approach which addresses them as linked processes would seem more productive than one which studies them in isolation.

Much has been made of the role of fitness and its association with psychological health; for example, Moses et al (1989) found that although fitness often accompanies the sense of well-being, it is not a prerequisite. Being physically active is seen as more important. This point is brought out in studies which show non-aerobic exercise to be as effective for psychological well-being as aerobic exercise, since only the aerobic component can be said to contribute to cardiovascular fitness (Doyne et al 1987, Martinsen et al 1989, Donaghy et al 1991). Thus, it is the engagement in physical activity rather than the enhancement of aerobic fitness which is associated with the positive mood shift. However, it must be said that the outcome of research on this topic is not consistent, and Scully and colleagues (1998) in their review do not feel the evidence is strong enough to declare the matter resolved.

There are no satisfactory answers to these questions, nor to the much debated topic of whether exercise actually causes improvements in psychological well-being. At present all that can be said is that an association exists between physical activity and psychological health (Mutrie 1997). Ruuskanen and Ruoppila (1995), in their survey of 1244 elders in Finland, suggest that exercise may promote a subjective sense of well-being, but go on to raise the question of the extent to which a sense of well-being might lead to continued physical activity. Such comments introduce a further dimension to the argument in the form of *direction of causality*.

Clearly, more work needs to be done to deepen our understanding of this issue.

DEPRESSION

The evidence associating exercise with relief from depression has been gathering strength over the last two decades and this association has been demonstrated in both cross-sectional and large-scale epidemiological studies (Mutrie 2001). The role played by physical activity and exercise in the management of mild-to-moderate depression may be an important one (Donaghy & Durward 2000, Paluska & Schwenk 2000) while positive effects may also extend to the more severe forms of the condition (Craft & Landers 1998). Lawler & Hopker (2001), however, are reluctant to conclude in favour of exercise (apart from short-term relief) on account of the poor quality of some of the research. In spite of such drawbacks, Mutrie & Faulkner (2003) find compelling evidence of a positive relationship between physical activity and mental health.

Exercise as a treatment for depression has not only been found effective but its results compare well with those of psychotherapy (Biddle & Mutrie 2001). Furthermore, when psychotherapy and drug intervention were added to exercise there was only a slightly larger, non-significant effect than with exercise on its own (Craft & Landers 1998).

Patients themselves have reported favourably on exercise: Scully and colleagues (1998) noted that some patients with depression rated exercise the most valuable component of the total treatment programme.

The effects of exercise on depression have been investigated among different population groups, one of which is the elderly. In the above-mentioned survey of Finnish elders, Ruuskanen and Ruoppila (1995) found a significant correlation between absence of physical exercise and attacks of depression. At the other end of the age range, Steptoe and Butler (1996), in their study among adolescents, demonstrated an association between vigorous exercise and antidepressant changes.

Although most studies have in the past indicated the superiority of aerobic over strengthening exercise, there have been increasing reports of the value of strengthening exercise as an antidepressant (Doyne et al 1987, Martinsen et al 1989, Donaghy et al 1991). Doyne et al compared the effects of aerobic and strengthening exercise programmes on women suffering from depressive disorders. After 8 weeks, depression symptoms were significantly reduced in both exercise groups, with no significant difference between them. More recently Singh et al (1997), in their study of 32 depressed elders, demonstrated that the depression scores of participants decreased significantly following a programme of resistance exercises.

Both aerobic and strengthening exercise were found to be useful for relieving depression in North et al's meta-analytic review (1990), as they were in the work of Biddle & Mutrie (2001).

Exercise as a preventive measure

Since exercise has been shown to confer substantial benefit as a treatment for depression, it has been hypothesized that it might also have some protective value in psychologically healthy members of the community. Weyerer and Kupfer (1994), reviewing work on physical activity and mental health, found evidence that exercise did help to reduce the risk of depression and that physically inactive individuals ran a significantly higher risk of depression than regular exercisers. Fox (2000a) supported this view.

Not all studies concur with this result, however. Cooper-Patrick et al (1997) undertook a prospective study on 973 middle-aged physicians to explore the preventive capacity of exercise, but results did not indicate that exercise reduced the risk of developing depression. It seems that no confident judgements can be made on the predictive value of physical exercise, although a trend suggesting a protective effect does exist (Donaghy & Durward 2000).

Depressive psychosis

More severe forms of depression are apparently not helped by exercise. There is no convincing evidence of effectiveness in this area (Smeaton 1995).

ANXIETY

Anxiety can refer either to an emotional state or to a personality disposition. The first is called 'state' anxiety, the second is 'trait' anxiety. State anxiety occurs as a temporary reaction to an event perceived as threatening; it refers to the experience of apprehension in a precise moment. Trait anxiety, by contrast, is characterized by the individual's tendency to view all neutral events as potentially stressful and to experience state anxiety as a response to them (Spielberger 1980). State anxiety tends to accompany most disorders and is a natural concomitant of adverse conditions. Some findings suggest that exercise training can help to relieve both forms (Donaghy & Durward 2000). For example, Taylor (2000) found that a small-to-moderate effect on state anxiety could be achieved by single sessions of exercise; reductions in trait anxiety, on the other hand, would require a longer period of exercise.

It is perhaps easier to accept that exercise (a high arousal activity) could relieve depression (a low arousal state) than that it could relieve anxiety, itself a high arousal state. Nevertheless, exercise has been fairly consistently associated with decreased levels of state anxiety (Scully et al 1998). The link is, however, a modest one. Donaghy & Durward (2000) rate the effect of exercise as low-to-moderate. The most persuasive results have been found in the field of generalized anxiety, where a marked treatment response often occurs. Martinsen (1990) found that little benefit was gained in the field of panic disorder or agoraphobia. However, this conclusion has subsequently been challenged by the findings of Broocks et al (1998) in their study of 46 outpatients with moderate to severe degrees of panic disorder, where symptoms were reduced by a programme of exercise. Although exercise (aerobic) was found to be less effective than medication (clomipramine), its effect after 10 weeks was significant.

With regard to specific anxiety disorders, such as panic, reviewers find the evidence inconclusive (Donaghy & Durward 2000) but the research base is small compared with that of depression. Future work will cast more light on this area where, in many instances, anxiety and depression occur in the same individual.

Both aerobic and resistance forms of exercise have been found useful. Weighing the evidence in the state of knowledge of 1998, however, it seemed that greater effects were obtained from aerobic than from non-aerobic exercise (Scully et al 1998).

SCHIZOPHRENIA

Faulkner & Biddle (1999) have reviewed 12 studies investigating the effects of exercise on the symptoms of schizophrenia. Exercise programmes typically consisted of 30 minutes three times a week and ran for periods ranging from 8 to 24 weeks. Most studies indicated some kind of benefit: depression scores were reduced in seven; aerobic fitness was improved in five; self-esteem was increased in one and psychotic symptoms were reduced in three.

In an area of limited research where much of it is characterized by methodological weakness, Faulkner & Biddle find it difficult to draw conclusions. However, they suggest that exercise may play an effective adjunct role in the treatment of schizophrenia, relieving depression, anxiety and negative symptoms on the one hand, and providing a possible coping strategy for psychotic symptoms, such as auditory hallucinations, on the other.

MOOD STATES

The effect of exercise on mood states has been widely studied, showing that both aerobic and strengthening exercise may be associated with enhanced mood. Both healthy and clinical populations can benefit, although the effect is greatest in clinical groups.

Many of these studies used the Profile of Mood States (POMS) (McNair et al 1971) as their measuring tool. This is a scale consisting of 65 items with six sub-scales: depression, tension, anger, fatigue, confusion and vigour. Slaven and Lee (1997) used the POMS to study the interaction of physical exercise and mood in 220 middle-aged women in order to assess the benefits of regular aerobic exercise as an alternative to hormone replacement therapy. Results showed that scores on the POMS were significantly more positive among respondents who exercised than among those who did not. Thus, it is suggested that regular exercise may help to protect women from symptoms of menopause-related distress.

Pre-menopausal women have also been shown to benefit in studies examining the effects of exercise on psychological symptoms of pre-menstrual tension. Favourable effects were reported in the review of Scully et al (1998), particularly when the exercise was aerobic, non-competitive and of moderate intensity.

SELF–ESTEEM

Self-esteem is a measure of the regard a person has for himself and can be defined as reflecting the individual's perceived self-worth and competence. Fox (2000b) defines it as a self-rating of how well the self is doing. Thus, self-esteem is fundamentally tied up with psychological well-being (Ch. 16, p. 142).

The self, however, is not a simple concept and can be viewed as having domain-specific components. One of these is the physical self where moderately strong correlations with global self-esteem across the lifespan have been demonstrated (Fox 2000c).

Does exercise improve self-esteem? Fox (2000a) has reported that an association does exist between physical activity and global self-esteem but it is a weak one. However, exercise seems to help most people view themselves more positively (Carless & Fox 2003).

Exercise programmes need to run for a minimum of 12 weeks before any change in self-esteem becomes measurable. Greatest benefit has been found to occur in those whose self-esteem was low to start with (Carless & Fox 2003).

It is not clear what mechanism is involved. Carless & Fox (2003) suggest that participation in physical activity might favourably influence physical self-perceptions which, in their turn, might lead to positive changes in global self-esteem. In this model the physical self is seen to play a mediating role between exercise participation and self-esteem.

Using the Physical Self-perception Profile, a scale devised by Fox (1997), Donaghy (1997) investigated different aspects of the physical self, such as perceived physical skills and physical appearance, in 158 problem drinkers. After a 3-week course of exercise, both aerobic and strengthening, participants showed an improved perception of their physical self-worth. Self-perceptions of their fitness and strength also showed an improvement which was maintained at follow-up 2 months later. There was a positive association between objective levels of fitness and strength, and participants' perceptions of these parameters.

It is not known, however, what effect such changes in physical self-perceptions may have on the global self-esteem of this population group or on their decisions to adopt a healthier lifestyle. Donaghy suggests that the sense of self-efficacy may be favourably influenced by the experience of exercise leading to a change in the perception of self-worth and creating the confidence to continue with physical exercise.

PROBLEM DRINKING

A condition which is often accompanied by high levels of depression and anxiety is problem drinking, where exercise is shown to have more to offer than relaxation. Exploring the benefits of different types of exercise, Donaghy and colleagues (1991) compared aerobic with resistance forms in 45 problem drinkers, using a control group who received a form of autogenic relaxation. The authors examined a wide range of outcome measures, among which were changes in psychological well-being. Results showed that both aerobic and strengthening exercises significantly lowered depression scores and also reduced anxiety scores, while the autogenic group showed no differences. Thus, it is suggested that aerobic and strengthening forms of exercise are effective in alleviating mood disorders in problem drinkers. This finding supports the view that exercise which promotes cardiovascular fitness is not essential for creating psychological benefit.

However, since alcohol misusers tend also to have low fitness levels, regimens which focus on aerobic aspects of exercise would seem to offer particular advantage (Donaghy & Mutrie 1999).

Reviewing studies which investigate the effects of exercise in the treatment and rehabilitation of the problem drinker, the conclusion has been drawn that physical exercise is indeed linked to improved fitness and strength and that this finding can be stated with some confidence. Regarding the psychological benefits of exercise with this clinical group, the evidence is, however, less strong (Donaghy 2003, Donaghy & Mutrie 1999).

SLEEP

Without sleep we can hardly be said to enjoy psychological well-being. Insomnia, however, has been found to respond favourably to exercise. In their sample of 29 healthy, sedentary men and women in late middle-age, King and colleagues (1997) demonstrated a significant improvement in global sleep score following a training programme consisting of four half-hourly sessions a week of brisk walking at an intensity of 60–75% HRmax for 16 weeks.

WOMEN'S HEALTH

Physical activity appears to be psychologically useful for young women who experience premenstrual syndrome (Scully et al 1998). Its benefits, however, extend to women at all stages of life. This includes the elderly. A recent study in a large cohort of Australian women in their 70s across a 3-year period demonstrated an association between physical activity and emotional well-being (Lee & Russell 2003).

DOSAGE OF EXERCISE

A general principle of exercise prescription is that it should be introduced gradually and progress by small stages covering a period of several weeks. This is to ensure that the activity designed to benefit the body is matched by the body's capacity to tolerate the exercise.

Dimensions of exercise

It is conventional to describe exercise in terms of its three dimensions:

- intensity
- duration
- frequency.

Intensity. Intensity, which can be high, medium or low, has received particular attention from researchers. Although results have not been consistent, there seems to be a consensus that moderate intensity activity produces the greatest benefit. 'Moderate', in the context of exercise, means that the exercise should be vigorous enough to create a physical effect but not so strenuous that the person feels unduly challenged. Extremely high intensities can have negative effects by inducing a degree of stress (Gauvin & Spence 1996).

The suggested superiority of moderate over high intensity exercise is illustrated in the work of Moses and colleagues (1989) who investigated the mood changes following exercise in 109 sedentary non-clinical volunteers. After 10 weeks of training, reductions in psychological tension were significantly greater in the moderate intensity exercisers than in the high intensity exercisers.

Although there have been studies which indicate the value of high intensity exercise (Tate & Petruzzello 1995), and studies in which no difference between moderate and high intensity exercise is found (King et al 1993), most investigations conclude in favour of moderate intensity exercise.

Low intensity exercise has also been shown to confer benefit, as Aganoff and Boyle (1994) demonstrated in their study of symptom reporting in middle-aged women. Significant improvements in the mood scores of the participants resulted from this kind of exercise. Low intensity exercise has also been associated with reductions in muscle tension as recorded in electromyographic readings (Sime 1990).

Amid conflicting reports therefore, it cannot be said with confidence that any one intensity level appears superior to the others. Because of this, Scully and colleagues (1998) take the view that the situation calls for a compromise whereby the individual is asked, on the basis of health and inclination and in consultation with professional advisors, to select his own goals. Such a strategy has the added advantage of increasing the participant's sense of commitment.

Duration. Regarding the duration of exercise sessions, literature reviews tend to indicate the benefit of 20–40 minutes (Gauvin & Spence 1996). This duration can be split into 10-minute segments and still provide benefit (Blair et al 1992), while in the case of anxiety, short 5-minute bouts can also have value (Scully et al 1998). One advantage of short exercise periods is that they can be fitted into break times, which makes them ideally suited for people suffering from work stress. In setting the duration much depends first on the nature of the exercise, in that lighter activities are easier to sustain for longer periods, and second on the physical health and age of the individual, which will affect his exercise tolerance.

Frequency. On the matter of frequency there are no fixed recommendations: programmes vary in their specifications from 3 to 7 times a week. Certainly a high frequency of practice is advocated, but whether 7 times a week confers more benefit than 5 times a week has not been established. Most researchers suggest that daily exercising has merit.

Optimum length of programme

The benefit derived from exercise programmes builds up over the weeks until it reaches a peak. In their review of the effects of exercise on depression, North and colleagues (1990) found that maximum psychological benefit peaked at 17 weeks, although some gain could be expected after just 4 weeks. Similar results have been found for anxiety.

When exercising for psychological health the programme chosen should be enjoyable, non-competitive and carried out in pleasant surroundings (Shephard 1997). There are, however, no official guidelines specific to exercise in this field. Published guidelines refer to physical health and come from institutions such as the Health Education Authority (HEA 1995) and the American College of Sports Medicine (Pate et al 1995). These are: 30 minutes of moderate intensity activity on most days of the week. Fox (2000a) suggests that a similar programme is appropriate in the field of mental health, adding that any exercise programme should match the needs of the individual.

Adherence to exercise programmes for psychological health

All exercise programmes are dependent on the willingness of the participants to carry out the procedure. Without their cooperation, the results will not have any meaning. In the field of therapeutic exercise, however, the adherence rate is not high. Reviewing estimations, Glenister (1996) finds it varies between 50% and 80% for short-term programmes. For long-term programmes it is lower still. Moreover, adherence to vigorous exercise programmes is lower than it is to moderate intensity programmes (Glenister 1996). There seems to be a generally low willingness on the part of people to carry out regular exercise, with only 10% of the population committed to it (Scully et al 1998).

CONCLUSION

Evidence mounts in support of the idea that physical activity is associated with psychological well-being (Biddle 2000). As the argument in favour of exercise gains strength, so the areas in which improvements take place become identified, such as mood, self-concept and work behaviour (Folkins & Sime 1981), self-esteem and cognitive function (Mutrie 1997) as well as depression, anxiety and stress (Gauvin & Spence 1996, Glenister 1996, Scully et al 1998). However, not all authors reach the same conclusions and this lack of consensus gives a guarded tone to the reviews.

The strongest evidence of benefit lies in the field of mild-to-moderate depression where symptoms are significantly reduced by exercise (Donaghy & Durward 2000). Moreover, benefits can be gained in as short a time as 1 or 2 months and can last for up to a year (Donaghy & Durward 2000). Findings in other areas tend to be less robust (Mutrie 1997, p. 306). In drawing conclusions, however, writers indicate the paucity of good quality data. Many of the studies contain methodological flaws which reduce their validity and, because studies use a variety of populations, a wide range of exercise modes and different measuring systems, it is difficult to make comparisons. Scully and colleagues (1998) point to such issues and emphasize the need for large-scale multidimensional experimental programmes, while Smeaton (1995) urges replication of existing work.

TOOLS FOR MEASURING EXERCISE INTENSITY

A standard measure of exercise intensity is the percentage of maximum oxygen uptake ($\dot{V}O_2max$). This requires skills and apparatus which may not always be available. Simpler to measure is the percentage of maximum heart rate (HRmax) and since the two scales bear a linear relationship to each other, the HRmax is the method commonly employed (Smeaton 1995).

HRmax is estimated by subtracting the person's age from the figure 220. In the case of a 40-year old individual this would be 180, representing his hypothetical maximum. If the programme requires a 60–65% HRmax level of intensity, then the pulse rate for this individual should be kept within the range of 108–117 during exercise.

This figure is appropriate for healthy individuals. People who are less fit, however, can take the figure of 200 instead of 220 as their starting point, and those under medical supervision should seek the advice of their doctor.

Criticisms of this method include the possibility of error within the age categories and difficulty in palpating the pulse for those unfamiliar with the practice (Birk & Birk 1987). An alternative method for determining exercise intensity has been

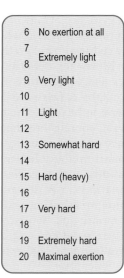

6	No exertion at all
7	
8	Extremely light
9	Very light
10	
11	Light
12	
13	Somewhat hard
14	
15	Hard (heavy)
16	
17	Very hard
18	
19	Extremely hard
20	Maximal exertion

Figure 14.1 The perceived exertion scale with ratings. (Borg 1998, with kind permission of the author.)

developed by Borg (1970, 1998). This researcher considers that the single best indicator of physical strain is the individual's own perception of exertion. This entails the integration of signals from all parts of the body including muscles, joints, pulmonary and cardiac organs and the central nervous system. For the novice this means concentrating on what Morgan (1981) has called the 'total inner feeling of exertion'.

Borg, a psychologist from Stockholm, devised a scale for rating this perceived exertion. It consists of descriptive phrases indicating the subjective response to different levels of exercise intensity (Fig. 14.1). The perceived exertion rating of 13–14 is seen as corresponding to 70% HRmax and the rating of 10–11 as corresponding to 60% HRmax. Thus, a glance at the scale helps the exerciser to judge the degree of effort required. Its sheer simplicity makes the scale attractive. Validity has been repeatedly demonstrated and high coefficients obtained (Borg 1998). Burke & Collins (1984) have found the scale to correlate strongly with oxygen consumption. Reliability has also been shown, but although coefficients have often been high, Bowling (2001) considers that more work still needs to be done. Negative criticisms include the possibility of discrepancies between subjective reports and physiological effects.

The scale can be used either on its own or in combination with pulse rate for assessing exercise intensity (Birk & Birk 1987).

PITFALLS AND RECOMMENDATIONS

In recommending exercise to participants, the health care professional needs to be aware of its hazards. Exercise can be excessive and beyond the capacity of the individual. There have been instances of muscles and tendons being injured and even death occurring in the course of exercise. It is important, therefore, to keep the activity within safe limits. The following points should be borne in mind:

1. Exercise should not be seen as a substitute for medical help in the presence of disease or suspected disease. People with cardiovascular problems should first consult their doctor before taking up exercise.

2. A medical examination is an essential preliminary for middle-aged or older people who wish to embark on activity at an unaccustomed level. Individuals who suddenly take up vigorous exercise would be seriously at risk if they had unrecognized cardiac problems.

3. Any programme of exercise should be introduced gradually and progress in small stages in order to allow the organs to adapt to the new demands. Walking or swimming are useful ways to start. Unaccustomed strenuous activity is potentially hazardous.

4. All exercise should be preceded by some kind of 'warming up' activity to prepare the muscles for action (Safran et al 1989). Warming up takes the form of mild activity such as running on the spot, or gentle contractions against resistance performed for 5 or 10 minutes. The effect of this procedure is to open up the blood vessels in the working part, thus protecting against ischaemia (inadequacy of local blood supply), which can occur in unprepared muscles.

Stretching has also traditionally featured in many 'warming up' programmes prior to exercise; however, the value of stretching in this context is now regarded with some doubt. A systematic review of studies examining the effects of stretching before exercise did not support the view that this intervention reduces the risk of injury and muscle soreness (Herbert & Gabriel 2002).

5. Cooling down is also important. During vigorous or moderate exercise a higher than normal proportion of the total blood volume circulates through the voluntary muscles. This state continues for some time after the exercise has come to an end, and causes a lowering of the blood pressure. It is potentially hazardous in the elderly, but should be guarded against even in the very fit. As a remedy, the exercise can be slowly reduced in intensity or, alternatively, some lighter activity such as slow walking can be performed to bring about a gradual return of normal blood distribution (Hough 2001).

6. Exercise should not be too strenuous. To be safe, exercise should be well within the capacity of the individual and performed regularly. The individual should never feel he is exercising to the limit of his strength. He should also know how to recognize signs of fatigue. Warnings of overwork in the form of chest pain or faintness, for example, should never be ignored (Allied Dunbar National Fitness Survey 1992).

7. While team sports and marathons can be fun, they involve a spirit of competition which may be stressful. Non-competitive activities, on the other hand, impose less pressure on the individual, who can pace himself in a way that takes account of his reactions.

8. In the case of older people, the exercise should be light and regular. Demands should be kept low since ageing organs do not have the reserves of strength or the resilience of younger organs. Aerobic work should not be too arduous, while resisted work for muscle strengthening should be seen as potentially hazardous because of the rise in blood pressure which accompanies it. In most other respects, older people derive the same benefit from exercise as younger people. They simply need to know when to stop.

9. The capacity of the individual to carry out exercise may be compromised by the drugs he is taking. It is advisable to check that these do not conflict with the effects of exercise. This applies particularly where high doses have been prescribed.

10. The cardiovascular benefit of jogging has to be balanced against the possible stress it imposes on the weight-bearing joints (US Preventive Services

Task Force 1989), although hard evidence of any association between running and the risk of osteoarthritis in weight-bearing joints is slight (Blair et al 1992). However, if there is a family history of joint problems, it may be advisable to consider an alternative form of aerobic exercise such as cycling or swimming.

11. Bone mineral density in athletes has been found to be higher than it is among people who take no exercise. However, exercise can be excessive and, in the case of young women in endurance sports such as long-distance running or ballet dancing, there can be a temporary reduction in the level of oestrogen, with resulting amenorrhoea (cessation of menstruation). If prolonged, this can lead to loss of bone. As soon as the excessively strenuous exercise stops or is lowered in intensity, however, the oestrogen level rises, menstruation returns and bone loss is halted.

12. 'Fatigue fracture' is a condition which sometimes afflicts rowers and long-distance runners. It is inclined to occur where the level of exertion markedly exceeds what is customary for the individual.

13. Exercise is contraindicated during any kind of fever and should be avoided during viral infections such as influenza.

14. It is possible to become addicted to exercise. Trainers and trainees need to be aware of this phenomenon and to control any trend in its direction.

The gradient of risk

Blair and colleagues (1992) refer to a gradient of risk across activity levels: the more intense and longer-lasting the exercise, the greater the risk it imposes. They emphasize the benefits of lower levels of activity since these are associated with reduced risk while yet conferring significant fitness benefit. Blair et al recommend a public health message which reads: 'A little exercise is better than none at all', rather than one which insists on minimum levels of exercise intensity.

While the advantages of exercise must be set against its potential hazards, most people derive benefit from it. It should, however, be carried out in a sensible manner (Royal College of Physicians 1991).

Further reading

Biddle S J H, Fox K R, Boutcher S H (eds) 2000 Physical activity and psychological well-being. Routledge, London

Biddle S J H, Mutrie N 2001 Psychology of physical activity: determinants, well-being and interventions. Routledge, London

Donaghy M, Durward B 2000 A report on the clinical effectiveness of physiotherapy in mental health. Chartered Society of Physiotherapy, London

Everett T, Donaghy M, Feaver S 2003 Interventions in mental health: an evidence-based approach for physiotherapists and occupational therapists. Butterworth-Heinemann, Oxford

Mutrie N 1997 The therapeutic effects of exercise on the self. In: Fox K R (ed) The physical self: from motivation to well-being. Human Kinetics, Leeds

Chapter 15

Breathing

INTRODUCTION

A wide variety of breathing routines have been proposed to induce relaxation, such as slow breathing, deep breathing, breathing meditation and abdominal breathing. Using the breathing system as a means of gaining relaxation is clearly an accepted approach. Moreover, the techniques are easy to learn and can be carried out anywhere – a fact which makes them available in the stressful situation itself.

In this chapter the respiratory mechanism is first described; exercises which induce relaxed breathing patterns are presented; there is a section on hyperventilation, and also one on the pitfalls of breathing exercises.

THE PROCESS OF BREATHING

Breathing is an automatic process governed by centres in the brain stem (pons and medulla). These activate the diaphragm and costal muscles to open the rib cage which expands in three directions: vertically, laterally and anteroposteriorly. Negative pressure in the pleural cavity pulls the lungs out, causing air to be sucked in. Relaxation of the same muscles results in the recoil of the thoracic structures and the expulsion of air. The respiratory organs are illustrated in Figure 15.1.

Oxygenated blood leaves the lungs bound for the heart which pumps it round the body where its oxygen is exchanged for waste products, amongst them carbon dioxide. These are carried back to the

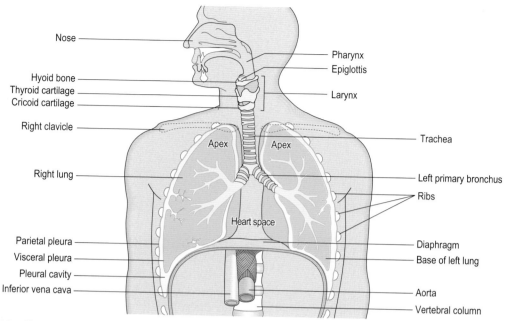

Figure 15.1   The organs of respiration. (From Waugh & Grant 2001.)

heart. The spent blood is then returned to the lungs where it gives up its carbon dioxide and collects a fresh supply of oxygen. The interchange of blood gases takes place in the alveoli (air sacs) which contain surfaces richly supplied with hair-like blood vessels through which the gases diffuse (pass through membranes). The direction in which the gases pass is determined by their concentration, i.e. they move from a situation of high concentration to one of low concentration. Thus oxygen passes from the air in the bronchial tubes to the blood, and carbon dioxide passes from the blood to the air in the bronchial tubes. Each breath makes a contribution to the process. Figure 15.2 shows the structure of a terminal bronchiole with its air sacs.

Chemoreceptors in the walls of the aorta and the carotid arteries help to control breathing and are sensitive to changes in the amount of carbon dioxide circulating in the blood (Waugh & Grant 2001). The levels of carbon dioxide influence physiological activity, and are conventionally represented in terms of the partial pressure of carbon dioxide ($P\mathrm{CO_2}$). The arterial $P\mathrm{CO_2}$ may range from 35 to 45 mmHg (4.7–6.0 kPa) in the healthy individual (Hough 2001). Carbon dioxide levels are measured using arterial blood gas samples or end-tidal

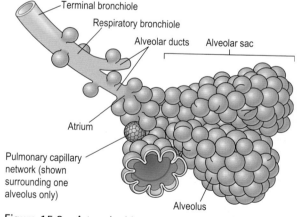

Figure 15.2   A terminal bronchiole with its air sacs.

airflow (air delivered at the end of exhalation and measured at the mouth or nostril); the results from either the blood or the airflow are very similar in normal lungs (Gardner & Bass 1989).

Overbreathing and underbreathing

Overbreathing leads to excessive loss of carbon dioxide and a lowered arterial $P\mathrm{CO_2}$ (hypocapnia); underbreathing to a build-up of carbon dioxide and a raised arterial P_{CO_2} (hypercapnia). A small rise (mild hypercapnia) is associated with lethargy and symptoms resembling those of parasympathetic dominance, i.e. relaxation (Slonim & Hamilton 1976).

RATIONALE OF BREATHING CONTROL

Most relaxation methods like imagery and muscle routines influence the autonomic nervous system by indirect routes. Breathing is different. It is directly linked to the system which controls physiological arousal. This adds to its potential as a means of inducing physiological relaxation (Lichstein 1988).

The kind of breathing which accompanies sympathetic arousal is quite different from the kind of breathing characteristic of parasympathetic arousal: the first tends to be fast and staccato-like, while the second tends to be slow and gentle. This connection between slow breathing and parasympathetic dominance has created a perception that slow breathing has stress-relieving properties and has led to its adoption as a relaxation technique (Sudsuang et al 1991). The approach is thus underpinned by physiological theory, but it also has cognitive elements in the form of the imagery which features in some of the exercises.

Its mechanism, however, is unclear. Lum (1981) proposed that slow breathing had a corrective effect on an abnormal pattern of breathing, while Garssen et al (1992) suggested that it may reduce stress for other reasons such as distraction.

BREATHING AWARENESS

This is a phrase which refers to the focusing of attention on the breathing pattern. It puts the individual in touch with the respiratory process and helps him to feel he has some control over it. As such it forms a useful introduction to the topic. Breathing awareness begins with an exploration of the movements of the chest and abdomen which accompany respiration.

EXPLORING RESPIRATORY MOVEMENTS

During the inspiratory phase the chest expands through all dimensions. Participants can confirm

this for themselves by carrying out the following exercises for which plenty of time should be allowed.

1. Lying or sitting

Place your hands on the lower edge of your ribs, fingertips a few centimetres apart. Feel your hands rise and separate as the air flows in, and recoil as it flows out.

2. Sitting with head and arms resting on a table

With movement in the front of the chest now restricted, you can feel the chest expanding backwards.

3. Lying or sitting

Place your right hand over the solar plexus (the soft part between the ribs and the navel) and your left hand over the front of your chest below the clavicles (collar bones). Notice what happens under your hands when you breathe. As the air enters, feel the expansion growing, first under your right hand, then rising through the chest to reach the area under your left hand. Explore that idea for a minute or two.

The emotional state

Breathing is also subject to a person's emotional state:

Imagine for a few moments a situation that makes you feel uneasy ... Next, imagine one in which you feel at ease ... Did you notice any change in your breathing pattern from one to the other?

Breathing in a calm individual is associated with relaxed abdominal muscles and is characterized by visible movement of the upper abdomen; breathing in a stressed individual is associated with a predominantly upper costal movement and often involves contraction of the shoulder girdle muscles. Calm breathing tends to have a slow rate; stressful breathing, a more rapid one.

SLOW BREATHING

As mentioned above, relaxation is associated with a reduced rate of breathing. The natural pace of respiration in a resting individual is a slow one, and since the oxygen requirement is low, breathing also tends to be rather shallow. The individual may occasionally take a deep breath and find it profoundly relaxing, but the natural tendency is for such a breath to be followed by the original pattern of slow and fairly shallow respiration. Certainly, the breathing of an unrelaxed individual is itself often shallow, but the difference between tense and relaxed shallow breathing is that the former occurs at a fast rate and is accompanied by tight shoulder muscles which restrict the natural movements of the thorax, whereas these factors are absent in a relaxed individual.

GENERAL POINTS REGARDING BREATHING AS A RELAXATION TECHNIQUE

1. Breathing should occur at the natural pace of the individual.
2. It should be seen in terms of 'letting the air in' rather than 'taking a breath'.
3. A smooth transfer should take place between inhalation and exhalation, and between exhalation and inhalation unless the exercise indicates otherwise.
4. Breathing through the nose is preferable to breathing through the mouth since the nasal passages both filter and warm the incoming air.
5. Although some exercises may emphasize particular aspects of the breathing cycle, the respirations should always be gentle.
6. Artificially deep breaths should not be repeated in close succession because they can lead to hyperventilation.

The above principles are incorporated into the routines described here. It is helpful when practising new forms of breathing control to adopt an attitude of quiet self-awareness rather than one which is intent on scrutinizing the performance (Van Dixhoorn & Duivenvoorden 1989).

BREATHING ROUTINES FOR RELAXATION

1. Abdominal breathing.
2. Breathing pouch.

3. Out tension, in peace.
4. Breathing meditation (1).
5. Breathing meditation (2).
6. Breathing with cue words (cue-controlled relaxation). This has been described in Chapter 8 (p. 71).
7. A yoga exercise.
8. Breathing 'chi'.
9. Sighing.

One breathing exercise is probably enough in one session. It can be repeated a few times, then dropped and taken up again later in the session. Allowing breaks between the exercises is a safeguard against overbreathing which may occur if the exercises are too enthusiastically carried out. Overbreathing or hyperventilation is discussed in a later section of this chapter.

ABDOMINAL OR DIAPHRAGMATIC BREATHING

This refers to the kind of breathing which emphasizes the downward expansion of the chest cavity. It is useful at this point to inform or remind participants of the role of the diaphragm.

The diaphragm is a sheet of muscle whose edges are attached to the lower ribs, creating a floor to the chest. In the resting state it is dome-shaped. Contraction of the diaphragm flattens the dome, thereby lengthening the chest and sucking in air. Relaxation of the muscle causes it to reassume its dome shape which helps to push the air out. But the diaphragm also forms the roof of the abdomen and, as such, its movements affect the position of the internal organs: as the contracting diaphragm presses down on the organs, it causes the abdomen to swell slightly. Similarly, as the relaxing diaphragm releases its pressure on the organs, the abdomen sinks back again.

To carry out an abdominal breathing exercise, the individual should first make himself as comfortable as possible, and spend a few minutes quietly resting. The following instructions may then be given:

> Spend a few moments running through a sequence of pleasant imagery ... then, as your mind relaxes turn your attention to your breathing ... lay one hand lightly over the solar plexus. Focus your

attention on this area. Start the exercise with a breath out ... a naturally occurring breath out. Notice a slight sinking of the area under your hand. Next, allow air to flow into the lungs, noticing the slight swelling which takes place under your hand. Then as the air is expelled, notice the area under the hand sinking back again. Allow the breathing to take place naturally.

Some writers teach abdominal breathing by urging pupils to 'think in and down' (Innocenti 2002). This helps to create a natural abdominal movement.

BREATHING POUCH

A variation of abdominal breathing, this exercise incorporates imagery. It is adapted from Everly & Rosenfeld (1981).

Concentrate on your breathing rhythm without trying to change it. Become aware of your upper abdomen swelling as you inhale and sinking as you exhale. Picture an imaginary, hollow pouch lying inside your abdomen ... as you breathe in, air travels down to fill the pouch, making the abdomen swell ... breathing out empties the pouch, causing the abdomen to sink back ... if you place your hand over your abdomen, you can feel gentle swelling and sinking taking place.

'OUT TENSION, IN PEACE'

Listen to your breathing without altering its pattern ... imagine your tensions being breathed out ... imagine them being carried away, a little at a time with each breath out ... and now, imagine that every time you inhale, you are breathing in peace, a little at a time with each breath ... breathe out tension ... breathe in peace ... gently breathing ... feeling peace flowing through your body ... always keeping your breathing natural...

BREATHING MEDITATION (1)

Let your mind follow the path of the breath, taking care not to change its pace or its rhythm. Think of the air flowing in through your nostrils, along your nasal passages, down your windpipe and into your lungs ... then, gently and smoothly turning, it is carried out along the same route ... turning again as

the air is drawn back in ... notice the feel of the air ... warm as it leaves, and cool as it enters ... continue on your own with this idea for a few minutes.

BREATHING MEDITATION (2)

This script illustrating 'breath mindfulness' is adapted from Lichstein (1988). It is particularly addressed to people with high blood pressure.

With your eyes closed, settle into your chair, couch or wherever you have chosen to be ... let your body lose its tension and let your mind gradually become calm by using some pleasant imagery ... allow your mind's eye to rest on the upper part of your abdomen ... be aware of it swelling and sinking as you breathe ... notice these breathing movements without trying to change them ... just observe them in the knowledge that your body takes full care of your breathing ... allow your breathing to continue on its own ... flowing gently and smoothly ... perhaps you can feel the rate getting slower ... this is because your resting body doesn't need so much oxygen as when you are active ... your heart rate also is lowered and your blood pressure falls, as a state of quiet settles on you ... allow yourself to enjoy this feeling of tranquillity ... let your mind continue to focus on your breathing for a few minutes longer.

BREATHING WITH CUE WORDS

This exercise is described under the name of cue-controlled relaxation in Chapter 8 (p. 71).

A YOGA EXERCISE (Quoted by Hough 1991)

Sit with your feet flat on the floor, and as you inhale, imagine the air being drawn in through the top of your head, travelling down through your body and passing out through your feet.

BREATHING 'CHI'

Breathe in the energy force, 'chi', and let it flow into the solar plexus ... then ... on the breath out ... let it flow to an area of your body that needs healing or soothing...

SIGHING

> Enjoy the feeling of being relaxed and notice your slowed breathing. As the air leaves your body on the next breath, let it go with a sigh ... Aaaaah ... and then resume normal breathing ... two or three breaths later, repeat the sighing sound...

EVIDENCE OF EFFECTIVENESS

Matsumoto & Smith (2001) report that relatively little research has focused on breathing as a specific approach. Among the few published works on the topic is the comparison study of Bell & Saltikov (2000). These researchers compared the effectiveness of the Mitchell method inclusive of diaphragmatic breathing with diaphragmatic breathing alone in 45 normal male participants. Using heart rate as an outcome measure, significant reductions were found in both intervention groups relative to the control condition of supine lying. However, no significant difference in effectiveness was found between the two groups themselves. In other words, diaphragmatic breathing appears to be an effective relaxation technique on its own and becomes no more effective by being presented in conjunction with the Mitchell method. In their analysis these researchers suggest that physiological benefits of the Mitchell method may be largely due to the component of diaphragmatic breathing and that the technique of Mitchell may be only as effective as diaphragmatic breathing on its own (Bell & Saltikov 2000).

An earlier study looked at the effects of focused breathing on recovery after cardiac surgery. Twenty-nine patients were trained pre-operatively in breathing routines. Investigating their reactions after surgery, Miller & Perry (1990) found significant decreases both in physiological responses and in pain reports compared to patients who did not receive the breathing instruction.

The research base is small, however, on this topic and no firm conclusions can be drawn.

HYPERVENTILATION

Exercises which succeed in slowing the breathing rate tend to reduce ventilation. This is a useful strategy to employ whenever a person is under stress, since stress tends to increase ventilation. Ventilation in a person under stress can be increased to such an extent that it disturbs body systems. At this level it is called 'hyperventilation'.

In the state of hyperventilation, a person overbreathes: that is to say, he processes a greater volume of air than is required by his body at that moment (Innocenti 2002). Thus, a hyperventilating person is one who is breathing in excess of body needs: taking in too much oxygen and releasing too much carbon dioxide. This results in reduced levels of carbon dioxide in the arteries and body tissues. The arterial P_{CO_2}, normally around 42 mmHg (5.6 kPa), can fall to as low as 26 mmHg (3.5 kPa) (Innocenti 1983). Since carbon dioxide is acid the pH value of the blood rises, creating alkalosis. This results in neuronal excitability, vasoconstriction and a widespread disturbance of the body chemistry.

Itself a symptom of stress, overbreathing thus creates symptoms on its own account, one of which is cerebral vasoconstriction (Gardner & Bass 1989). This is related to symptoms such as:

- dizziness
- headache
- visual disturbance.

Other symptoms listed by Gardner & Bass include:

- paraesthesia (tingling) caused by alkalosis
- chest pain caused by coronary vasoconstriction
- palpitations caused by paroxysmal dysrhythmia
- anxiety and/or panic attack caused or aggravated by misattribution of physiological symptoms.

The breathing pattern of a hyperventilating person displays irregularities which may include any of the following (Hough 2001):

- rapid breathing, rising in some cases to 30 or more breaths a minute
- sighing, yawning, excessive sniffing
- halts in the breathing cycle
- marked movement in the upper region of the chest
- difficulty getting the breath.

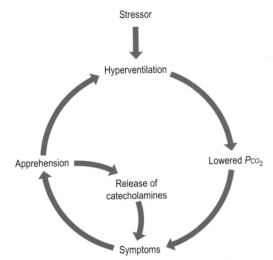

Figure 15.3 The cyclic pattern of hyperventilation.

These symptoms are collectively referred to as 'the hyperventilation syndrome'. Many of them resemble the symptoms of sympathetic nervous system activity. The apprehension they create can itself release catecholamines which reinforce the initial symptoms, setting up one vicious circle within another as shown in Figure 15.3.

Contrary to what might be supposed, the overbreathing does not lead to a greater availability of oxygen because the hypocapnia causes vascular changes which result in a decreased amount of oxygen being transferred to the tissues (Lum 1981).

The condition may be acute or chronic. Acute hyperventilation, which occurs in some people during moments of extreme stress, can give rise to marked symptoms. In chronic hyperventilation, however, there are often few visible symptoms: a process of adaptation appears to take place where the respiratory control mechanism undergoes 'resetting' to a lower level of P_{CO_2} (Gardner & Bass 1989, Gardner 1992). However, in order to maintain this level, the respiratory drive must be increased, i.e. the individual must take deeper than normal breaths or suffer chest discomfort.

Although there is no conclusive way of testing for chronic hyperventilation, an indication of the state can be gained from simple tests. Three are described below:

- Provocation test: the individual is asked to overbreathe rapidly for about 2 minutes. This not only reproduces symptoms which he is able to recognize if he is a hyperventilator, but also demonstrates to him that he has some control over them. This test should not, however, be carried out where the individual is suffering from cerebral vascular disease or where there is a history of epilepsy, and should be conducted only under medical supervision if heart disease is present or suspected. Therapists need also to be aware of the possibility of strong feelings being released in the course of the test (Hough 2001). However, the test in its current form is falling out of use since it has been found that about 25% of non-hypocapnic people also display a positive result (Innocenti 2002).

- The individual is asked to hold his breath. Difficulty in holding it more than a few seconds suggests that he might be hyperventilating (Hough 2001).

- The Nijmegen questionnaire (Van Doorn et al 1982): this contains a list of 16 subjective symptoms (Fig. 15.4). The individual marks the appropriate boxes and the values are added up to give a final score. This is expressed as a fraction of 64 which is the maximum score. If he scores above 23 he is considered to be suffering from hyperventilation syndrome. Validity has been reported but is not conclusive, and until further evidence emerges, the scale is considered only as a useful component of the screening process rather than as a decisive single tool (Van Dixhoorn & Duivenvoorden 1985, Vansteenkiste et al 1991).

TREATMENT

Breathing re-education

The individual is first made aware of his existing breathing pattern which is then gradually replaced by a new one through a process of gentle re-education. Treatment is aimed at raising the levels of dissolved carbon dioxide in the arterial blood and reprogramming the respiratory centre to trigger inspiration at these higher levels (Innocenti 2002).

	0 Never	1 Rarely	2 Sometimes	3 Often	4 Very often
Chest pain					
Feeling tense					
Blurred vision					
Dizzy spells					
Feeling confused					
Faster or deeper breathing					
Short of breath					
Tight feelings in chest					
Bloated feelings in stomach					
Tingling fingers					
Unable to breathe deeply					
Stiff fingers or arms					
Tight feelings around mouth					
Cold hands or feet					
Palpitations					
Feelings of anxiety					

Figure 15.4 The Nijmegen questionnaire (Van Doorn et al 1982). (From Hough A. 1996 Physiotherapy in respiratory care, 2nd edn, p. 209. With kind permission from Stanley Thornes.)

This can be achieved by modifying the breathing pattern in different ways:

1. altering the rate and depth, making the breaths slower and/or shallower
2. holding the breath for a few seconds
3. changing the composition of inhaled air by rebreathing exhaled air.

Altering rate and depth. When people are asked to reduce their rate of breathing they tend to take deeper breaths. This will not change the arterial $P\text{CO}_2$ level. If it is to be changed, the interaction of rate and depth needs to be considered. When reducing one, the other has to be held constant if the $P\text{CO}_2$ is to be raised. The individual can be reminded that slowing the rate means that the same volume of air is passing through, only travelling more slowly. A rate of 10–12 breaths a minute is a useful first target (Hough 1996). This can be reduced as the condition improves.

Breathing cycles which address rate and volume are introduced (Innocenti 2002). For instance, a cycle for slowing the breath might consist of a gentle breath in followed by a slowed breath out. Counting strategies can be incorporated, for example, counting 'one … two …' on the breath in and 'one … two … three … four …' on the breath out.

For reducing the volume of air that passes through the lungs, short breath holds can be used. Innocenti suggests using them in an intermittent manner throughout the day. Apart from this, a regularity of breathing pattern is aimed at throughout the treatment and an abdominal form of breathing encouraged (Innocenti 2002).

In the early stages of re-education, controlled breathing may create air hunger because the brain continues to maintain a high respiratory drive. Later however, following daily practice, the respiratory centre will begin to make the necessary adaptation (Rowbottom 1992).

Breath holding. If, during re-education, this feeling of air hunger becomes too great, the individual may sometimes find himself taking an excessively deep breath. This, of course, further lowers his $P\text{CO}_2$ and temporarily worsens his condition. As a corrective measure, one breath hold is recommended lasting 5 or 6 counts (2 or 3 seconds), performed following the breath out. This compensates for the preceding unnaturally deep breath (Innocenti 2002).

Changing the composition of inhaled air by rebreathing exhaled air. Air is made up of a variety of gases of which oxygen contributes 21% and carbon dioxide 0.04% (Wilson 1990). However, this applies only to the air which enters the lungs. The air which leaves the lungs contains a lower proportion of oxygen and a higher proportion of carbon dioxide (exhaled air contains about 4% carbon dioxide). If a person in a hyperventilated state, i.e. with a low arterial P_{CO_2} rebreathes his own exhaled air, the condition will be temporarily corrected. A convenient way of doing this is to breathe into a paper bag (25×30 cm) previously filled with fresh room air, with the neck of the bag held firmly over the nose and mouth. Powell and Enright (1990) suggest rebreathing 4 or 5 times, taking a rest, then repeating the process if necessary. Hough (2001) emphasizes that the rebreathing should be gentle, while Innocenti (2002) urges the individual to maintain an upright position, i.e. sitting or standing, so that if he should lose consciousness, he would automatically drop the bag.

The hyperventilating person may feel that the bag procedure draws attention to himself when used in a public place. A convenient, although less effective alternative is to cup the hands over the nose and mouth and, without releasing the hands, continue to breathe into them.

Rebreathing exhaled air is useful in acute hyperventilation and particularly if symptoms rise to panic level. Where symptoms are chronic, however, rebreathing will do little more than temporarily relieve them (Gardner & Bass 1989). Treatment of chronic hyperventilation should focus on the re-education of normal breathing patterns (as above).

Education

People who habitually overbreathe need to understand that their symptoms are the result of a normal chemical reaction to stress. It occurs to some extent in everyone, particularly during crises. For certain individuals, however, it may become a habit, which they can be helped to overcome by correcting the breathing pattern and learning to identify the precipitating factors.

Relaxation

Because of the association between anxiety and hyperventilation, relaxation has a part to play, both as a preliminary to breathing re-education and as a component of stress management.

Home practice and self-management

Training the respiratory centres of chronically hyperventilating individuals to accept higher levels of P_{CO_2} takes time. Only practice can restore a normal breathing pattern. This practice consists of slow, smooth, shallow, abdominal breathing performed for about 15 minutes, three times a day (Hough 2001, Innocenti 2002). In addition to the therapeutic programme, there are other strategies which can help to slow the breathing rate such as humming and reading aloud (Hough 2001).

People who hyperventilate may also need to examine environmental features which trigger or aggravate their condition, and to deal with them in an appropriate way.

In their study of hyperventilating individuals, Pinney and colleagues (1987) demonstrated that a programme of education, relaxation and abdominal breathing helped to relieve the condition in 94% of participants.

DISCUSSION

Cowley (1987) ... wn that 50% of those who ... entilation syndrome also ... . It is, however, often difficult ... een hyperventilation in ... attack. Similar symptoms ... being a result either of ... ation of the sympathetic ... 986). Some researchers ... n interaction between ... lity which is supported ... acks to decline follow- ... n respiratory control ... Clark (1986) does not ... s being the cause of ... ors predominate in ... erventilation occurs, ... lily sensations must ... nt and interpreted

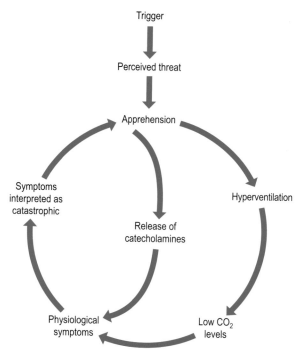

Figure 15.5   How hyperventilation might interact with cognitive factors to create a panic attack.

in a catastrophic way for panic to develop. Figure 15.5 illustrates this idea.

Breathing retraining has been shown to result in a slower breathing rate, a decrease in anxiety and a reduction in the frequency and intensity of panic attacks (Han et al 1996).

PITFALLS OF BREATHING EXERCISES

1. Breathing exercises for inducing relaxation should not be seen as a substitute for medical treatment where a disorder exists. They may, however, be used as a complement if the physician or physiotherapist agrees.

2. The individual should never feel he is straining or forcing the breaths; they must always feel comfortable.

3. Dizziness during the exercises is probably a symptom of hyperventilation, i.e. the exercises are being performed too deeply or too quickly. Remedies may be found in the section on hyperventilation. Alternatively, the individual could take a rest from the exercise. It is useful if the instructor describes the condition of hyperventilation at the outset.

4. Since individuals vary in their breathing rates, routines imposed by the instructor are not recommended in a group situation. The instructions can be phrased in such a way that participants individually decide on a pace that suits them.

5. Although slow, abdominal breathing can be an effective way of inducing relaxation, it may not suit everyone. In particular, people who suffer from air hunger for whatever reason, may not find it helpful to manipulate their breathing rate.

6. Although people who suffer from panic disorder have been shown to derive benefit from relaxation, a few individuals occasionally report the occurrence of panic attacks during periods of relaxation. Two possible explanations are offered here. One comes from Hough (2001), who points out that relaxation weakens the psychological defences and may allow disturbing feelings to rise to the surface.

An alternative explanation is put forward by Ley (1988) who suggests that if a person who is currently hyperventilating begins to relax, he lowers his metabolic rate. This reduces his production of carbon dioxide. If he does not make a corresponding reduction in ventilation, his hypocapnia will increase and his symptoms become more marked.

Further reading

Hough A 2001 Physiotherapy in respiratory care: an evidence-based approach to respiratory and cardiac management, 3rd edn. Nelson Thornes, Cheltenham

Innocenti D M 2002 Hyperventilation. In: Pryor J A, Prasad S A (eds) Physiotherapy for respiratory and cardiac problems: adults and paediatrics, 3rd edn. Churchill Livingstone, Edinburgh

SECTION 3

Cognitive approaches to relaxation

Chapter 16

Self-awareness

INTRODUCTION AND RATIONALE

'Being aware' or 'being conscious' convey similar ideas. Their use when applied to the self, however, is very different. Being aware of the self is defined as 'the tendency to focus attention on the private aspects of the self' (West 1987). This signifies a process of self-exploration; a getting-to-know one-self; recognizing one's strengths and weaknesses. Being conscious of the self as we use the phrase in everyday language, on the other hand, implies the sense of being 'painfully aware of being observed by others' (Burnard 1991). A person who is self-conscious sees herself as being critically scruti-nized by the observer, and in this role allows herself to be turned into an object. The result of self-consciousness is embarrassment; the result of self-awareness is self-knowledge.

Increased self-knowledge comes from listening to ourselves: to who we are, what we are and how we are (Tschudin 1991). It relates to questions such as 'Am I the person I want to be?' and if not, 'What is stopping me becoming that person?' or 'Why don't I allow myself to develop to my fullest?'. The answers help us to understand ourselves. The better we know ourselves, the easier it is to make decisions which further our life plans. Without this knowledge, we may find decisions being made for us.

Self-awareness also puts us in touch with our outward behaviour, and the way others may be responding to it. In this way, self-awareness can enhance our personal relationships.

The notion of self-awareness is fundamentally linked to the notion of living in the present, responding in the here-and-now, and being aware of the present moment, since that is where we express ourselves and make our impact on life. Of course, we need to take into account lessons learned from the past and goals set for the future, but it is all too easy to dwell on these and let the present take care of itself. This can lead to our losing whatever control we had of it. Being aware of the self helps us perform in the present.

Greater control of our lives, enhanced relationships and improved self-knowledge all contribute to our peace of mind. Self-awareness exercises can thus be seen as relaxation techniques.

Authors have structured self-awareness in different ways. Stevens (1971) divided it into three parts: an outer world of sensory information; one inner world of feelings (visceral and emotional); and a second inner world of mental activity (thoughts and images). Burnard (1992) sees the internal part as corresponding with Jung's four functions of the mind (thinking, feeling, sensing and intuiting), to which he adds a visceral component which includes muscle tension and bodily relaxation. The external part refers to what other people see: our verbal and non-verbal behaviour together with other aspects of the way we present ourselves.

To Tschudin (1991), the inner world consists of thoughts and emotions and the outer world of people and environments with a 'go-between' world relating to the senses. A composite view is presented here (Fig. 16.1). The inner aspect includes thinking, intuition, emotions and bodily sensations which include those of muscle tension; the outer aspect refers to the way we relate to other people; and the intermediate area is concerned with the five senses.

Self-awareness exercises are essentially of the mind, being concerned with the thoughts in the head. The approach is thus underpinned by cognitive theory. Exercises presented here are adapted from Stevens (1971), Burnard (1992) and Bond (1986).

EXERCISES IN SELF–AWARENESS

AWARENESS OF THINKING STYLE

We have different ways of thinking: sometimes we think in a vertical or focused way as when doing arithmetic. At other times our thinking may be more inclined to a lateral style, as, for instance, when we are engaged in creative work. We also have our own personal styles of thinking: some people tend towards a cause–effect style, others to a broader canvas style.

Other modes of thinking relate to the self-concept and self-esteem (Ch. 14, p. 122). For example, thinking strategies which direct the individual into areas likely to lead to successful outcomes are associated with high self-esteem, while those which direct her into areas with a low probability of success tend to be associated with low self-esteem (Fox 1997, p. 116). Self-esteem can also be promoted by attributing successful outcomes to one's own efforts and poor outcomes to external factors over which one had no control (Blaine & Crocker 1993).

Or again, thinking can be influenced by the individual's locus of control (Ch. 3, p. 26): an internal locus with its accompanying sense of self-reliance seems to be related to high self-esteem, whereas

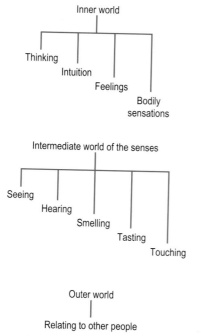

Figure 16.1   Aspects of the self.

an external locus seems to be related to lower levels of self-esteem (Fox 1997, p. 118). Although our self-esteem owes much to value systems set up by the culture and society we belong to, it is also governed by our use of self-serving strategies, such as the way we present ourselves (Carless & Fox 2003). To Fox, low self-esteem is more a defect in the use of self-enhancement strategies than a reflection of any deep sense of disregard.

The individual can review her own style in the following manner:

> Take a few moments off to make a list of the thoughts that are going through your mind and the dialogue that accompanies them. Write them down. Repeat this twice later in the day. Compare the items on your three lists and notice if a pattern emerges. Is some particular thought claiming your attention? If so, how do you approach it? Do you see it as a problem to be solved or do you let it dominate you? If you are trying to solve it, are you using a focused method or are you keeping your mind open and receptive to fresh ideas? Both approaches are useful. Do you have a tendency to favour one more than the other?
>
> Do you tend to think in ways which enhance your self-esteem such as steering the self in directions likely to lead to success? Or do you tend to cling to areas where success is less likely to occur? Do you make a point of interpreting outcomes in ways which show yourself in the best possible light, or do you let negative interpretations assert themselves?
>
> Again, do you see most problems as being surmountable and, to some extent, within your control? Or do you, generally speaking, feel yourself to be a pawn in the hands of fate and a victim of events?
>
> This is an opportunity to examine your attitude towards yourself and to ask if it is serving you well.

AWARENESS OF INTUITIVE POWERS

Our glorification of the rational has all but eclipsed the imagination in everyday affairs. We distrust intuition or, at best, give it short shrift. Our belief in the undeniable value of logical thinking does not, however, mean we must stifle the imagination, and those who underestimate its power may do so at their peril for it communicates with the inner self.

> Sit quietly and allow yourself to become relaxed. Follow your breathing, and next time you breathe out, release all your tension in a long sigh. Scan your body, checking that all your muscles are relaxed. Imagine yourself in a place of beauty and peace. Allow your thoughts to drift in and out. Focus on a matter that has been claiming your attention recently ... keep it light ... there's no compulsion to resolve it at this moment ... just listen to yourself ... tune into yourself ... be receptive to any ideas that float into your head ... listen to your gut feeling; you can judge its merits later ... just be open to yourself ... When you are ready, bring your visualization to an end.

AWARENESS OF FEELINGS (EMOTIONS)

The capacity to use our mental abilities is strongly influenced by the emotional state of the individual, whose thinking brain can be overwhelmed, even paralysed by the emotional brain (Goleman 1996). Goleman emphasizes the importance of self-awareness in this area.

To focus on emotions need not be seen as self-indulgence. Rather, it is a form of self-examination which can provide us with insights and perhaps indicate useful paths of change. While our emotions may be said to enrich our lives on the one hand, they give us trouble on the other; some feelings can be so strong they cloud our judgement and others may be so uncomfortable we repress the thought that gives rise to them.

Heron (1977) reminds us that society urges us to control rather than express emotion, and this, he claims, blocks our development as full human beings. Anger and grief are two examples where this occurs. He sees the handling of emotions as a skill and has developed a model which identifies four aspects of this skill. They consist of the degree to which we:

1. are aware of our emotional patterns
2. express ourselves in controlled or spontaneous ways
3. share our feelings
4. use catharsis to move forward.

1. Awareness of emotional patterns

We need to recognize our feeling patterns and tendencies to react in certain ways. Only when we are aware of them can we see how they may be influencing our behaviour.

2. Control or spontaneity

Many situations require us to hide our feelings, but there are other occasions when a more spontaneous response is called for. Whether we express our emotion or hold it back is governed not only by the circumstances but also by our general inclination. Some individuals have a tendency to respond in one way rather than another. If so, are they aware of it?

3. Sharing our feelings

Self-disclosure is part of the process of deepening a relationship, and this applies whether the individual is making the disclosure or listening to another making hers. Although the sharing of feelings involves taking a risk, the relationship is unlikely to develop without it. Most relationships are enriched by some degree of self-disclosure; the extent to which it occurs depends partly on the nature of the relationship and partly on the inclination of the individual. Is she *inclined* to share her feelings?

4. Releasing emotions in a process of catharsis

This aspect of emotional skills provides a safeguard against the bottling-up of emotions. If emotions are not expressed or dealt with at the time they are aroused, they may get repressed. In this latter case, a subsequent environmental trigger may stir them up and lead to inappropriate behaviour of two kinds: first, we may over-react if we see the issue as a safe channel in which to let off the pressure of our repressed emotions, or second, we may under-react, having trained ourselves to keep a tight rein on our feelings at all times. Either way our response is a maladaptive one. The process of catharsis helps to free the individual from the tyranny of unresolved emotions. Heron lists three elements of cathartic release:

1. Letting-go of feelings. This can take place in a controlled way such as going for a jog or doing a workout; it can also be achieved in less restrained ways such as shouting into a pillow or kicking a cushion.

2. Gaining insights. The release of emotions may be accompanied by intuitive insights which deepen

the individual's understanding of the situation and of herself.

3. Decision making. If emotional release has cleared her mind of its burden, and newly found insights have enriched her perceptions, the individual is better able to plan and carry out constructive changes to her life and solve the problems which stand in the way.

A self-awareness script based on Heron's model is presented below.

> Spend a few minutes considering your feeling patterns ... do you tend to react in characteristic ways? ... what are these? ... for example, do you tend to hold back your feelings or do you make spontaneous responses? ... can you think of occasions when you have used one or the other? ... and to what effect? ... (pause)...
>
> Do you tend to share your feelings or are you reluctant to trust people? ... have you been let down in the past by sharing your feelings? ... if so, has it affected your readiness to trust others? ... (pause)...
>
> How do you deal with situations which make you angry? ... do you answer back (as the occasion permits), or do you tend to bottle up your feelings? ... having bottled them up, are you able to find ways of releasing that pent-up anger? ... if so, do you feel more content afterwards? ... think of occasions when you have used catharsis...

AWARENESS OF THE BODY

From time to time, the body needs attention. In between, we spend periods of varying length without giving it a thought. Breathing, digestion, skin sensations can all be ignored; muscle tension also passes unnoticed. If we are interested in reducing muscle tension, it can be useful to make a point of listening to the body occasionally.

> Allow your thoughts to focus on your body. Notice any sensations, such as stomach rumblings, joint discomfort, itches or the tendency to sigh ... things you normally disregard as you concentrate on your work. Perhaps you are also ignoring feelings of tension in your muscles, in your back, your shoulders, your face or your writing arm ... try focusing on those areas and releasing the tension ... realize that you could just as easily increase it ... try for a

moment deliberately exaggerating the tension in the muscles ... notice that you have the power to switch it on or off ... simply by making a conscious effort you can increase or decrease those feelings of tension. Explore that idea for a few moments.

AWARENESS OF THE ENVIRONMENT

This aspect of the self is concerned with information from the five senses: sight, sound, smell, taste and touch. Much of this activity never gets through to our consciousness, which may be to our advantage if we are concentrating on a piece of work. However, it is through our senses that we experience our environment and are able to relate to the world.

Sit on your own. Allow the breath out to carry all your tensions with it. Bring your mind to focus on what is happening around you: the sounds inside the building and outside ... the smells of the kitchen/office/shop/ classroom/factory ... the taste of the coffee you just drank ... the arrangement of the furniture in the room ... the colour of the decoration ... the temperature of the room ... the feel of the chair underneath you, the pen or the peeler in your hand ... focus on each one separately for a few moments. If you are driving notice the countryside. If you are waiting in a bus queue pick out the different sounds in the street ... if you are walking to the letterbox, notice the front gardens along the way...

Notice how the exercise has the effect of taking you away from your preoccupations and giving you an acute experience of the present moment.

AWARENESS OF THE WAY WE RELATE TO OTHERS

People can only know about us from what we show of ourselves: our appearance, general demeanour and what we say. These are outer aspects of the individual, and disclose much or little of the inner self depending on the level of intimacy. All that can be known about a person is what she consciously or unconsciously reveals, so that what we reveal is important since it establishes our identity in the world. Our behaviour, whether verbal or non-verbal, creates us as individuals in other people's eyes.

Verbal behaviour refers to the actual words spoken. Non-verbal behaviour includes aspects of speech, such as tone of voice, timing, emphasis, accent (paralinguistic features), as well as facial expression, eye contact, gesture, posture, physical proximity, clothes and appearance (Argyle 1978). The way we respond within the interaction provides a further level of behaviour: how we prompt, cut in, and listen.

Assertiveness

We also define ourselves by our readiness to be assertive or not (Ch. 1). Assertiveness involves knowing how to advance our life goals while respecting the interests of other people. Put another way, it means insisting on having our *own* interests respected while other people advance *their* goals. For example, are we able to refuse a request which we feel is unreasonable?

Do you find it easy to say 'No' to a request in a situation where saying 'Yes' makes you feel you are being taken advantage of? Can you think of an occasion when this occurred? How did you react? Were you happy with the outcome? If not, how did you feel? In your imagination, go back to the occasion. Recreate the scene and rescript your part with you saying 'No'. What effect does this have on the other person? What effect does it have on you? Now ask yourself why you said 'Yes' in the first place? How would you deal with a similar request in the future?

Promoting a relationship while retaining a feeling of self is one of the social skills. This feeling of self is tied up with our self-esteem, i.e. the degree to which we feel we have worth. Low self-esteem is linked with non-assertive behaviour; high self-esteem with assertive behaviour. To increase her assertiveness, the individual needs to recognize her personal strengths and qualities.

Bond (1986) illustrates these points in her models of non-assertive and assertive behaviour. In the first, the individual is locked in a negative cyclic pattern of behaviour, while in the second, she has established herself in a more positive behavioural pattern (Fig. 16.2). In order to break out of the first and move to the second, she has to intervene at some point in the negative cycle. She has to question the appropriateness of the role she is playing and explore new possibilities. Such intervention

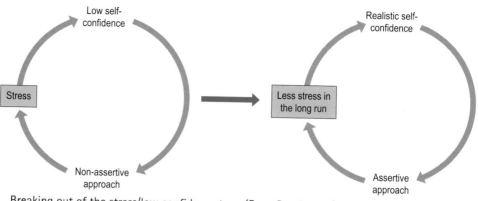

Figure 16.2   Breaking out of the stress/low confidence trap. (From Bond 1986.)

over time will tend to make her behaviour more assertive and result in more rewarding interpersonal experiences.

A script for an individual assessing her own assertiveness (or non-assertiveness) might run as follows:

> Allow yourself to feel relaxed before you begin. Run through a relaxing procedure until you feel very calm and tuned in to yourself. Let your thoughts focus on a person you know ... someone you are not close to ... someone with whom you have had difficulties but are obliged to see from time to time...
>
> Let your mind gently focus on this person ... let her take shape ... notice how she looks: her expression ... what she is wearing ... spend a little time creating her presence ... then see yourself also, including your expression, posture and clothes, as you, in your mind's eye, greet this person.
>
> Observe your actions ... do they strike the right note? ... is the conversation balanced in the sense that neither person is acting aggressively to the other's submissive behaviour? ... if it is unbalanced what, if anything, do you think you should do about it? ... it may be that you feel your behaviour is appropriate ... on the other hand, you may wish to modify your style, to make it more assertive ... you will know best what is needed in the situation...
>
> If you decide to modify your style, consider ways in which you might begin ... test these out in your imagination ... notice how your new behaviour feels ... spend a few minutes mentally experiencing the scene...

BENEFITS AND PITFALLS OF SELF–AWARENESS EXERCISES

Exercises such as those described above can heighten our awareness of ourselves and the way we relate to other people. We also, in the process, deepen our self-knowledge. Through self-awareness exercises we learn to 'listen' to the self in all its aspects, and to tune in to its nuances. Self-awareness exercises, by their emphasis on 'exploring, experimenting, experiencing', thus lead us to a better understanding of ourselves (Stevens 1971).

The pitfalls of self-awareness include the following:

1. Regularly engaging in introspection may result in a tendency to become self-centred.

2. The determined pursuit of self-understanding may lead some people to take themselves too seriously, even to the point of losing their sense of humour. This is misuse of the self-awareness concept.

3. Getting to know oneself can be a painful process, while changing oneself is difficult. Our efforts are, however, rewarded by the discovery that we have more power than we realized to control our lives: a thought which itself engenders a sense of calm.

As a relaxation technique, self-awareness might be said to be at the other end of the scale from distraction (the diversion of attention away from the self). Each is effective on its own, but together they complement one another: self-awareness protecting the individual from the hazards of denial, while distraction protects her from too much introspection.

Further reading

Fox K R (ed) 1997 The physical self: from motivation to well-being. Human Kinetics, Leeds

Freshwater D (ed) 2002 Therapeutic nursing: improving patient care through self-awareness and reflection. Sage, London

Goleman D 1996 Emotional intelligence. Bloomsbury, London

Chapter 17

Imagery

CHAPTER CONTENTS

INTRODUCTION AND RATIONALE

Imagery has already been mentioned during discussion of passive relaxation, breathing, the Alexander technique and self-awareness. Here imagery is considered in its own right.

Achterberg (1985) defines imagery as 'the thought process that invokes and uses the senses'. Sight, sound, smell, taste and touch modalities can all be involved in this activity, which may take place in the absence of any external stimulus. It could be said that imagery is thinking in pictures as opposed to thinking with words.

The importance of the image was underlined by Aristotle who said that without it, thought is impossible. Einstein also found imagery an essential component of thought. It is particularly associated with the creative function of thinking. However, we are forming images all the time, whether making plans for the future, remembering items from the past or creating fantasy in realms beyond our experience.

How can imagery relieve stress? A cognitive explanation was advanced by Dossey (1988) who suggested that imagery brings about a change in the individual's perceptions. Many researchers, on the other hand, consider that the mechanism lies in the distraction created by the pleasant imagery which can divert the mind from intrusive thoughts. There are also physiological explanations, for example, McCance & Heuther (1998) proposed that pleasant images could trigger the release of endorphins and create an analgesic effect; and Melzack & Wall (1983) put forward their theory whereby pain messages are blocked from consciousness by a 'gate' mechanism which shuts them off when the sensory channels are loaded with other information (which may include imagery).

Although the precise mechanism of imagery is unknown, it is believed to involve the right cerebral hemisphere. This chapter contains a short discussion on the concept of laterality which is followed by a section on the unconscious mind. Examples of different kinds of imagery will be found in a later part of the chapter.

LATERALITY

The cerebral cortex is divided into two hemispheres, each of which has four lobes: frontal, parietal, temporal and occipital. Research indicates that the hemispheres have specialized roles (Fig. 17.1). One side, usually the left, is believed to process logical thought and language. It is involved in linear, analytic and rational thinking, reading, writing and mathematical activity and is normally the dominant hemisphere. The right hemisphere is seen as dealing with information of a non-rational nature, being concerned with creative thinking, fantasy, metaphor, imagery, dreams, analogies, intuition and emotion, including feelings of stress and is normally the non-dominant hemisphere. However, it is believed to acquire dominance during altered states of consciousness, i.e. states of mental functioning which seem different to the individual from the ordinary pattern experienced by her (Atkinson et al 1999). Deep

relaxation is one such state. Others include dreaming, drug-induced states, hypnosis, meditation, daydreaming and guided imagery. During these states, the influence of the left brain is reduced, which allows material from the right hemisphere, normally hidden, to become accessible. Thus, the altered state is seen as providing a path to the interior of the self.

Lyman et al (1980) claim to have found a connection between images and emotions, having shown experimentally that emotionally charged situations are more likely than neutral ones to be accompanied by imagery. They posit a direct relationship between the right hemisphere (which is associated with imagery) and the autonomic system (which governs the physiological responses associated with emotion).

The link between imagery and physiological processes can be demonstrated by imagining a lemon (Barber et al 1964):

> Visualize its exterior shape, colour, scent and texture; then slice it across the middle, look at the pale, glistening flesh, squeeze it gently and watch the juice dripping from it; take the cut end to your mouth and lick it. Notice your mouth watering.

Electromyographic recordings also demonstrate associations between visualization and physiological activity: positive imagery has been shown to lower muscle tension levels and negative imagery to raise them (Jacobson 1938, McGuigan 1971).

In applying these findings it is suggested that a useful approach to stress relief and relaxation is through methods which involve the right hemisphere (Davis et al 2000).

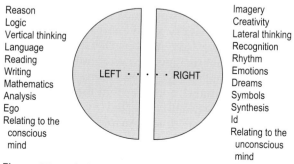

Reason	Imagery
Logic	Creativity
Vertical thinking	Lateral thinking
Language	Recognition
Reading	Rhythm
Writing	Emotions
Mathematics	Dreams
Analysis	Symbols
Ego	Synthesis
Relating to the	Id
conscious	Relating to the
mind	unconscious
	mind

LEFT · · · · · RIGHT

Figure 17.1 Left and right hemisphere activities. (Adapted from Shone 1982.)

THE UNCONSCIOUS

Freud (1973) viewed the unconscious as a repository of repressed fears and unresolved emotions. It thus represented aspects of ourselves which we wished to forget. Its contents were only available in certain states such as dreaming, when the conscious mind was less dominant. A Jungian view of the unconscious, however, saw it as also containing the seed of infinite new possibilities deriving from insight, intuition and inspiration (Jung 1963, Fordham 1966). Thus, while Freud viewed it in negative terms, Jung's view was primarily positive.

Whatever their theoretical position, writers in general agree that the unconscious operates not with the language of logic, but through pictures, emotions, senses, symbols and imagery, i.e. the concerns of the right hemisphere. Hidden and elusive, the unconscious does not lend itself to direct investigation, either from the scientist or from the self-analysing individual. It is this quality of elusiveness that moves Jung to speak of the difficulty in penetrating one's own being. His archetypal figures (earth mother, wise man, persona, shadow, anima and animus) are the expression of attempts to find new ways of gaining access to the unconscious.

The inner guide

Arising out of these ideas is the concept of the 'inner guide': a mental construct that links the individual with her inner self. In its role as channeller of information from the unconscious, the inner guide may be seen as the personification of the intuitive self. It can take forms other than those of archetypal figures and may appear as any person or animal whose attributes have appealed to the individual's imagination.

Typically the inner guide evolves in the mind during a session of deep relaxation, using an imagined setting of rich sensory quality. Oyle (1976) suggests a place of peace and beauty such as a mountain lake or a natural grotto, while Ferrucci (1982) prefers an Alpine peak reached after an arduous climb. A figure is conjured up; it advances slowly. The visualizer welcomes the approaching figure, noticing everything about it: what it looks like, how it is dressed, who if anyone, it resembles. A dialogue ensues. Ferrucci warns against the possibility of the guide being no more than a self-deceiving fantasy and suggests criteria for testing its authenticity:

- does it bring answers which come from the self?
- does it bring understanding?
- does it carry a sense of rightness?
- does its message make sense in the light of reason and morality?
- will its advice stand up in real life situations?

Even after acceptance of the guide as authentic, its advice should always be scrutinized and not blindly accepted. Although the guide is an aspect of the inner self, it may not be working in the individual's best interests. On the other hand, too sceptical an attitude will tend to generate fewer ideas than a trusting one.

The individual need not feel restricted to one guide, and may find it useful to have one male and one female, each supplying complementary wisdom. A hazard of working with a number of inner guides, however, is that the personality may come to be seen as a collection of separate entities when the aim of the exercise is to achieve integration.

Any meeting with an inner guide should be rounded off with words of gratitude, respect and appreciation as this helps to strengthen the individual's respect for her inner self. Continuity also is important and may be established by a contract to meet on another occasion.

THERAPEUTIC EFFECTS OF IMAGERY

Imagery can be used in a therapeutic sense to promote the following:

1. *Self-development and psychological change.* These effects are expanded in Chapter 18.
2. *Relaxation.* Zahourek (1988), working in a nursing context, sees imagery as a therapeutic tool which can reinforce the message to relax.
3. *Healing.* This is an area not covered in the present work.

PROCEDURE OF A THERAPEUTIC IMAGERY SESSION

RELAXATION

For the imagery to be effective, the individual should first be in a state of relaxation. Fanning (1988) regards relaxation as 'an absolute prerequisite' of effective imagery. The individual may use any method she finds helpful, but passive approaches are seen as being the most appropriate (Achterberg 1985). Thus relaxation is a precondition as well as a result of therapeutic imagery.

INTRODUCTORY REMARKS TO PARTICIPANTS

As with other approaches, a short passage of explanation is necessary.

> Imagery is about building pictures in the mind. The pictures can be pleasant or unpleasant. The first kind induce a feeling of calm, the second, of unease.
>
> The relaxing effect of pleasant imagery is partly due to the distraction it creates from stressful thoughts. Daydreaming is an example of this kind of imagery. However, the imagination can also bring us nearer to our inner selves, and this aspect of it is used to help people discover new possibilities within themselves, thereby enriching their lives. This kind of imagery is more structured than daydreaming.
>
> You'll find it helpful to make yourself relaxed before you begin.

EXERCISES IN IMAGERY

Exercises which use different kinds of imagery are then presented. They may include any of the following:

- Single sense
- Imagery as symbol
- Imagery as metaphor
- Colour imagery
- Guided imagery.

TERMINATION

A session of imagery should be gradually brought to an end. First, the image is deliberately allowed to fade. Then the visualizer slowly brings her attention back to the room in which she is lying, and in her own time opens her eyes. In the next few minutes she gives her limbs a gentle stretch and then resumes normal activity.

EXPLORING SINGLE SENSES

Some people find it easier than others to conjure up images. Not only do people differ in the vividness and clarity of the images they create, but they also differ in their ability to control the image once formed (Finke 1989). Image-making is thus a skill with more than one facet.

There is some evidence to suggest that image-forming can be improved with practice, although the extent of any such improvement has not been determined (Kosslyn 1983, Lichstein 1988). Nevertheless, exercises are often used in the belief that they help to develop innate potential. A difficulty in imaging should not, however, be seen as a deficit but rather as a manifestation of the many ways in which human beings differ from one another. People who report difficulty in forming images may also describe a sensation which fulfils the same function in their thought processes.

For those who wish to explore their capacity to create images, however, the following exercises are presented. They use the modalities of sight, sound, smell, taste, touch, temperature and kinaesthetic sense. A total of 15–20 seconds can be spent on each item.

Sight

Visualize:

- a shape: circle/triangle/square
- an oak tree
- a snail
- a sailing boat
- a button
- a strand of hair.

Sound

Since auditory images tend to be less dominant than visual ones, it can be useful, when evoking the former, to surround oneself with an imaginary mist or darkness which swallows up any visual images and releases sounds in isolation. Imagine:

- the wind blowing through the trees/through river sedges/through sheets on a clothes line
- the ring of your telephone
- different people calling your name
- horses' hooves on different surfaces: cobblestone/tarmac/hard sand/deep mud
- scales played on the piano
- traffic starting off
- water flowing along a rocky stream bed/lapping on a lake shore/cascading from a height.

Smell

Slowly conjure up, one by one, the following smells:

- thyme trodden underfoot
- petrol fumes
- newly baked bread
- hyacinth scent
- chlorine
- new mown grass
- vanilla.

Taste

Imagine the taste of:

- sprouts
- figs
- banana
- mayonnaise
- grapefruit
- toothpaste.

Touch

Let other sensory images fade as you turn your attention to those of touch. Evoke the following tactile images:

- shaking hands
- standing barefoot on loose/dry sand
- running your fingers over satin/velvet/sacking
- brushing past fur
- holding a smooth pebble
- threading a needle.

Temperature

Imagine sensations of heat and cold:

- drinking a hot liquid
- sunlight falling on your arm
- moving from a warm room to a cool one
- holding an ice-cube
- stepping into a warm bath.

Kinaesthetic sense

This sense is the perception of body movement. Feel yourself engaged in a form of activity:

- swimming
- running on grass
- sawing wood
- throwing a ball
- climbing a sand dune
- hanging a coat on a peg
- stirring syrup.

Imagery drawn from all sense modalities

Fanning (1988) suggests an exercise which draws on all the above sense modalities:

> Take a fruit that you like, say an orange. Feel its texture ... weight ... size ... notice its shape ... colour and surface markings ... is it firm or soft? ... smell it ... then dig your nail into the peel and begin to tear it off. Listen to the faint sound of the tearing. As you peel the orange, notice how the flesh gets exposed here and there, releasing a new smell. Separate the segments and put one in your mouth ... bite through its juicy flesh ... feel the sensation of the juice running over your tongue ... recognize the taste of orange...

From the above exercise it can be seen that variety of sensory detail helps to build a vivid mental image. When we visualize a scene we usually draw on more than one sense modality, and we can make the scene still more vivid by adding further sensory information. Images of sight, sound, smell, texture, temperature and the sensation of body movement can all be used to enrich the mental picture. Guided imagery (p. 157) develops these ideas.

SYMBOLIC IMAGERY

Jung (1963) writes that symbols serve to connect us with the unconscious; they are keys which can unlock the deeper parts of the psyche. Symbols also feature in the writings of Assagioli where he notes the tendency for people to project meaningful ideas onto them. One of Assagioli's best known examples is his visualization of a rose (1965), paraphrased below:

> Picture in your mind a rose bush ... see its root ... its stem ... its leaves. Crowning the stem is a rose in tight bud. See it folded inside its protective sepals. As you watch, the sepals begin to roll back revealing the closed flower, firmly and intricately packed ...

gradually, the petals begin to unfold and as they do, you may feel a blossoming also taking place within you ... the rose continues to open and as you gaze at it, and smell its perfume, perhaps you can feel its rhythm resonating with your own rhythm ... stay with the rose and as it opens further revealing its centre, allow an image to take shape – one that represents whatever is creative and meaningful within you ... focus on the image ... and let it speak to you...

The symbol is seen here as a phenomenon to be experienced rather than decoded. It is suggested that by identifying with the symbol, the individual can discover new aspects of herself. This idea has been developed by Ferrucci, a student of Assagioli's. Two examples of Ferrucci's visualizations (1982) are presented below (in slightly altered form).

The fount

Imagine a rocky cleft in which a natural spring rises. It is a warm summer day. See the bubbling jet of water sparkling in the sunlight ... listen to its gurgling and splashing ... the water is clear and pure ... cup your hands and drink from it ... imagine the liquid travelling down your throat and into your body ... in your mind's eye step into the spring and feel the water flowing over you ... your feet, legs and the whole of your body ... imagine it also flowing through your thoughts ... and through your emotions ... feel the water cleansing you ... let its purity unite with your purity ... let its energy become your energy ... and as the fount continues to renew itself, feel life within you also renewing itself...

The bell

Picture a meadow on a warm day. Perhaps you are lying in the soft grass, surrounded by scented wild flowers. In a nearby village church, a bell begins to peal. The sound it makes is pure and clear and as it reaches you, it seems to arouse within you a deep, hidden joy ... the sound fades for a moment as the wind changes ... then ... it returns ... carried back to you, this time with renewed force ... filling the air and echoing through the valley ... and as you listen, the sound seems to vibrate inside you ... resonating with your own melody ... and awakening new possibilities within you...

THE USE OF METAPHOR

Imagery lies at the heart of metaphor. Metaphor itself, by describing one thing in terms of another, offers a fresh approach; a new and more telling interpretation.

Three items which illustrate the use of metaphor in relaxation imagery follow. In each one, the individual identifies with the image.

The rag doll

Sit in an armchair. Close your eyes. Take one deep breath low down in your chest. Then let your breathing set its own rhythm ... listen to it ... and as you listen to it, imagine a rag doll ... see its soft floppy arms and legs ... its lolling head ... its slumped body ... inert ... immobile.

Now, try seeing yourself as that rag doll. Conjure up a feeling of being slumped ... the weight of your arms dragging your shoulders down ... your head rolling into the chairback ... your face expressionless ... your jaw relaxed ... feel the passive quality of the rag doll ... and as you continue to sit there ... enjoy the feeling of being passive...

The fragment of seaweed

Lie down in a quiet place. Close your eyes. Breathe in deeply once ... then relax into the rhythm of your natural breathing...

Picture a length of seaweed, rich, dark green, leafy seaweed, floating in the shallows. Air pockets keep it buoyant and allow it to bob up and down. As it floats, it changes shape, drawn this way and that as the currents swirl beneath it ... pulling it ... twisting it ... stretching it ... bunching it...

Now, picture yourself as that piece of seaweed ... notice how limp your body feels ... your outstretched arms and legs gently swept to and fro ... imagine the wave passing underneath you ... lifting you up as it rises, and lowering you as it dips, but always buoying you up ... feel your body giving to the movement of the water...

The jelly

Settle yourself in a peaceful place. Close your eyes and listen to your breathing ... listen to it getting calmer with every moment that passes...

> Imagine a jelly not quite set. It has been turned out of its mould and stands, holding itself together but not yet firm. Every time the plate is moved, it wobbles.
>
> Now, think of yourself as that jelly. You are standing on a dish, and every time someone knocks the table, a ripple runs through you. You yourself are not able to initiate the movement; only others can do that by bumping into your table or moving your dish ... and, every time this happens, you wobble. One bump, and you wobble several times ... imagine you are about to be bumped into ... feel your body limp ... let all the tension go out of it ... let yourself become a wobbly jelly...

TRANSFORMATIONS

Images can also undergo transformations: harsh images can give way to smooth ones. Fanning (1988) shows how negative emotions, represented by harsh images, can be influenced to move in a more positive direction, when the harsh images are transformed into smooth ones.

> Imagine the sound of discordant music ... listen to its harsh tones ... and as you do, let your painful thought express itself in terms of the dissonant notes ... feel the mood of your difficulty resonating with the sound. Then gradually allow the image to undergo a transformation ... follow the music as it slowly resolves into harmonies ... and, as the harmonies fill the air, experience the beginnings of a change in your feelings...

Other examples of negative imagery resolving into pleasanter forms are:

* sour lemon juice into sweet lemon sorbet
* sandpaper into silky fabric.

Both come from Fanning (1988). The next two are drawn from Davis et al (1988):

* a screaming siren into a woodwind melody
* the glare of a searchlight into the soft glow of a lamp.

Four of the sense modalities (taste, touch, sound and sight) are represented in these examples. The fifth, smell, is illustrated below in the transformation from:

* burning rubber into smouldering pine logs.

The above are simply examples. The most effective imagery is that which the individual creates for herself, choosing the context to which she can best relate.

DISTANCING

The distress caused by unpleasant events can be overwhelming. Moreover, the intensity of the emotion aroused by them may cloud the individual's judgement. In order to gain a more objective view, she may find it useful to draw back from the scene mentally: in effect, to distance herself. Certain images promote the feeling of being able to put a distance between herself and the situation:

* a leaf floating downstream
* clouds moving across the sky
* helium-filled balloons rising
* bubbles being blown away
* a train receding along a straight track.

COLOUR

People say they have favourite colours. Is this because certain colours make them feel good? And is this governed by the association that those colours have with pleasant events in their lives? It is generally believed that red is a stimulating colour and blue a soothing one but to what extent is the preference for one over the other tied up with the mood of the moment? Such notions might help to explain why a person does not always choose the same colour. Or does she simply become sated with one colour and feel the need to replace it with another (as in decorations, clothes, etc.)? These are psychological considerations, although the aesthetic aspects of colour give the topic a further dimension.

However, in the present context we are concerned with psychological aspects. Certainly colours can create strong effects. Some of these can be explored through exercises in colour imagery. The following example is adapted from the work of an autogenic therapist, Kai Kermani (1990).

> With your eyes closed let the word 'colour' float into your mind. The word may first evoke one particular colour although others will quickly follow.

Take the one that first appears. Stay with it. Let it develop in any way it wants to: flooding your field of vision, appearing in patches, little flecks or any other arrangement. Concentrate on the colour in a passive way, letting it speak to you. Does it remind you of anything? Does it trigger any special feelings or memories? If it has no effect on you, try 'stepping into' it and allowing it to surround you ... notice any effect it now has on you ...

After a few minutes, or when you are ready, allow the colour to draw itself away from you. In your mind's eye, watch it resuming the form it had in the beginning.

If colour can indeed influence our mood, then colour visualization could have particular value. We could mentally surround ourselves with single colours to gain specific effects, soothing our feelings when we are anxious and raising our mood when we are depressed. Single colours are again explored in the following two exercises.

Imagine finding yourself in a room decorated exclusively in a colour of your choice. See the entire room in this one colour, the walls, ceiling, paintwork, carpet, upholstery. If you have difficulty, try going through the motions of painting the walls and hanging the curtains. Totally immerse yourself in this colour and notice the effect it has on you ... does it relax you or give you a lift? ... why did you pick it? ... what associations does it have for you? ... stay with it long enough to absorb its full effect ... then let it fade.

Now picture yourself in a room decorated in a colour you don't like ... Surround yourself with this colour, let it permeate your consciousness (so long as it doesn't disturb you, in which case stop the exercise) ... Ask yourself why you dislike this colour and what effect it is having on you ... When you are ready, let the colour fade and be replaced by the colour of your choice before ending the visualization.

(It is preferable to end colour imagery sessions with a colour that the visualizer feels comfortable with, in order to carry away a rewarding sensation.)

Ernst & Goodison (1981) present a sequence in which colour flows to and from the visualizer. It is reproduced here in modified form:

First relax yourself using any method you find works for you. Close your eyes if they are not already closed. Let your mind be as still as possible. Pick a colour that feels right for you. Pick it spontaneously and see it before your eyes. You can picture it as brushstrokes of paint, coloured cloth, tinted smoke or coloured atmosphere. Let it extend all round you. Notice its quality, its tone and be aware of any associations it has for you. Feel yourself relating to this colour, harmonizing with it, becoming infused with it. Imagine yourself absorbing the colour through every pore of your skin until your body is filled with it ...

Now ... let the colour begin to radiate from you ... feel yourself releasing it ... making it expand all round you until it gradually comes to fill the room you are in. As you continue to generate more colour, see if you can fill the building you are in ... pause for a moment ... then slowly begin to draw the colour back, first from the building ... then from the room ... watching it get more condensed ... until it gathers in a cloud around you ... feel yourself bathed in this colour ... now ... absorb it back into your being ... into the very organs of your body ... pause again ... then watch it drawing itself away from all parts of you ... feel yourself being emptied of the colour. Convert it back to the paint, cloth or smoke in which it started. Be aware of how you feel after doing the exercise. Notice any effect it had on you.

CHAKRAS

In Hatha Yoga vital energy is seen as being focused in specified areas of the body known as 'chakras'. These are situated at:

- the base of the spine
- the lower abdomen
- the navel
- the heart
- the throat
- the brow
- the crown of the head.

Each chakra is associated with one of the colours of the spectrum: the base of the spine with red, the lower abdomen with orange, the navel with yellow, the heart with green, the throat with blue, the brow with indigo and the crown of the head with violet.

Kermani (1990) presents a passage of healing imagery based on the chakras, which is reproduced here in slightly altered form:

> See yourself lying in a natural setting of your choice. The sun is shining and it is warm and pleasant. Look around you ... build the scene. What plants are growing? Do they have a scent? What sounds can you hear? Feel the sun on your body. Imagine its rays bringing warmth to all parts of you. Imagine also the light broken up into its component parts so that it lies in a coloured spectrum across your body: warm red rays falling on your legs and hips, relaxing and warming them; orange rays casting a gentle light over your lower trunk; a soft yellow light glowing across your stomach; green rays casting a soothing light over your heart; blue light bathing your throat and lower face, a cool indigo light falling on your brow and violet light around your head.
>
> Picture a ray of blue light travelling from each eye ... allow these twin rays to carry away any tension ... carrying it into the vastness of space ... as it recedes, feel yourself relaxing ... finally, a silver light appears ... let it gather up all the colours and ... as it does, let it draw away any remaining tension from your body, dissolving it and leaving you in a state of deep calmness ... imagine the silver light spreading around you to form a circle ... allow the circle to include others who also wish to share this peace. They stay for a few moments and as they leave, you notice they have left a gift for you ... it is a gift which you will recognize...
>
> When you are ready, gently allow the scene to fade ... slowly, bring your attention back to the room in which you are lying. Feel the floor beneath you as you open your eyes.

WHITE LIGHT

The Rosicrucians, a brotherhood formed during the Renaissance, regarded white light as a symbol of guidance, inspiration and healing. The idea has been developed by Samuels & Samuels (1975):

> Take yourself in your mind's eye to a place that is special for you. Imagine it filled with brilliant white light ... let that light flow through you ... filling your body and your mind ... healing you ... strengthening you ... renewing you.

GUIDED IMAGERY

DEFINITION AND DESCRIPTION

Guided imagery is a therapeutic technique which uses the imagination to achieve desirable outcomes such as decreased pain perception and reduced anxiety (Ackerman & Turkoski 2000). It has been described as an inner communication involving all the senses and is believed to form an emotional connection between the mind and the body (Tusek & Cwynar 2000). The method can be used in most situations of pain and distress and is a useful adjunct to conventional medical and psychiatric treatments (Tusek & Cwynar 2000).

The visualizer conjures up a naturalistic scene, often of her own choosing, and moves around within it, noticing particularly its sensory content. A meadow, forest, beach or garden makes a suitable setting. Within this context, it is helpful to introduce a path and for three reasons: it can suggest a goal, provide a passage for the inner guide, or simply carry the visualizer through the scene.

Where imagery is being presented to a group, it is convenient for the instructor to decide on a particular scene and to suggest its basic structure. For example, if a meadow is decided on, the instructor can suggest other features such as a stream and a backdrop of distant hills. The time of year and the weather can make the scene more vivid. The visualizer is asked to notice the scents and sounds as well as the appearance of the scene. It is left to the instructor as to how much information is offered. The participant fills in the detail.

The following paragraphs (adapted from Lichstein 1988) give the flavour of guided imagery:

> Please get comfortable and close your eyes. As your mind becomes more peaceful, your body will also lose some of its tension. I am going to ask you to imagine a scene which you find pleasant and relaxing. Take a moment to choose the setting...
>
> Let your scene take shape ... do not force it in any way ... just allow it to form by building its sensory detail ... create it visually ... making it as vivid as you can ... imagine the sounds that accompany it ... the scents that float in the air ... the textures that surround you ... feel the warmth of the sun on your skin ... find a path and experience the

sensation of moving through the scene … feel the tension leaving your body … feel it being carried away each time you breathe out … and enjoy the peace and calm of the scene you've created …

For those who are looking for more specific scenes, three examples follow: a sunny beach; a country meadow; and a scented garden. (If the trainee suffers from hay fever, the first item is the best choice.)

A sunny beach

Imagine a stretch of shoreline … make it rocky or smooth as you like … notice the ground underfoot, is the sand wet and hard or is it dry and soft? … if the sun is shining perhaps you can feel its warmth on your skin … and see the light dancing on the water … perhaps you can smell the sea air as it fills your nostrils … what sounds can you hear? … the gulls calling? … the waves breaking? … a motor chugging? … you may decide to take a walk along the beach and, as you travel, notice how the scenery changes … perhaps rocks begin to break up the surface of the beach, with pools beneath them … you might feel you want to dip your hand into one of them … and are surprised to find how warm this shallow water is …

A country meadow

Picture yourself in the country … perhaps you are in a field in early summer … notice how long the grass is … notice also how green it is … are there wild flowers growing in it? … which ones? … can you smell their scent rising up? … and is there a gentle breeze? … enough to rustle the leaves on the trees? … you may decide to wander along a narrow sheeptrack … and as you cross the ground, perhaps you can hear the sound of water … if it's a stream, notice how it runs … whether smoothly or bubbling over rocks … and how soon does it swing out of sight? …

A scented garden

Let your mind conjure up the scene of a beautiful garden … notice the way it is laid out … the trees, shrubs and flower beds … perhaps it has just rained … a gentle summer rain … can you smell the air, warm and moist? … in your imagination notice the scents around you … is it honeysuckle? … or is it thyme? … or perhaps it's newly mown grass … you may decide to walk through the garden, along a path which perhaps carries you under some trees … notice how cool it is in their shade … and how warm when you step out into the sunlight again … notice also the trees which line the path … and the texture of their bark … in your mind's eye reach out to touch one of them … was it smooth or deeply incised? …

EVIDENCE FROM RESEARCH

Imagery is a safe and non-invasive technique which does not require elaborate equipment. As a coping tool for reducing anxiety and stress, it has been found useful (Donovan 1980, Hamm & O'Flynn 1984, King 1988) and Dossey (1988) finds it can reduce psychological stress in a healthy working population. With hospital patients guided imagery has been used to enhance patient experience, resulting in significant decreases in anxiety, pain, narcotic consumption, side effects, financial costs, care and length of stay (Tusek & Cwynar 2000). However, imagery alone has rarely been studied as a treatment (Luskin et al 2000). It is often combined with muscle relaxation techniques in the treatment of clinical conditions. For example, Cupal & Brewer (2001) found significantly less pain and re-injury anxiety following a course of relaxation and imagery among individuals undergoing rehabilitation after anterior cruciate reconstruction; and Johnson (2000) showed that the mood levels of competitive adults with long-term injuries could be significantly raised by relaxation and guided imagery.

Cancer pain is another area where the combination of these two techniques has been studied. In the conclusion of her review article, Wallace (1997) found that relaxation and imagery appeared to reduce the sensory experience of pain. The evidence in their favour is not strong but it is suggested that the combined techniques have a place as an adjunct to other forms of treatment.

The use of imagery as a tool for promoting relaxation is supported by the work of Haas & Axen (1991) who showed that the behaviour of alpha waves becomes altered during sessions of therapeutic imagery. Further evidence of the benefit of the approach may be found in Chapter 27, where many of the trials involve the use of imagery and help to justify its widespread use in the clinical field.

PITFALLS

A list of the pitfalls relating to imagery can be found at the end of Chapter 18 (p. 170).

Further reading

Zahourek R P 1997 Relaxation and imagery: tools for therapeutic communication and intervention. Alternative Health Practitioner 3(2): 89–109

Chapter 18

Goal-directed visualization

CHAPTER CONTENTS

DEFINITION

In their book *Seeing with the Mind's Eye*, Samuels & Samuels (1975) describe a technique using imagery which has two phases, receptive and programmed. In the receptive phase, the individual passively listens to her inner self, drawing on her own wisdom. In the programmed phase, she engages in an active and deliberate thought process for the purpose of improving a situation or resolving a problem in her life. It is based on the assumption that, by repeatedly experiencing an outcome in the imagination, we increase the likelihood of it taking place in real life.

The Samuels' work has been developed by Achterberg (1985), Simonton et al (1986) and others in areas of medicine and healing; and by Shone (1984) and Fanning (1988) among others in areas of self-development and relaxation. Since in this book we are concerned with the latter area, the definitions of Fanning and Shone are appropriate. Fanning describes this kind of imagery as 'the conscious, volitional creation of mental sense impressions for the purpose of changing oneself'; Shone refers to it as a mental experience which helps to bring about desired outcomes. Implicit in both definitions is the notion of a goal.

How does this form of imagery differ from other forms? One answer is that it is more explicit than techniques which rely on metaphor and symbolism; it is also more purposeful than reverie states such as daydreaming. How is it different from talking to yourself, reflecting, and giving yourself advice? It may not *be* very different, but it does seek to offer a structured, step-by-step approach.

RATIONALE

The mechanism of visualization as a method for enhancing well-being is incompletely understood. However, its success is often explained by the belief that the body cannot distinguish between the event as experienced and the event as imagined, a notion which is supported by a finding that the same physiological responses occur in each case (Dalloway 1992). As a result, therapeutic responses can be learned and practised in a safe environment, from which it is proposed, they can later be transferred to the event in real life; if not wholly transferred, at least their likelihood of occurring is strengthened (Dalloway 1992).

Thus, tasks perceived to be difficult can lose some of their threat after being visualized with a successful outcome. This is mental rehearsal, a procedure which allows the individual to familiarize herself with the feared event and, in her imagination, to achieve her goal. Impending stressful events such as athletic competitions and performances of various kinds can be approached in this way (Farmer 1995).

THE METHOD

The method, which incorporates other techniques such as progressive relaxation and guided imagery (Chs 4 & 17) lends itself to a variety of conditions and situations of which smoking cessation is one and this topic is considered in some detail. The chapter opens with a general description of the procedure under the following headings:

- position
- preparatory relaxation
- special place
- receptive visualization
- positive self-statements or affirmations
- programmed visualization
- termination
- an additional technique.

POSITION

The visualizer lies down in a comfortable position in a dimly lit, warm room, free from noise and interruption. She closes her eyes.

PREPARATORY RELAXATION

Imagery is preceded by a short session of relaxation, since relaxation is generally regarded as a precondition as well as an effect of visualization. Its role here is to create a 'state of balance, quietude and peace, free of negativity' (Ryman 1994). It allows the mind to be receptive to new information and tends to enhance the formation of images (Tusek 2000). The technique employed can be chosen by the individual, although Achterberg (1985) suggests that passive forms of muscle relaxation are more appropriate than tense–release, which she claims is ineffective for imagery work. Slow, gentle abdominal breathing will also help to induce deep relaxation. The visualizer may recite appropriate phrases such as 'My mind is calm and clear', 'I am open to images that will help me'.

Although this preliminary relaxation is common practice, there is little evidence to support its value as a facilitator of imagery (Lichstein 1988). Indeed, there are those who claim the opposite, i.e. that a totally relaxed body is accompanied by a mind devoid of images (Jacobson 1938). If muscular relaxation clears the mind of images, how can it also promote them? Lichstein (1988) refers to this as a matter yet to be resolved. Perhaps the answer lies in finding a level of relaxation which is deep enough to release tension but not so deep that images cannot form.

SPECIAL PLACE

Lying quietly, the visualizer builds an imaginary scene or 'special place' as a retreat for relaxation and guidance (Davis et al 2000). The scene is rich in sensory images of sight, sound, smell, taste, texture, temperature, and gives her a feeling of peace and tranquillity. A beach, meadow, lake or forest all offer possibilities. The visualizer is encouraged to imagine how the body would feel in the special place, emphasizing sensations like sinking into springy turf or soft sand. Some time is spent initially setting the scene so that it can easily be recreated in subsequent visualizations. Since imagery is a right hemisphere activity, the constraints of logic do not apply. Thus, the special place may contain any figment of the imagination which the visualizer finds useful, as for example, a permanent sunset in the background, a viewing screen in a forest clearing or a crystal ball in a mountain spring. It is in such a scene that the inner guide could appear (Ch. 17, p. 151), and so there should be a clearly defined way in.

Some people prefer an indoor special place such as an attic room or a garden shed; others like to have both, using them on different occasions. There is no right or wrong way: whatever works for the individual is right.

RECEPTIVE VISUALIZATION

The visualizer imagines herself in her special place. This is where she can feel in tune with herself and where she will be likely to gain insights. She is in a state of mind that allows her to listen to the part of herself which is normally beyond conscious awareness. It is a passive state of mind which in some ways resembles daydreaming, but differs from the latter in that the visualizer is asking specific questions of herself (Samuels & Samuels 1975). Whether she is making a choice, sorting out a conflict, uncovering motivations or exposing automatic thoughts, the receptive visualization is a way of allowing intuitive insights to be released and inner wisdom to be revealed.

The visualizer should be advised that if uncontrollable or unpleasant feelings which she is not ready to deal with arise, she can walk away or distance herself in some other manner. She can also end the visualization. Otherwise she quietly tunes in to her unconscious. If ideas do not flow, the inner guide can be called and asked for advice (Ch. 17, p. 151).

An example of a receptive visualization script is given below. (Allow 10 or 15 minutes for it.)

Lie down. Get yourself comfortable and close your eyes. Run through a relaxing procedure until you feel very calm. Visualize yourself lying in your special place. Evoke its atmosphere by mentally experiencing its sights, sounds, smells and textures.

Feel at home there. Let your attention gently focus on the item that preoccupies you ... just keep an open mind ... quietly listen to the thoughts that flow through it ... if you are stuck, call on your inner guide ... listen to the wisdom your inner guide brings ... realize that it is your own wisdom, coming from your deeper self ... spend a few minutes listening to yourself...

When you are ready, end your visualization and gently bring your attention back to the room.

Write down any ideas that came to you. Consider them. Have you gained any insights? Do you want to change your way of handling this situation? Are there more positive ways of dealing with it?

Receptive visualizations can be repeated as often as they continue to provide insights.

POSITIVE SELF–STATEMENTS OR AFFIRMATIONS

The positive self-statement, often referred to as an affirmation, helps the visualizer to see herself as being capable of realizing her aspiration and achieving her goal. Inherent in the affirmation is the suspension of self-doubt. Examples include the following:

- I believe in myself.
- I am in control of my life.
- I can achieve my aim.

While the above statements are of a general nature, additional affirmations relevant to the matter in question can also be composed. Thus, for a person wishing to become more relaxed, the following statements may be included:

- I feel calm.
- I am at peace.
- I can cope in stressful situations.

Positive self-statements need to be short, in the first person and in the present tense; the best ones are those composed by the individual herself (Fanning 1988). When repeated, they act like self-hypnotic suggestions, influencing the individual's view of herself in a positive direction, and adding force to the positive images of the programmed visualization (described below).

PROGRAMMED VISUALIZATION

General comments

In this phase, the individual may work on images that emerged during the receptive phase, turning them over and trying them out in different forms in her imagination. When she finds the most effective solution to her problems, she visualizes herself as instrumental in achieving it. Actions are imagined which allow her to feel herself displaying the qualities she wants to possess. Goals are mentally reached with the individual operating as their successful agent. By daily repetition, the new images of herself start to blend with her self-image, tending to generate still more positive internal dialogue and, in the manner of a self-fulfilling prophecy, increasing the likelihood of the desired outcome in real life.

Sometimes, while in the programmed stage, the visualizer gets 'stuck'. In this case, returning to the receptive stage may help to clear the block.

On other occasions, the receptive and programmed phases may not be clearly separated. Not all visualization work falls neatly into receptive and programmed categories, and individuals should not feel under pressure to structure them separately if one continuous visualization seems more appropriate. There is no set pattern for the programmed visualization: the topic itself will determine the style.

Procedure for programmed visualization

The preliminaries are similar to those for receptive visualization, that is, the person relaxes herself using cue-controlled relaxation (Ch. 8, p. 71) or passive muscular relaxation (Ch. 7).

She then evokes the scene of the situation she wants to resolve, whatever it might be. (This is not the special place but a real-life situation.) Again, rich sensory detail is essential to bring it to life. Time spent building the scene enables her to experience it more keenly. She then works on the item, experimenting with it until she finds a good solution which she then enacts in her imagination. She plays a role which succeeds.

The tone of the programmed visualization is demonstrated in the following passage:

Let your thoughts become quiet and bring your attention to focus on your goal. Believe in your capacity to reach it ... don't dwell on the difficulties; just think of the result. If there are problems, see them as a challenge ... feel an eagerness to achieve ... to be a person who has reached that goal ... feel yourself in the part ... imagine yourself as having arrived ... congratulate yourself for getting there ... enjoy it...

TERMINATION

When the visualization is over, the procedure is brought to an end with a termination on the following lines:

If you are ready, gradually bring your attention back to the room you are in ... slowly count one ... two ... three ... and, as you open your eyes, feel yourself alert and refreshed.

Goal-directed visualization thus consists of the individual opening herself to her own wisdom (receptive phase), and then using it in her imagination to bring about the desired outcome (programmed phase).

ADDITIONAL TECHNIQUE

'Distancing', i.e. drawing back from the scene to examine her actions, is a technique which allows the visualizer to gain a more objective view. In an imaginary viewing screen or crystal ball she watches her behaviour patterns; how she copes with situations and relates to other people.

This approach may reveal maladaptive responses she might be making. She then modifies those responses and reruns the film in a way which leads to a successful outcome. The next move is for her to step into the scene in her imagination, in order to experience the skills she observed herself displaying on the screen.

RELAXATION AND GOAL–DIRECTED VISUALIZATION

It can be seen that relaxation is related to goal-directed visualization in a variety of ways.

- It is used as a preparatory measure to induce a state of mind conducive to visualization.

Before the individual begins her visualization, she should first become relaxed.

- It may be experienced as a secondary effect following mental rehearsal in which the individual sees herself successfully coping with an activity which has hitherto been associated with stress.
- A need for relaxation may be created while the goal is being achieved, such as during the struggle to withdraw from cigarettes or tranquillizers.

Goal-directed visualization is thus not a primary method of inducing relaxation, but it does have close links with it.

APPLYING THE METHOD OF GOAL-DIRECTED VISUALIZATION

Unlike most other methods described in this book, goal-directed visualization addresses the specific problems of a person. This feature is seen in both the receptive and the programmed components. Thus it is not possible to present a model script without a clear understanding of the background.

A key factor in the success of any plan is the motivation of the visualizer. While for some individuals this is not a problem, others may need encouragement. One way of fostering motivation is to make the goals specific. For example, having a timescale for a smoking abstinence plan defines it more clearly. Creating subgoals or intermediate stages is another useful strategy, since they act as stepping stones along the way. This has the effect of making the ultimate goal seem easier to reach, as well as providing rewards at intervals. Smoking one less cigarette a day can constitute a subgoal; so can taking one more step to a person recovering from leg injury. Difficulties can be considered in advance and ways of solving them worked out (Fig. 18.1).

Samuels & Samuels (1975) advise the individual not to confide her visualization to anyone who may not share her faith in the wisdom of the goal and in her capacity to reach it. Unshaken belief is vital for her success.

Of course, participants in some groups may be too demoralized to begin; they may feel they have little future; they may be angry or depressed. These are valid reactions which call for modification of the method and perhaps referral to a specialist agency. In general, however, the approach can be a useful one.

Although it is difficult to construct a model script without specific knowledge of the problem concerned, an attempt is made here to provide an example.

The reader is reminded of the principal items in the method.

Receptive visualization. The individual tunes in to her own wisdom.

Self-statements. She reaffirms herself through positive internal dialogue.

Programmed visualization. She works on a plan for the future in which she sees herself surmounting

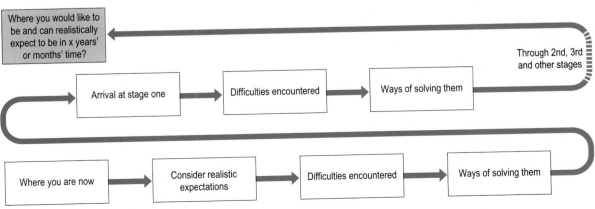

Figure 18.1 Setting goals.

obstacles, realizing possibilities and achieving goals. The keynote of this stage is seeing the self as succeeding.

VISUALIZATIONS FOR PEOPLE WHO WANT TO GIVE UP SMOKING

It could be argued that smoking has more to do with relaxation than smoking abstinence has, and many people become smokers because they perceive cigarettes as being a source of mental calm. However, many such people may then wish to quit smoking. Quitting is associated with stress, which means that the same people may be seeking an alternative means of obtaining relaxation. Health care professionals increasingly find themselves faced with groups of people who are struggling to give up cigarettes and for whom relaxation training has been prescribed. Although any of the methods in this book might help, a method which directly addresses the problem would seem to have particular advantages.

Within a single group of people who wish to reduce their smoking habits, there may be a wide variety of aspirations: one person may want to cut down from 40 cigarettes a day to 20, another may want to give up altogether. They may also have different ideas as to how to go about it: one may want to reduce by one cigarette a day, another may want to make a more abrupt change. Or again, the group may consist of people who are looking for ways of avoiding relapse after having successfully given up smoking. The following visualization (adapted from Fanning 1988) is designed for people who have decided to give up altogether.

Receptive visualization

Lie or sit in a position which you find comfortable. Close your eyes. Allow yourself to unwind. (The instructor presents either passive relaxation or slow breathing.) As your body and mind become calm, let your special place take shape in your imagination. Notice the sights, sounds and smell of the place. Put out your hand and feel the textures: the grass, the rug, the pine needles, etc. ... feel that you are there ... lying peacefully ... tuned in to yourself.

Gently bring your mind to focus on your smoking habit. Explore your feelings about it. Why do you smoke? Perhaps you hadn't thought about it before, just taken it for granted. In your mind's eye, take out a cigarette and light up ... what does it do for you? ...

Run through different situations during the day when you feel the need of a cigarette ... start with breakfast time ... what prompts you to reach for the first cigarette? ... then follow yourself to work ... smoking on the journey ... at work in your coffee break ... after the midday meal ... again in the afternoon ... on the way home ... to round off the evening meal ... last thing at night ... do you notice if you smoke for different reasons? ... do you get different rewards from smoking? ... when do you find you particularly want a cigarette? ...

Bring your visualization to an end when you are ready ...

The visualizer may feel she smokes for different reasons at different times. Some of the reasons why people smoke are:

- to feel reassured
- to relieve boredom
- to feel soothed
- to feel relaxed
- to give her hands something to do
- to give herself a lift
- to reward herself
- to keep her weight down.

She decides which of these apply to her and is then urged to think of alternative ways of meeting these needs:

- For reassurance, she tells herself she does not need a crutch.
- To relieve boredom, she gets out a crossword puzzle.
- To feel soothed, she reminds herself of the love of her partner.
- To feel relaxed, she runs through a relaxation sequence.
- To give her hands something to do, she carries a small, rounded pebble which she rolls in her hand.
- To give herself a lift, she remembers the prize she won for cookery/essay-writing/athletics last year.
- To reward herself, she buys the salmon roll instead of the cheese roll.

- To keep her weight down, she eats an orange instead of a second helping of potatoes, or goes for a walk/workout, etc.

Positive self-statements or affirmations

The individual cultivates a view of herself as a healthy non-smoker by composing a few positive self-statements which she recites regularly to herself:

- I am healthy
- I am a non-smoker
- I have the strength to control my habits
- I value the time when I am not smoking

Additionally, she is gentle with herself for occasionally breaking her resolve:

- I can forgive myself for occasionally breaking my resolution.

Some people find it helpful to have one strong reason for changing their behaviour and to focus on this one idea whenever they feel in danger of weakening.

Programmed visualization

This takes the form of a mental rehearsal of coping activities which may focus on the goal itself (the end result) or on the means of achieving it (the process) (Ryman 1995). The example below is mainly concerned with the process.

At the start of the session the instructor can offer passive relaxation or relaxation through abdominal breathing.

> Lie down and spend a few minutes relaxing quietly. Imagine yourself at the beginning of a normal day. Run through every moment when you think you might want to light up. Have an alternative way of dealing with every urge to smoke. Start with the moment when you would have the first cigarette of the day ... evoke the scene using sensory detail to bring it to life ... really live the moment in your imagination ... feel yourself craving a cigarette, then promptly use your alternative strategy ... and as you do so, encourage yourself with your positive self-statements...
>
> Move on to the next moment when you would want to light up ... and the next and so on ... making each moment come alive by recreating the scene as

> vividly as you can ... employing alternative strategies and encouraging yourself with positive self-statements ... remind yourself of the benefits of giving up smoking: clear lungs, no cough, extra change in your pocket ... and if you feel your resolution weakening, remind yourself why you made it in the first place.
>
> Continue through the day, appreciating the experiences that not smoking opens up to you: the taste of your food ... the garden scents ... the fresh smell of your clothes ... and the easy way you climb the hill. See yourself as someone who doesn't smoke...
>
> At some point, feel your stress levels rising as something goes wrong at work ... you weaken and take out a cigarette ... but after a couple of puffs you stub it out ... allow yourself to feel pleased that you could have a slight relapse but not let it interfere with your determination to conquer your habit ... see yourself continuing to carry out your resolution and succeeding ... see yourself as someone who can cope without resorting to cigarettes...
>
> When you are ready, bring your visualization to an end with a count of one ... two ... three ... open your eyes ... look around you ... stretch your arms and legs ... and in your own time prepare to resume normal activity.

Some visualization therapists include an aversion component as a further incentive to give up smoking. This could take the form of images of dirty ash trays, blackened lungs, stained fingers or smoky atmospheres. Aversive measures work for some people; other people simply switch off if the image becomes too unpleasant.

The benefits of programmed visualization come from daily practice: the constant repetition of a routine in which the individual sees herself as successful in the task she has set herself. The above example is offered as a guideline or starting point from which the health care professional may wish to develop her own script. Alternatively, participants can be encouraged to compose their own visualizations, since the most effective ones are those designed by individuals for their own use (Fanning 1988).

Where motivation needs strengthening, the following additional visualization may be found useful:

> Find a quiet moment. Relax yourself and close your eyes. Imagine the house in which you expect to be

living 10/5/2 years from now. Go inside … explore it … what does it tell you about the occupant: yourself? … who else lives there? … try identifying with your older self … notice how it might feel to be that older self … at work … at her hobby … with her family … then, try looking back at yourself as you are now … do you have anything to say to yourself? …

When you are ready, allow your visualization to fade … slowly, bring yourself back to the present … counting one … two … three … as you open your eyes…

EVIDENCE OF EFFECTIVENESS OF IMAGERY IN CHANGING SMOKING BEHAVIOUR

Many formal smoking cessation programmes have been shown to have high success rates which have typically reached levels of 70% or over (Feldmann & Richard 1986, Schwartz 1987, Wynd 1989). This success has been attributed to different components of the programmes: education, stress reduction, cognitive-behavioural strategies and relaxation imagery.

The relapse rate, however, also tends to be high. Shiffman (1985) believes that relapse occurs when individuals lack the coping skills to continue their abstinence. Such coping skills include:

- behavioural strategies:
  - removing oneself from a scene in which others are smoking
  - using distraction techniques
  - practising relaxation
- cognitive strategies:
  - using pleasant imagery to divert oneself from the thought of smoking
  - creating images of improved health.

Because relaxation imagery has been successfully used for smoking cessation, Wynd (1992) employed it in the prevention of relapse. Her controlled study of 84 quitters covered a post-cessation period of 3 months. At the end of that period, 72% of participants were still abstaining from smoking.

The effectiveness of training people to provide smoking cessation programmes was investigated by Silagy et al (1994). They reviewed eight randomized controlled trials in which the performance of health care professionals trained in smoking cessation interventions was measured against that of an untrained control group. Results showed a modest but significant increase in the number of quitters attending the trained participants compared with those attending the untrained controls. Thus, training is seen to increase the skills of those who provide smoking cessation programmes, leading to a higher level of success. The authors consider that further improvement in client outcome would require changes in health service policy which gave greater prominence to prevention.

Some recent work has focused on the experience of craving and how this can be influenced by different kinds of imagery; for example, whether standard images evoke urges to smoke of more or less intensity than self-created images (Conklin & Tiffany 2001). The answer would help to determine the degree to which craving is dependent on environmental factors, such as seeing other people smoking. Research has produced conflicting outcomes and the issue has not been resolved. This is partly owing to the different ways individuals react to smoking cues (Niaura et al 1998) and the various ways in which these cues can be presented (Conklin & Tiffany 2001).

OTHER APPLICATIONS OF GOAL-DIRECTED VISUALIZATION

Goal-directed visualization can be used in a wide range of situations and conditions associated with stress, for example:

1. performance fear
2. sport and athletics
3. anger
4. problem solving and decision making
5. eating disorders
6. phobia and panic disorder
7. alcohol and substance misuse
8. cancer
9. pain.

From insights gained during the receptive phase, a realistic solution can be worked out. This solution can then be mentally rehearsed during the programmed visualization, and a successful outcome experienced in the imagination.

Performance fear

The programmed visualization can be used to take the individual through every moment of the event whether it is a stage performance, a speech or similar activity. The scene becomes familiar to her. She mentally experiences all possible occurrences and develops coping strategies for dealing with them. Above all she experiences the successful achievement of her goal. This has the effect of building and maintaining her confidence.

Sport and athletics

Physical skills have a psychological dimension which is served by imagery in two ways, one cognitive, the other motivational (Paivio 1985). In the cognitive one the player imagines successful routines in the game and rehearses appropriate strategies in her imagination. This leads to a strengthened integration between the physical and the psychological elements of skill and helps to refine performance. In the motivational one, attention is given to the feelings of arousal and affect which accompany performance. The player trains herself to channel her emotional energy in positive directions such as imagining the experience of winning. In this way, the sensations of stress, pain and anxiety associated with the activity can be reduced.

A third type, healing imagery, is also practised by athletes following injury (Sordoni et al 2002) (see Ch. 27, p. 236).

Visualization has been employed to great effect in the field of sport and athletics, with numerous research findings supporting its use. The classic study was performed by Richardson (1969) who showed that basketball players who spent 3 weeks simply visualizing their throws achieved almost the same level of improvement (23%) as players who spent the time practising throws with a ball and whose level of improvement was 24%. A control group whose members did neither showed no improvement.

Further discussion of this topic can be found in the work of Blumenstein et al (1997).

Anger

For an individual who wishes to reduce her tendency to become angry, alternative and preferred courses of action can be mapped out (Ch. 3, p. 28). The programmed visualization is employed to familiarize the individual with her capacity to respond in these preferred ways. Relaxation and positive self-talk play a prominent part (Fanning 1988).

Problem solving and decision making

A receptive visualization can be used to collect ideas for solutions. After weighing them up, the unrealistic ideas are discarded and the realistic ones retained. Possible results are then predicted both in the short term and in the longer term. These are then considered for their merits and disadvantages which together form the basis of the individual's final choice. Having picked what she considers to be the best solution, the individual mentally puts it into effect, experiencing its successful outcome in a programmed visualization. Figure 18.2 illustrates the process from identification of the problem to adoption of the best solution.

Vissing & Burke (1984) found that individuals who regularly practised visualization when faced with problems had more success at solving them than those who did not.

Eating disorders

In the case of people wishing to lose weight, alternative strategies may be found to take the place of eating. These are incorporated into daily programmed visualizations in which the individual sees herself successfully carrying out her plan (Fanning 1988). In the course of it she builds an image of herself as someone who looks nice whatever size she is, but has chosen to lose some weight. Any diet she is following should be medically approved.

Anorexia calls for more specialized treatment.

Phobia and panic disorder

Programmed visualizations allow the sufferer to see herself overcoming fear and mastering the situation. They are often performed in a hierarchal fashion, i.e. a list of situations from low to high threat is drawn up. The individual starts with the lowest and, taking each one in turn, mentally goes through the experience of overcoming her fear, using slowed breathing, relaxation techniques and

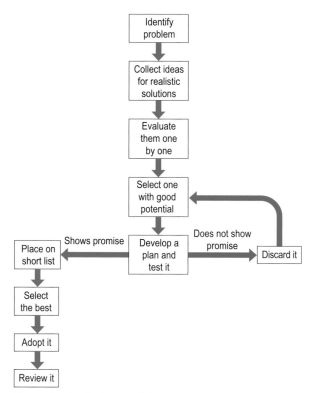

Figure 18.2   Problem solving.

positive self-talk. This method is known as desensitization and was first introduced by Wolpe in 1958.

Alcohol and substance misuse

In programmed visualization the individual mentally rehearses the successful achievement of her goal using positive self-talk and alternative strategies (p. 166). She also finds ways of relaxing herself during the period of dose-tapering and beyond.

Cancer

Imagery in this context can be used in a number of ways. In one of these attention is focused on reversing the physiological changes produced by the tumour. Mental pictures of the cancer cells being attacked by white blood cells are created by the visualizer. The scene is made as vivid as possible by casting the cancer cells as villains. They can play any role which the visualizer chooses, such

as for example, enemy infiltrators. In this scenario, the white blood cells could be represented as a vast army which slowly and inexorably overpowers the intruders and destroys them. The scene is imagined in every detail and the exercise repeated at frequent intervals.

It has been shown that heightened immune responses can occur in patients with cancer who have practised relaxation and healing imagery compared with those who have not practised these techniques (Gregson et al 1996).

Pain

Imagery is used as a therapeutic aid in some types of pain, although it should never be viewed as a substitute for medical attention. It can, however, be a useful coping device for minor ailments, such as aches in different parts of the body, where techniques such as transformations (Ch. 17, p. 155) can sometimes help the individual to get through difficult patches. Its use as adjunctive therapy in some forms of intractable pain is a specialized area not covered in the present work.

COMMENT

It is believed that the individual's performance in real life is enhanced by having mentally viewed herself in a goal-achieving light. Perceiving herself to be a winner is one of the central ideas of *Psycho-cybernetics*, in which Maltz (1966) writes of the mechanism within us which needs to be constantly presented with unqualified success goals in order to function as a success mechanism.

PITFALLS OF IMAGERY AND GOAL–DIRECTED VISUALIZATION

A cautious attitude is advised when using imagery. Pitfalls include the following:

1. Visualization should never be allowed to take the place of medical help. People suffering from mental or physical symptoms should consult their doctor, and those already receiving medication should let their doctor know of their intention to use relaxation and imagery techniques.

2. Imagery and visualization methods may not be suitable for people suffering from severe mental disorders. Imagery is particularly inadvisable for people who have difficulty in separating fantasy from reality and for those who experience hallucinations. Ackerman (2000) refers to the inadvisability of using imagery when taking medication for a thought disorder.

3. People differ in their ability to form images for reasons which have yet to be established (Kosslyn et al 2001). For those who find it difficult, a muscular approach might be more useful. On the other hand, since visualization is thought by some to be a learnable skill, practice may increase proficiency (Dalloway 1992).

4. Goals, which should be set by the individual herself, need to be attainable. To set goals that are out of the individual's reach will only create additional stress.

Goals may also be set too low to be constructive, as occurs in individuals whose self-esteem has crumbled. Exceptionally low self-esteem can make a person feel she does not deserve success and joy. A first step would be to help her to value herself.

Working towards a goal often entails the need to change. The individual, however, may not want to change, and although she would like to reach the goal, she may place obstacles in its path.

5. Since imagery tends to put people in touch with deeper parts of themselves, strong emotional reactions such as anger, resentment, guilt and frustration may be experienced. Weeping is fairly common. If it occurs, the instructor can reassure the distressed participant on the following lines:

> It's all right to weep here … it often happens … it shows how deeply relaxed you are … and how truly in touch with yourself.

Insofar as the participant is working through previously repressed material, weeping may have positive value for her. The instructor, on the other hand, may find the reaction difficult to handle. Such an incident would be a matter for discussion with the supervisor (Ch. 2, p. 19).

Zahourek (1988) likes to warn participants at the outset that deep-seated emotions may be released during imagery. Larkin (1988) suggests to participants that they need acknowledge only those emotions they feel comfortable with. This is not to disclaim ownership of their feelings, but rather to allow time for them to be accepted.

Mildly disturbing thoughts can be reduced in intensity by blurring the image, letting it recede or dissolving it in white light. For severely disturbing thoughts, the image should be cancelled and the visualization terminated.

In a study that rated the occurrence of different negative reactions, it was found that intrusive thoughts had the highest frequency, followed by disturbing sensory experiences and the fear of losing control. The frequency of such effects bore no relation to the therapist's experience (Edinger & Jacobsen 1982).

6. By contrast, intruding images can be so attractive that the visualizer is lured in their direction, away from the original goal. This is daydreaming; it differs from therapeutic forms of imagery in that it is unstructured and tends to be remote from reality. (This is not to say that daydreaming is without psychological benefit, since it is essentially a self-affirming strategy (Singer 1975). Some people, however, daydream to the extent of having difficulty in relating to the real world.)

7. A participant may be so depressed that he or she is harbouring thoughts of suicide. Any mention of taking his or her life must be viewed seriously and the person urged to seek professional help.

8. Occasionally, an individual may experience feelings of unreality. These can be dealt with by a grounding technique such as feeling the floor underneath her (Ch. 20, p. 184). If, however, the feeling is strong, the image should be allowed to fade, and the visualization brought to an end.

9. It is not the object of the exercise to create a hypnotic trance. Neither is it likely that one will occur. However, since some individuals are more susceptible than others, the possibility exists that the instructor may inadvertently create one. When a person is in a hypnotic trance, the power of suggestion becomes greater. That being so, the instructor needs to be aware of the phenomenon of post-hypnotic suggestion.

Post-hypnotic suggestion results in the individual blindly carrying out injunctions outside the trance situation. For example, a statement such as: 'When you go home you will assert yourself' would be indiscriminately applied. This would leave no room for reassessment of the situation which might, in changing circumstances, call for a modified approach.

Any suggestion which could be applied inappropriately outside the relaxation session should be avoided. Generally speaking, however, post-hypnotic suggestion is not a problem since the individual tends to resist any exhortation that runs counter to her personal goals and moral principles (Lynn & Rhue 1977).

Larkin (1988) has useful advice for the health care professional who is offering imagery and is concerned to avoid hypnotizing the client: suggestion should be indirect, incorporating words like 'can', 'may', 'might' and 'perhaps'. Larkin emphasizes the importance of presenting the client with options, so that the suggestion finally adopted comes from the client herself.

However, if the instructor is in doubt as to the effect of her words, she can terminate the session with a cancelling statement (Shone 1982) on the lines of:

> Before you bring your visualization to an end, cancel any suggestion you do not wish to take effect in your waking life.

As mentioned earlier, it is unlikely that unintentional hypnosis will occur.

10. As part of the visualization procedure, the individual constructs new self-statements. One of these may be ill-conceived. The visualizer needs to be alerted to this possibility and to the importance of cutting out any such self-statement.

11. Certain colours can have a powerful and unexpected effect on a person. The antidote for such an experience is to substitute white light for the offending colour, while at the same time attaching a message of calmness to the white light. If, however, the effect of the colour is very strong, the visualization should be brought to an end.

12. Jung felt that too much emphasis on the inner world could take a person away from everyday happenings, and that it was important to ground oneself in something solid such as work or family.

13. Occasionally, a participant has difficulty returning from his visualization. Repeating the termination procedure usually resolves the problem. Another device is to include in the termination procedure some reference to feeling alert and refreshed.

When techniques are being learned and applied, one cannot count on instant success. As with any new skill, the most that can be expected is a trend in the desired direction. Frequent practice, however, strengthens this trend.

Further reading

Gawain S 1995 Creative visualization: use the power of your imagination to create what you want in your life. New World Library, California

Ryman L 1994 Relaxation and visualization. In: Wells R J, Tschudin V (eds) Wells' supportive therapies in health care. Baillière Tindall, London

Chapter 19

Autogenic training

ALTERED STATES OF CONSCIOUSNESS

An altered state of consciousness is often referred to as a 'trance'. It has been described as a condition in which critical faculties are suspended and the 'limits of … a person's … usual frame of reference and beliefs temporarily altered … making her … receptive to other patterns of association and modes of mental functioning' (Erickson & Rossi 1979).

The classic trance is the hypnotic trance, induced by procedures which create intense focal awareness, such as concentrating on a swinging pendulum. The participant becomes highly responsive to suggestion: 'the process whereby the individual accepts a proposition put to her by another, without having the slightest logical reason for doing so' (Hartland 1971). This is often described as 'uncritical acceptance'. Outwardly, the trance resembles drowsiness and dozing and is accompanied by a general reduction of muscle tone and a dilatation of the capillaries; the person is, however, awake and highly focused, although she may lose awareness of her surroundings.

Hypnosis may also be self-induced, in which case the individual herself governs the trance and plants the suggestions. The attention is again turned inwards, although this trance is described as a light one, in which the individual retains awareness of her surroundings, being conscious of herself in all her senses (Rosa 1976). She does not, however, reflect on herself (Rosa 1976), which is to say that she does not distinguish between the self as subject (the 'I') and the self as object (the 'me') (Mead 1934).

Incomplete understanding of the mechanism of trance makes it difficult to draw further distinctions between trance states of differing depth. Some writers see altered states of consciousness as separate entities, different in kind from each other, while others view them as lying on a continuum between sleep at one end, and wakefulness at the other. The latter view suggests that the altered states represent varying grades of trance, different only in degree and all part of the same entity (Barber 1969, 1970).

HISTORY AND INTRODUCTION OF AUTOGENIC TRAINING

Autogenic training (AT) is an approach derived from self-hypnosis. It dates from the 1930s, when Johannes Schultz, a psychiatrist working at the Berlin Neurobiological Institute, discovered that some patients had learned to put themselves into a light trance by concentrating on images of heaviness and warmth. Even more interesting was the fact that they had seemed to benefit in terms of their mental health. Schultz called this self-generated trance state 'autogenic', and proceeded to develop a therapy based on it.

The goal of the procedure was attainment of this autogenic state, achieved by means of given phrases recited by the pupil. These phrases, by their imagery and autosuggestion, created what was called the 'autogenic shift'; a shift in the participant away from a stressed state towards the state known as autogenic. Exactly what, however, was the autogenic state?

A prominent exponent of the method, Luthe (1965), has described the autogenic state as being linked to drowsiness. In this work Luthe considers the nature of this 'drowsiness' and its relation to hypnosis, but without reaching any conclusion. These matters have still to be resolved. Today AT is an established approach, but since the trainee is active in her own treatment, it is generally regarded as a relaxation technique rather than a form of hypnosis.

What, however, is the difference between hypnosis and relaxation? Zahourek (1985) answers the question by pointing out that hypnosis purposefully aims at producing a trance; hypnosis also emphasizes therapeutic suggestion. In relaxation, by contrast, there is no striving for a state of trance, and any suggestion made is under the control of the individual herself who, as a human being, is constantly making suggestions to herself anyway. Certainly, some of the devices used in relaxation, i.e. passive concentration, self-suggestion and imagery, are closely related to hypnosis, but they are not confined to that practice; and their effective use does not require the full knowledge of a formal hypnosis training (Zahourek 1985).

Imagery and autosuggestion form part of most relaxation approaches (Larkin 1988); indeed, many would say there are elements of suggestion in all stress reduction methods (Barber 1984). To ensure that they are used responsibly, however, it is necessary for the health care professional to have clear goals, to use techniques designed to promote those goals and to be aware of the hazards involved.

Davis et al (2000), addressing their book particularly to those who 'work with people who are in stress' (itemizing doctors, nurses, therapists, teachers and supervisors), present step-by-step directions for mastery of different approaches, one of which is self-hypnosis. They claim that no cases have been reported, even among the most inexperienced practitioners, of harm resulting from self-hypnosis (Davis et al 2000). This is an important point because, although self-hypnosis is not one of the methods contained in this book, there is no strict demarcation between self-hypnosis and relaxation. Pitfall number 9 in Chapter 18 (p. 171) is relevant to this discussion.

RATIONALE

AT is not underpinned by any theory; rather, it is based on principles of suggestion. It is claimed that the recited phrases, following many repetitions, create a light trance which increases the suggestibility of the participant and helps to promote a natural healing process. Possible explanations include the Freudian notion of lowered mental defences allowing communication with the interior. The method also has cognitive and physiological elements: cognitive ones in its attention-focusing phrases, and physiological in the induced sensations of warmth which associate it with the parasympathetic branch of the autonomic nervous system, and a reduction of physiological arousal. The sensations of warmth are also associated with an improved blood flow which brings with it an augmented supply of oxygen. This can benefit a variety of conditions including rehabilitation following injury and recovery from surgery as well as providing relief from stress and anxiety.

In their search for an underlying mechanism, Henry et al (1993) suggest that AT may be re-establishing a balance between the sympathetic and parasympathetic systems.

DESCRIPTION

Autogenic training teaches the body and the mind to relax. It is based on four requirements.

1. Reduced external stimulation, i.e. a quiet environment with dim lighting.
2. An attitude of passive concentration, described in the booklet advertising the autogenic training course as a state of mind which is relaxed, non-striving and unconcerned with the end product. This means not forcing any change, rather, just letting the exercise work (Achterberg 1985); an 'allowing' rather than a 'doing' (Rosa 1976). If, while engaged in passive concentration, distracting thoughts enter the mind, they can be ignored or gently dismissed. Thoughts which carry insightful images, however, can be seen as a valuable product of the exercise. Passive concentration may be said to exist in other approaches such as meditation and some forms of progressive relaxation.
3. The repetition of relaxation-inducing phrases based on six main themes:
   a. heaviness in the arms and legs
   b. warmth in the arms and legs
   c. calm and regular heartbeat
   d. calm breathing
   e. warm solar plexus
   f. cool forehead.

These phrases are repeated to emphasize their effect and to draw the client's attention away from the external environment. Suggestions of heaviness can be intensified by images of lead, while those of warmth can be deepened by images of sunshine or warm water (Rosa 1976). The first two themes are frequently presented on their own (by clinicians and researchers alike), although it is not known at what cost to the overall relaxation effect (Lichstein 1988).

4. Mental contact with the body part to which the phrase refers.

Central to AT is the principle of client control: the trainer describes the method, but it is the trainee who carries it out. To reinforce this notion, the phrases are styled in the first person. The instructor reads the relevant phrase using a slow and soothing tone and the trainee repeats it mentally or vocally three times. About 30 seconds are assigned to each phrase and a further 35–40 seconds for continued focusing of attention by the trainee. After working through the allotted phrases a cancellation procedure is carried out as a safeguard against any deep-trance state. The whole routine is then repeated three times. This marks the end of the lesson and leads into a discussion and debriefing session for which the trainees are seated (see Ch. 2, p. 17).

Schultz & Luthe (1969) worked slowly through the schedule, taking 6 months to complete the instruction. The need to save time and money has, however, led to reductions in length, and now the full programme is presented in a few weeks.

The phrases themselves may be interspersed with relevant messages, for example, 'I feel at peace' or 'I am relaxed', as in the following version which is adapted from the works of Kermani (1990) and Lichstein (1988).

PROCEDURE

INTRODUCTORY TALK TO TRAINEES

A short description prepares the trainees who should be seated:

> Autogenic training has been shown to help people overcome feelings of anxiety. It creates a state of extreme calmness which helps people to be in touch with deeper parts of their mind. The mind becomes more receptive than normally. Individuals can suggest changes to themselves which they feel may enhance their lives.

The method consists of short phrases describing sensations of heaviness and warmth in the limbs. I'll be reading them out and as I do I'd like you to focus your attention on each in turn, repeating the phrase three times under your breath.

An important feature of this approach is that you should feel passive and casual about it; avoid forcing any response to occur. Let the sensations of heaviness and warmth arise on their own, rather than making an effort to bring them about. If other thoughts intrude, just bring your attention back to the phrase; focusing on it will help to weaken their hold on you.

I'd like you now to settle into a relaxed position (lying or reclining) for the exercises ... please close your eyes ... imagine yourself in a place that makes you feel relaxed ... perhaps a warm, sunny meadow...

THE EXERCISES

The trainer proceeds with a short scanning procedure designed to relax the body; it is presented at the beginning of each lesson (Ch. 7, p. 64).

Lesson 1

Begin with the dominant arm.

I feel at peace.
My right arm is heavy.
My right arm is heavy.
I feel at peace.
My right arm is heavy.
My right arm is heavy.

The trainer asks participants to continue to think about the heaviness in their right arm as they lie in the sunny meadow. After a few minutes the trainer carries out the cancellation procedure:

When you are ready, slowly allow yourself to become aware of the room. Open your eyes. Let them scan the interior of the room. Make a few fists. Bend and stretch your limbs. Tell yourself you are now feeling fresh and alert.

This is followed by the first of three repeats of the same routine. When these come to an end there is a discussion and debriefing session with the participants in a seated position (Ch. 2, p. 17).

Lesson 2

I feel at peace.
My left arm is heavy.
My left arm is heavy.
I feel at peace.
My left arm is heavy.
My left arm is heavy.

Think of your arm being heavy as lead.

Lesson 3

I feel at peace.
Both my arms are heavy.
Both my arms are heavy.
I feel at peace.
Both my arms are heavy.
Both my arms are heavy.

See yourself lying in the meadow, with your arms resting heavily on the lush grass.

Lesson 4

I feel at peace.
My right leg is heavy.
My right leg is heavy.
I feel at peace.
My right leg is heavy.
My right leg is heavy.

Think of your leg being heavy as lead.

Lesson 5

I feel at peace.
My left leg is heavy.
My left leg is heavy.
I feel at peace.
My left leg is heavy.
My left leg is heavy.

Lesson 6

I feel at peace.
Both my legs are heavy.
Both my legs are heavy.
I feel at peace.
Both my legs are heavy.
Both my legs are heavy.

Feel your legs sinking into the ground.

Lesson 7

> I feel at peace.
> My arms and legs are heavy.
> My arms and legs are heavy.
> I feel at peace.
> My arms and legs are heavy.
> My arms and legs are heavy.

Continue to focus on the feeling of heaviness in your arms and legs, as you imagine yourself lying in a sunny meadow.

Lessons 8–14

These are similar to Lessons 1–7, but warmth is substituted for heaviness. The effect can be augmented by images of the sun's warmth.

Lesson 15

> I feel at peace.
> My arms and legs are heavy and warm.
> My heartbeat is calm and regular.
> My heartbeat is calm and regular.
> I feel at peace.
> My heartbeat is calm and regular.
> My heartbeat is calm and regular.

Lesson 16

> I feel at peace.
> My arms and legs are heavy and warm.
> My heartbeat is calm and regular.
> My breathing is calm.
> My breathing is calm.
> I feel at peace.
> My breathing is calm.
> My breathing is calm.

Lesson 17

The abdomen phrases are omitted for people with any kind of abdominal inflammation.

> I feel at peace.
> My arms and legs are heavy and warm.
> My heartbeat is calm and regular.
> My breathing is calm.
> My abdomen is warm.
> My abdomen is warm.
> I feel at peace.
> My abdomen is warm.
> My abdomen is warm.

Lesson 18

> I feel at peace.
> My arms and legs are heavy and warm.
> My heartbeat is calm and regular.
> My breathing is calm.
> My abdomen is warm.
> My forehead is cool.
> My forehead is cool.
> I feel at peace.
> My forehead is cool.
> My forehead is cool.

Images of cool air streams may be created to reinforce the feeling of a cool forehead (Samuels & Samuels 1975).

HOME PRACTICE

Written handouts enable trainees to practise at home. This home practice is essential and builds up the skill of being able to respond readily to the phrases. Eventually, a single key phrase will have the capacity to switch on total relaxation.

Exponents insist that the six basic phrases remain unchanged. The choice of imagery, however, is left to the participant; a sunny beach, a heated bath, or a favourite chair in front of a log fire may be used as alternatives to the warm meadow scene. Having chosen her scene, however, the participant should remain with it throughout the training period.

During the trance state the trainee may introduce self-affirming statements or affirmations. These can express confirmations of her worth or may reinforce her determination to make certain changes in her behaviour. The phrases 'I feel at peace', 'I am relaxed' or 'I feel calm' are examples of affirmations for people who want to reduce their stress levels. Such personal maxims are most effective when kept short, simple and when expressed in the first person and in the present tense. Other examples, adapted from Davis et al (2000), are:

- I believe in myself (for those lacking in confidence).
- I have control over what I eat (for compulsive eaters).

- Smoking is an unhealthy habit (for people who wish to quit smoking).
- My mind is quiet and serene (for anxious individuals).

Certain physiological problems can be addressed through 'organ-specific formulae' such as:

- My throat is cool (for a troublesome cough).
- My feet are warm (for a tendency to blush).

The trainee will incorporate particular phrases according to her personal requirements. AT should not, however, be viewed as a substitute for medical attention.

OTHER AT EXERCISES

AT also includes meditative exercises which involve colours, objects, concepts and personalities.

Other exercises known as 'advanced' belong to an area described as therapy rather than training, and are beyond the scope of this book.

EVIDENCE OF EFFECTIVENESS

Kanji & Ernst (2000) have reviewed the evidence and in their findings they suggest that AT does reduce stress and anxiety. Medium to large clinical effects have been found after treatment with AT and these tend to be stable at follow-up and to exceed placebo effects (Stetter & Kupper 2002). The meta-analysis of Stetter & Kupper shows that benefit has been found in psychological disorders such as anxiety, mild to medium depression and functional sleep disorders. Positive effects have also been observed in psychosomatic disorders such as tension headache, migraine, essential hypertension, coronary heart disease, asthma, Raynaud's disease and certain kinds of pain.

In the case of tension headache, Spinhoven et al (1992) demonstrated a significant reduction in its incidence among people receiving AT and self-hypnosis, compared with people on a waiting list. This result could not have been due to any greater effectiveness of self-hypnosis, since the same researchers also compared AT with self-hypnosis and found them to be of equal efficacy. In the case of asthma sufferers, significantly greater benefit was found in a group practising AT than in

supportive group therapy with which it was compared (Henry et al 1993).

Kanji (2000) studied the effectiveness of AT as a pain-reliever in conditions such as headaches, migraines, childbirth, back pain, heart pain and cancer pain, and found the approach to be useful. This researcher proposed that AT be introduced into the treatment of a wide range of pain-allied disorders where it could help to reduce the need for analgesic drugs.

In the field of anxiety disorders AT has been compared with progressive relaxation and found to be significantly superior in terms of EMG decreases and effects on symptoms (Takaishi 2000). A further finding from this study indicated that the patients judged AT easier to carry out than progressive relaxation. This suggests that an approach which involves passive listening, i.e. AT, may be a more effective route to relaxation than one which demands active concentration, i.e. progressive relaxation, for people experiencing anxiety-related disorders.

Not all results, however, are positive and many are equivocal. Weighing the evidence comparing the effectiveness of AT with that of other approaches, Stetter & Kupper (2002) find AT to be about equal. This accords with Lichstein's view that AT phrases seem to carry no more power as relaxants than phrases employed in other relaxation approaches (Lichstein 1988).

Results should be viewed with caution since the methodological quality of the individual studies varies widely (Stetter & Kupper 2002). Despite such drawbacks, however, it can be said that AT is an effective relaxation technique in most conditions associated with stress, either as a preventive measure or as an adjunct to conventional treatment (Broms 1999).

AT also has the advantage of being available to individuals experiencing conditions where movement is painful, such as arthritis, and conditions where movement is not possible, such as paralysis.

PITFALLS OF AUTOGENIC TRAINING

1. The phrase inducing abdominal warmth should be deleted for people suffering from abdominal inflammation (Rosa 1976).

2. AT is not suitable for children under 5 years of age nor for people lacking motivation.

3. Trainees should be advised to keep their personal formulae realistic. Creating unattainable goals will only lead to disappointment.

4. In the unlikely event of the phrases causing distress, the messages of heaviness and warmth can be reversed, i.e. the limbs can be made to feel light and cool; alternatively, the procedure can be stopped.

The pitfalls of visualization (Ch. 18) are also relevant (p. 170); points 1, 2 and 9 particularly, should be noted.

Further reading

Bird J, Pinch C 2002 Autogenic therapy: self-help for mind and body. Newleaf, Ireland

Kermani K S 1996 Autogenic training. Souvenir Press, London

Lichstein K L 1988 Clinical relaxation strategies. John Wiley, New York

Rosa K R 1976 Autogenic training. Victor Gollancz, London

Chapter 20

Meditation

INTRODUCTION

The word 'meditation' is used to describe varied states of inner stillness. It is also used to describe different methods of attaining those states. Again, the many schools of meditation all have their own interpretation. Thus, with no universally agreed meaning, attempts to define the word founder. Common to all interpretations, however, is the concept of emptying the mind of thought, that is, letting go the preoccupations that make up the mind's chatter.

If there is a general aim in meditation, it might be described as non-attachment, although some writers such as Fontana (1991) feel that to have an aim at all tends to destroy the result since any kind of goal-setting calls on rational powers and left-brain activity (Ch. 17, p. 150).

Meditation could perhaps, therefore, be seen as an opening of the self to reveal its inner world, while at the same time conveying no hint of determination since that would be alien to the meditative state.

People come to meditation for many reasons:

- to find peace
- to achieve awareness
- to gain enlightenment
- to find themselves
- to empty the mind
- to experience true reality.

Since relaxation is one of the effects of all these pursuits, meditation is a relevant topic for inclusion in a book such as this.

Originating in the East, meditation is an integral part of the Hindu, Taoist and Buddhist religions. In the West versions have been created which are simpler, and these have, for the most part, evolved from Zen and Yoga. The material presented here is of a non-religious form and comes from a variety of modern sources, notably the work of Fontana (1991, 1992).

It has been pointed out that meditation is both a state and a method. As a state, it is one in which the mind is stilled and listening to itself. The meditator is relaxed but at the same time alert.

As a method, it consists of focusing attention on a chosen stimulus. This concentration is sustained but effortless and has the effect of detaching the meditator from external life events on the one hand and from her own mental activity on the other. Thoughts may enter her head, but instead of examining their content, she allows them to drift away.

This attitude has been described as one of passive concentration, and it implies that the meditator has a relaxed attitude while, at the same time, giving attention of the kind that is without criticism or judgement. Mental functions, such as thinking and evaluating, are inappropriate since they are processed by the left brain; rather, the meditator should cultivate what in Zen is called a 'don't know mind', that is, a mind which is open and receptive to new, undreamed-of possibilities. Past and future associations are shed. The mind is emptied of all thought save awareness of the stimulus.

In common with hypnosis and daydreaming, meditation is an altered state of consciousness. Fontana (1991) distinguishes it from other altered states, seeing it rather as a rediscovery of normal consciousness since it takes the individual to the core of the self.

The meditator does not fall into a trance, become drowsy or surrender control; on the contrary, she is in a state of heightened awareness, alert, aware of her surroundings and securely focused on the present moment.

Passive concentration, referred to above, is also a feature of autogenic training and receptive visualization, although not of programmed visualization which, as it is involved with the achievement of goals, is essentially a left brain thinking activity and therefore remote from meditation. However, to say that meditation excludes the analytical thinking process does not imply that meditators consider left-brain activity to be of lesser value: analytical thinking is an essential human function. But its tendency generally to dominate mental activity has the effect of devaluing its counterpart, the imagination. Meditation enables the individual to redress the balance.

RATIONALE

It is claimed that meditation helps to quieten the mind and reduce the effect of stressful thoughts. It can thus contribute to a state of relaxation.

A number of theories have been put forward to account for the effect of meditation on the individual. Of these, Banquet's (1973) shift in hemispheric dominance is widely accepted. His research suggests that during meditation the left cerebral hemisphere loses its dominance, resulting in a more influential right hemisphere than occurs in everyday life. As a result, linear, verbal thinking plays a less prominent part, allowing intuitive, wordless thinking to express itself. By this means the individual may come to know and understand herself better and acquire a new peace of mind.

BENEFITS OF MEDITATION

Devotees of meditation claim that they benefit greatly from its practice. These are some of the advantages:

- A better understanding of the self is achieved through meditation. That is, through meditation the individual becomes more aware of herself and more receptive to the insights that arise from her deeper being.
- A new sense of relaxation and inner peace can be derived from meditation.
- The process itself promotes a clearer mind and improved powers of concentration. These extend outside the meditation session.
- The individual, by discovering her inner self, is able to live more in harmony with herself.
- By developing a sense of detachment, the individual comes to accept that many of her unpleasant emotional reactions are no more than short-lived bodily sensations created by her thoughts.

- The emphasis on self-awareness helps the individual to live in the present and to value the here-and-now. When the mind is concentrated in the moment, it becomes keenly alert.

A PROCEDURE FOR MEDITATION

INTRODUCTORY REMARKS TO THE NOVICE MEDITATOR

A few words describing the procedure are required before starting the first session.

> Meditation is an ancient method of quietening the mind. The method you are about to experience is a non-religious form. It is concerned with focusing the attention on different phenomena such as the breath, a visual object or a repeated phrase. The effect of the meditation will be to make you feel very peaceful. At no time will you lose consciousness or be controlled by any outside force. The state you reach will be entirely created by you. It is best to come to meditation without expectations; rather, to have an attitude which makes you content to be in tune with yourself.

A MEDITATION SESSION

A session may be seen to have four components:

1. attention to position
2. a winding-down procedure
3. concentration on a chosen stimulus
4. return to everyday activity.

Attention to position

In an environment that is quiet and warm, the meditator takes up a sitting or a lying position. Sitting is preferred since some people tend to fall asleep when lying down. The individual may sit in a straight-backed chair, sit cross-legged on a cushion on the floor, or take up the lotus position (cross-legged with each foot resting on the opposite thigh). This position can be very uncomfortable for people who are not used to it; even in the East it has never been obligatory if the novice found it unbearable.

Whichever sitting position is chosen, the hands rest on the thighs, with the fingers gently curled or arranged in traditional symbolic postures. The head should be held in a relaxed position directly above the spinal column to release the neck muscles from strain while the eyes may be closed or slightly open.

Winding–down procedure

Participants are asked to direct their thoughts inwards.

The meditation session is preceded by a check for muscle tension, i.e. each participant checks all her muscle groups to make sure they are as relaxed as possible. It is often referred to as scanning and may be introduced in the following way:

> I am going to ask you to check that your muscles are as relaxed as possible. Starting with your feet, notice any tension … then move up to your ankles, shifting them slightly if they are not relaxed … now your legs … and your hips … settle them into the chair or the floor. Continue up through your body to your shoulders, letting them drop down. Allow your arms to fall comfortably, with your fingers free of tension. And now your head: relax your jaw and let your tongue rest in your mouth … let all the muscles in your face feel smoothed out. Allow yourself to unwind, and as you unwind, feel in tune with yourself … listening to yourself … just being you … experiencing what it is to be you … being aware how it feels, without delving into reasons, explanations or even words…

Irritating sounds or bodily discomfort may interrupt the meditation. Davis et al (2000) suggest 'softening' them by purposely giving them attention for a few moments instead of pretending that they do not exist.

Concentrating on a chosen stimulus

'All meditations are built upon … concentration and tranquillity' (Fontana 1992). The individual quietly focuses attention on the chosen stimulus which may take the form of breath watching, gazing at a visual object or chanting a mantra. The purpose of the stimulus is to hold the attention of the participant.

This may be difficult at first since the mind is used to being engaged in a constant stream of images, memories and associations, all competing with one another. It will not help the individual to fight these distractions, but if she can accept their presence and continue her concentration on the stimulus, they will become weaker. Some people find it useful to regard intruding thoughts as clouds drifting by, or leaves floating down a stream. The attention is then gently brought back to the item under focus.

The result of this meditation may be nothing more than a respite from stress for the individual. On the other hand, as the focused mind enters a state of clarity and tranquillity, a deeper part of the self may be reached whereby new insight is gained (Fontana 1991).

Any hint of depersonalization may be counteracted by a process known as 'grounding' or bringing the individual back to the here-and-now. It involves encouraging the meditator to return her attention to some form of body awareness. Fontana (1991) suggests concentrating on the breathing, while Titlebaum (1988) emphasizes the value of feeling the ground. The following passage is adapted from Titlebaum (1988):

> Be aware of the ground beneath you. Feel it taking the weight of your body. Feel it supporting you. Notice the parts of your body which touch the ground or are in contact with the chair, if you are sitting. Concentrate on the sensations you are getting from these contact points and feel safely tethered to the ground.

The duration of the session should depend on the experience of the meditator; 5 minutes is considered enough for the novice, 15–20 minutes for the experienced practitioner.

Return to everyday activity

The return to everyday activity, also known as arousal or termination, is a sequence which brings the meditation to a close:

> When you are ready, let your meditation come to an end. If your eyes are open, remove your gaze from the point of focus. If your eyes are closed, allow the point of focus to fade until it disappears. Let it go with a feeling of gratitude towards it. Then turn your attention to your breathing, slowly counting three or four natural breaths.
>
> To help your muscles regain their tone, try slowly moving the body round in small circles before you get up. A few gentle stretches will also enliven the muscles.

Home practice

Regular practice enhances the benefits gained from meditation. Lichstein (1988), reviewing the evidence, refers to numerous studies which indicate a direct association between the number of hours spent practising and the beneficial effects of meditation.

FOCAL POINTS FOR MEDITATION

Items on which the attention may be focused cover a wide range of objects, sounds and other phenomena. Included in this section are the following:

- the breath
- visual objects, e.g. circle, mandala, candle, china bowl
- parts of the body, e.g. space between the eyes, crown of the head, big toe
- mantras.

Concentration on the breath is mentioned first for a number of reasons (Fontana 1991):

- it is constantly available
- it has a rhythmical quality
- it is directly linked to the autonomic system
- it symbolizes the life force.

THE BREATH

The practice of counting the breaths, with one count for every outbreath, is commonly used as a stimulus to hold the attention. On reaching the count of 10, the meditator reverts to 'one' again, and continues the process for 5 minutes. The breaths should be natural and unhurried. Other forms of breathing meditation consist of focusing the attention on parts of the body involved in respiration such as the tip of the nose or the moving abdomen.

The tip of the nose

In the passage below the meditator concentrates on the tip of her nose. It is assumed that she has already gone through a winding-down procedure (see above). Plenty of time should be allowed between the sentences.

Let your attention focus on your breathing and in particular, on the tip of your nose, that curved piece of cartilage that separates your nostrils. If you like, touch it with your fingertips to increase your awareness of it ... then concentrate on the feeling of air passing from the outside into your nostrils ... notice how cool it is ... notice also the warmth and moistness of the air that leaves your nostrils ... allow your breathing rhythm to be completely natural as you focus your attention on the tip of your nose ... feel the sensation of air being drawn in ... sweeping into your nostrils and, in its own time, passing out again ... if outside thoughts intrude, gently return to the sensation at the tip of the nose ... continue to focus your attention on that point ... feel your senses converging on that one spot.

On another occasion the meditator might wish to adopt a different focus as in the next passage.

The moving abdomen

Here, a counting procedure is combined with focusing attention on the abdomen.

Gently turn your attention to your breathing. Begin by noticing it in a general kind of way, then slowly bring your mind to focus on the movement of your abdomen ... keep your attention fixed on the movement of your abdomen ... swelling as the air is breathed in and sinking as it is breathed out ... allow the air to pass in and out quite naturally while you are concentrating on the abdominal movement. Do not try to influence the breathing rhythm but let yourself flow with it ... if your mind wanders, gently bring it back to the swelling and sinking abdomen ... counting the breaths helps to hold the attention ... one count for every breath out ... and when you get to 10 or lose count, start again. Please continue on your own.

VISUAL OBJECT

Visual concentration on an object, sometimes referred to as gaze meditation, offers varied possibilities. Almost any object can become the focus of attention but typically the object is chosen for its symbolic value or its neutral associations: a geometric shape, a candle or a flower all have these characteristics.

The circle

A circle has the following symbolic qualities:

- It has substance in that it may be solid.
- It has emptiness in that there may be nothing inside it.
- It has motion in that it can roll and spin.
- It has stillness in that it may come to rest.
- It has wholeness by virtue of enclosing all its parts within it.
- It has continuity in that any point along its circumference is both the end and the beginning.

If a circle is chosen as an object for meditation, the instructing meditator may produce one by drawing a thickedged ring about 30 cm (1 foot) in diameter, emphasizing the centre with a dot, and hanging it on the wall. It should be level with the eyes of the seated participant, who positions herself at a comfortable distance from it (Fontana 1991).

The following script can then be used.

Let your gaze fall on the centre of the circle and then remain there ... consider the circle simply as a shape and let it speak to you in intuitive terms rather than in words ... try to keep your gaze focused on the centre while at the same time absorbing the whole image ... do not examine it, but feel yourself experiencing it ... maintain the visual experience without reacting to it ... feel the image extending around your point of focus ... be aware of its extremities as your mind flows from the centre to the edges and from the edges to the centre ... if your attention should wander, gently bring it back to the centre point ... spend several minutes gazing at the image.

The mandala and the yantra

These serve a sacred purpose in the Buddhist religion. Their complexity, beauty and harmony enrich their symbolic quality and make them the supreme focal object for visual meditation. Although created for use by devotees, they can be meditated on at any philosophical level, and examples are shown in Figures 20.1 and 20.2. The mandala generally contains representations of living things while the yantra is predominantly geometric.

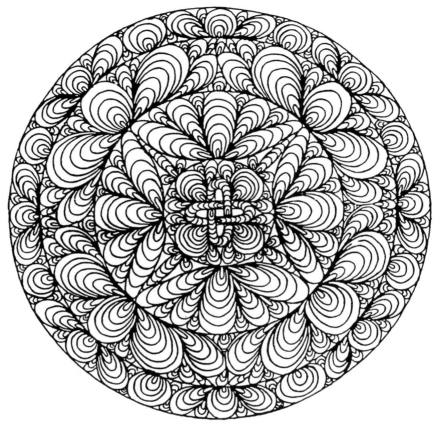

Figure 20.1 A mandala. Reproduced from The Stream of Consciousness by Pope & Singer (1978) with permission from Plenum Publications.

Both enclose symbolic motifs arranged in concentric rings around a clearly defined central point. This point symbolizes the inner self on the one hand and divine consciousness on the other, while the enclosing circles represent the cycle of life and the notion of Nature forever renewing herself. Thus the mandala/yantra stands for the personal as well as the transpersonal, for change within permanence, for life both in the present and in eternity, while affirming the fundamental unity of all things.

The candle

As mentioned above, the visual image can be used in different ways to clear the mind of thought. For instance, while the individual is gazing at the object, she can intermittently close her eyes and allow the image to recreate itself in her mind, as in the following meditation on a candle burning in a darkened room:

> Let the lighted candle hold your attention ... settle your eyes on the upper part of the wax column rather than the flame itself ... sit without moving while you gaze at it ... focus on it in a relaxed but constant way, letting the image fill your mind ... continue for at least a minute ... Now close your eyes. Notice that the image of the candle prints itself in the darkness ... hold the shape in your mind's eye, accepting any change of colour ... if it slips to one side, gently bring it back ... continue to focus on it until it fades ... then open your eyes and resume your gaze on the candle ... continue, repeating the sequence in silence for several minutes.

The image that appears behind the closed eyes is known as the 'after-image' (see Box 20.1).

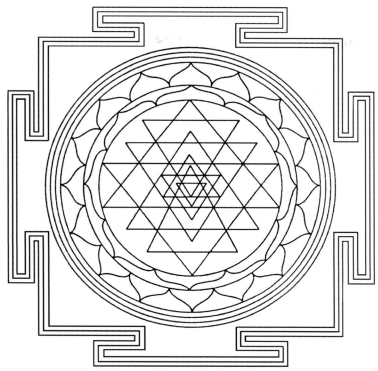

Figure 20.2   A yantra. Reproduced from The Elements of Meditation by Fontana (1991) with permission from Element Books.

When the gaze is fixed on a particular point for about a minute and the eyes are subsequently closed, the phenomenon of the after-image occurs. This is the negative representation of the object stared at. It immediately begins to fade and after about 20 seconds or so has disappeared. It is a physiological reaction which occurs when the retinal cells get fatigued. Experiencing the after-image is quite different from recreating forms in the imagination, a practice which belongs more to visualization than to meditation.

If the meditator is in doubt as to what she is seeing behind her closed lids, there are two questions she can ask herself:

1. Does the image fade or disappear within 20 seconds? If so, it is likely to be an after-image.
2. Can she scan the image, i.e. trace its outlines? If every time she moves her eyes to trace the outline the image moves too, it is behaving like an after-image (Samuels & Samuels 1975).

A china bowl

Certain objects lend themselves to a more exploratory approach. A flower or a piece of porcelain fall into this category. For instance, Davis et al (2000) suggest a china bowl:

> Settle your gaze on the object ... take it all in ... after a few moments, allow your eyes to travel over the object, tracing its lines ... noticing its colours ... its decoration ... and the way it glistens ... do not dwell on who made it, how or for what purpose, but see it simply as a shape ... experience its visual qualities as if you were seeing it for the first time ... if your mind wanders, gently bring it back to the object...

PARTS OF THE BODY

Other body parts as well as the breathing organs can be used to provide a focus of attention. This kind of meditation is a feature of yoga, where energy centres (chakras) are represented by the base of the spine, the lower abdomen, the navel, the heart, the throat, the space between the eyebrows and the crown of the head. After meditating on the sites in this order, the physical energies are said to be transformed into spiritual energies.

Yoga is a separate subject, and no attempt is made here to present it. However, the symbolic nature of the chakras makes them suitable sites for meditations outside yoga. Two examples are given here: the space between the eyebrows and the crown of the head.

The space between the eyebrows

Behind closed lids, let your eyes turn upwards and settle on the space between your eyebrows ... relate to it ... recognize its closeness to your brain ... feel its central position ... imagine viewing it from the outside ... then, imagine viewing it from the inside ... continue to focus on that one spot ... feel drawn to it ... and consider that, as the space between your eyebrows is part of you, so you are part of that space.

(Pause)

If outside thoughts drift into your mind, mentally blow them away and return to your point of focus ... to the space between your eyebrows.

The crown of the head

With your eyes closed, focus your attention on the crown of your head, concentrating on it in a passive way ... let your inner eye be drawn to it and held there ... see it from the outside, noticing how it appears ... then imagine it from the inside, from under the dome of your head...

(Pause)

Symbolically as well as literally, it represents the highest part of you ... if thoughts intrude, let them be carried away ... let them drift away from you as you gently return your attention to the crown of your head ... feel yourself identifying with it ... experiencing it ... feel yourself uniting with all that is highest within you.

On a simpler level, any part of the body can serve as the stimulus, for example, the big toe.

The big toe

With your eyes closed, your legs uncrossed and your muscles relaxed, draw your attention to your right big toe. See it in your mind's eye ... move it gently to make its presence felt ... notice how it feels when you move it ... focus on the sensations you get from bending and stretching it ... be aware of the feel of the sock or stocking over it, or of the shoe restricting it ... think of it carrying the full weight of the body ... think of its strength as well as its mobility ... if unwanted thoughts intrude, gently bring your attention back to the toe ... focusing on the toe...

MANTRAS

A mantra is a verbal stimulus which can be used to concentrate the attention. Traditionally it embodies an ancient, sacred truth whose meaning may reveal itself to the meditator during the process of concentration. A well-known example is the Sanskrit word 'om' which is said to represent the primal sound. Pronounced like 'home' without the 'h' (Smith & Wilks 1988), the sound can be intensified by stretching the syllable to form a ... oo ... mmmm (Fontana 1991). It is the *sound* of the mantra that has particular value for the novice meditator, although its meaning may also be contemplated at a later stage. The following piece is adapted from a passage in Fontana (1991):

Breathe in gently and as you let the air out, recite the word om: a ... oo ... mmmm. Feel the sounds vibrating within your body: feel the 'a' ringing in your belly, feel the 'oo' resonating in your chest and the 'mmmm' resounding in the bones of your skull ... let these sounds provide a focus for your attention ... link them into your natural breathing rhythm ... keep the breathing calm and slow and avoid any inclination to deepen it ... after 10 breaths, gradually reduce the volume of the sound until the word is spoken under your breath ... lower it further ... keep your attention focused on the mantra ... eventually, you will come to a point where your lips cease to move and the syllables lose their form so that you are left with just an idea ... feel it clinging to your mind ... united with it ... if thoughts intrude, turn them into puffs of smoke and let them be blown away.

Many other sounds or words can act as mantras, e.g. 'peace', 'harmony', 'calmness', or phrases such as 'God is love' and 'here-and-now'. It does not matter if the word has a meaning, since constantly reciting it will tend to divest it of that meaning, although the word may still retain its aura. It is advisable, however, to choose a word that has no emotional associations for the user, and one that is unlikely to stir up her thoughts. While the main purpose of the mantra is to hold the meditator's attention, its rhythmic repetition also has a soothing effect.

On the other hand, a mantra may be picked expressly *for* its meaning. In this kind of meditation the mantra is not reflected on philosophically so much as experienced. It is identified with, rather than analysed.

Lichstein (1988) compares mantra chanting with dwelling on the muscles in progressive relaxation (Ch. 4) and to the silent recitation of phrases in autogenic training (Ch. 19) and points out that in addition to their inherent relaxation properties, they all share the capacity to divert the attention from stressful thoughts.

Transcendental meditation

An approach which sets great store by the mantra is transcendental meditation (TM). Its central feature is the contemplation and repetition of a Sanskrit mantra bestowed by Maharishi Mahesh Yogi who brought the movement to the West in 1959. As well as gathering many disciples, TM attracted a great deal of research: from several hundred studies it emerged that TM created significant physiological changes associated with relaxation. However, lack of controls and the use of self-selected (volunteer) participants weakened the validity of some of these findings.

Proponents of TM insist on the mantra being chosen with ceremony and in secrecy by a master teacher, although this practice has not been shown to be any more effective than one which uses simple words (Benson 1976).

EVIDENCE OF EFFECTIVENESS

Electroencephalographic changes during meditation suggest a state of decreased arousal in the cerebral cortex. This supports the view that mental activity is reduced (Fenwick 1987). Certainly, meditation has been found effective in reducing tension, and as Lichstein (1988) points out, can often lead to deep states of physiological and phenomenological relaxation. However, it is unclear how much more effective it is than any other relaxation practice. Research findings are inconsistent; some point to the superior benefit of meditation, while others, such as that of Holmes et al (1983), are unable to show that meditation is any more effective at lowering physiological arousal than ordinary rest.

There is no Cochrane review on meditation at the present time (Cantor 2003). Existing research revolves mainly around TM which has been studied extensively and in a variety of populations, often comparing the approach with progressive relaxation (Cantor 2003). A series of trials has been conducted in the area of hypertension showing positive effects from TM. One of these, a study of older African Americans, compared TM with progressive relaxation and a control group who were given education. Reductions of both systolic and diastolic blood pressures in the meditation group were found to be significantly greater than those in the progressive relaxation group (Schneider et al 1995). Similarly, Barnes et al (2001) demonstrated significant decreases in systolic blood pressure following a 2-month daily course of TM in a randomized controlled trial of 35 American adolescents. These results are in line with those of a review conducted earlier, which suggested that several cardiovascular risk factors could be reduced by TM (Sharma & Alexander 1996).

Although many of the trials investigating the therapeutic effectiveness of meditation have produced positive results, a high proportion of them are flawed. In the absence of more rigorous testing, Cantor (2003) does not, therefore, find the evidence in favour of meditation to be strong.

The proposition that meditation produces a unique state of consciousness has been put forward, but there is no evidence to support it.

PITFALLS OF MEDITATION

These can be found at the end of the following chapter.

Further reading

Fontana D 1991 The elements of meditation. Element, Shaftesbury

Fontana D 1992 The meditator's handbook: a comprehensive guide to eastern and western meditation techniques. Element, Shaftesbury

Ozaniec N 2003 Teach yourself meditation. Hodder Educational, London

Sivananda Yoga Vedanta Centre 2003 The Sivananda companion to meditation. Gaia Books, London

Chapter 21

Benson's method

CHAPTER CONTENTS

THE RELAXATION RESPONSE

In the 1970s, the physiologist Herbert Benson, who was studying aspects of high blood pressure at Harvard's Thorndike Laboratory, was approached by a group of transcendental meditators who believed that their meditations could lower their blood pressure. Unconvinced, Benson at first discouraged their idea but he later changed his mind. He and his colleagues then began to carry out a series of investigations which revealed that transcendental meditation (TM) was accompanied by marked physiological changes: there were reductions in the heart rate, breathing rate, oxygen consumption, blood lactate levels and, of particular interest to Benson, blood pressure. These changes reflected diminished activity in the sympathetic nervous system.

One study demonstrated drops in systolic and diastolic pressures from group averages of 146 and 93.5 mmHg respectively (borderline high pressure) to 137 and 88.9 mmHg (within normal range), following several weeks of practising TM. Oxygen consumption was found to be reduced by 10–20% within the first 3 minutes of meditation. (It is interesting to compare this result with work on the sleeping state where the oxygen consumption was found to be reduced by only 8% and not before the person had been sleeping for 4 or 5 hours.) These were impressive findings, particularly in the case of the blood pressure recordings which were not made during actual periods of meditation. The participants, however, were volunteers who had already applied to join a transcendental meditation course to reduce their blood pressure. This would suggest that their motivation was high.

Extensive study of other meditation practices led Benson to the belief that the above effects were not confined to the practice of TM, but were the result of certain key elements common to all meditation practices. He set out to identify these elements, seeing them as responsible for eliciting what he called 'the relaxation response', or a state of decreased psychophysiological arousal. To Benson (1976), this was 'a natural and innate protective mechanism' that opposed the effects of the stress response. Viewed in these terms, the relaxation response appeared synonymous with parasympathetic nervous activity.

The key elements that Benson (1976) identified were:

- a quiet environment
- a comfortable position
- a mental device such as a word to focus on
- a passive attitude.

THE KEY ELEMENTS

Quiet environment.   In the ideal setting there is an absence of any background stimulus, pleasant or unpleasant.

Comfortable position.   Benson does not insist on any particular position since he feels that discomfort might draw the attention away from the mental device. The meditator should be allowed to choose her own position. She can, however, be too comfortable and tend to fall asleep; the orthodox lotus position (Ch. 20, p. 183) is thought to have been introduced partly to prevent that happening. For the same reason Benson does not recommend a lying position.

Mental device.   Since his studies had shown that TM was not unique in its ability to lower physiological arousal, Benson concluded that any repetitive, monotonous stimulus capable of holding the attention, could fulfil the function of the Sanskrit mantra, i.e. that any emotionally neutral object, sound or other phenomenon could be used as a focal point of attention. Benson chose the word 'one', which has similar qualities of resonance to the primal sound 'om', but he felt the choice of word or words was best made by the individual herself. He refuted the idea that the mantra's meaning added to its effect.

Passive attitude.   Passive acceptance is an essential feature of the approach. A 'let it happen' attitude should be adopted. Benson regards the passive attitude as 'perhaps the most important element in eliciting the relaxation response'. Distracting thoughts may intervene but they should be ignored and the meditator's attention returned to the recited mantra.

RATIONALE

By focusing the attention on a particular object, word or concept in a sustained and effortless way, meditators are able to detach themselves from daily events and induce a mental stillness. This stillness is reflected in reduced physiological responses, that is, diminished activity in the sympathetic nervous system (Benson 1976). Both cognitive and physical elements are present: the first relating to the focusing of attention on the mantra, and the second to the role of the breath. The theory underpinning the method is a unitary one in that the meditation creates a general, integrated calming effect. Although the participant is engaged in the cognitive activity of focusing on the mantra, the effect on the system is global. This led Benson to coin the phrase 'relaxation response'.

PROCEDURE

INTRODUCTORY REMARKS TO PARTICIPANTS

A few words explaining the method are addressed to novices who should be seated.

> The relaxation method you are about to learn is a non-religious version of meditation. It has a very simple form, requiring that you sit comfortably in a quiet place; that you focus your attention on the word 'one' and that you adopt an attitude which is accepting and unconcerned.
>
> These conditions will help you to experience what is called the relaxation response; a state which research shows is associated with reduced physiological activity. That means the heart rate will become slower and the blood pressure will fall.

You'll notice that you feel calmer than usual and the whole sensation will be a pleasant one.

At no time will you lose consciousness or be controlled by an outside force. The state you reach is one which you will have induced in yourself.

INDUCTION

When participants are ready, the induction sequence itself is carried out. The following version is adapted from Benson (1976). The '10 minutes' indicated can be extended to 20 as the meditator becomes more experienced.

Settle comfortably in whatever position you have chosen, and close your eyes. Relax all your muscles, starting with your feet and ending with your face. Feel yourself deeply relaxed.

Notice the rhythm of your breathing. Let the air in through your nose, allowing the breaths to take place quite naturally. Each time you exhale, recite the word 'one' under your breath. Repeat the word slowly every time you breathe out. If thoughts intrude, try to ignore them, and continue repeating the word 'one'.

Avoid any inclination to judge how successful you are being. Keep your attitude passive, and allow relaxation to occur in its own time. Please continue for 10 minutes...

When you are ready to end your meditation, continue to sit quietly for a few minutes with your eyes closed, then for a few minutes longer with them open.

FEATURES OF BENSON'S METHOD

As shown above, the induction is short and simple. Benson writes that his method carries little embellishment. Perhaps he made it too simple; in excluding all but the essentials, he may have overlooked the value of ceremony and ritual, which are important factors for some individuals (Carrington 1984, Lichstein 1988).

In identifying what he considered to be key factors, Benson's purpose was not to create a rival approach, but to devise a standardized technique which could be used in scientific investigation.

Apart from that, his method is very similar to transcendental meditation except that the word 'one' replaces the Sanskrit mantra and the process is entirely secularized (Lichstein 1988).

The emphasis placed on 'passive attitude' recalls the 'passive concentration' of autogenic training (Ch. 19). It is also not far removed from the quiet observation that characterizes progressive relaxation (Ch. 4). It would seem that, underneath their varying procedures, the approaches are saying much the same thing (Lichstein 1988), and that in their psychophysiological effects, they are all evoking the relaxation response.

In common with the authors of other methods, Benson stressed the importance of regular practice, to be carried out once or twice a day. When practising at home, people are urged not to use an alarm, but to guess when it is time to end the meditation.

EVIDENCE OF EFFECTIVENESS

Since 1974 Benson and colleagues have carried out a series of experiments to test the effectiveness of his method, but it has not so far been possible to replicate the marked physiological effects produced in the early studies (Eisenberg et al 1991). However, compared to transcendental meditation, little research has been carried out on Benson's method. What results are available are inconsistent.

Kerr (2000) has critically reviewed the literature and finds that reductions in both psychological and physiological responses to stress have been shown following a course of relaxation response meditation, although greater consistency has been found in the psychological responses. These responses are marked enough to give meditation a role to play, particularly in the field of coronary heart disease and hypertension, where the approach increasingly features in both prevention and treatment (King et al 2002). Among other psychosomatic conditions where benefit has been demonstrated is irritable bowel syndrome. Keefer & Blanchard (2000) found Benson's method moderately effective in a group of 21 men and women with the disorder.

Lichstein (1988) is persuaded that, in his concept of key elements, Benson did in fact discover a truth, but one whose mechanism is far from being understood.

PITFALLS OF MEDITATION

1. Meditation is not suitable for people in acute psychotic states. Nor is it advised in seriously disturbed individuals as it might trigger psychotic episodes. Such people may, however, benefit from other efforts to relax them as they tend to experience high levels of stress (Faulkner & Biddle 1999, Cantor 2003). People suffering from milder forms of mental illness, who wish to practise meditation, should first discuss it with their doctor or psychologist.

2. Meditation should not be used as a substitute for medical treatment. Individuals who may be already receiving medication should inform their doctor of their wish to study meditation since the effects of one may influence the other (McCormack 1992).

3. Although the central idea of meditation is to keep the mind focused and aware, it does occasionally happen that an individual loses the sense of who and where she is, or develops the feeling of being 'outside her body'. These are trance-like states of disorientation and depersonalization. In this event, a grounding strategy similar to the one referred to in Chapter 20 (p. 184) may provide a remedy. Altered states associated with a sound stimulus, e.g. a mantra, are more likely to lead to trance than those associated with other stimuli such as breathing. The instructor can safeguard against disorientation and depersonalization by regularly reminding participants to keep their attention focused on the stimulus (Fontana 1991).

4. Meditation creates an altered state of consciousness. The novice will not know in advance how she will respond. It is therefore recommended that, to begin with, sessions be kept short, that is, 5 minutes in length. This can be increased to 15 or 20 minutes for those with experience but not exceeded, as it is possible to meditate too much and run the risk of getting out of touch with day-to-day life. Benson (1976) reports that none of the participants in his studies displayed ill effects after meditating for 20 minutes twice a day.

5. The breathing meditations in Chapter 20 do not seek to interfere with the natural breathing rate or rhythm. However, the mere request to become aware of the breathing can result in a slight alteration of its rhythm. It is therefore suggested that, before attempting breathing meditations, the reader become familiar with the section on hyperventilation in Chapter 15 (p. 134).

6. Benson (1976) believed that it was better to practise meditation before a meal than directly after it. He considered that the process of digestion, by drawing the blood to the viscera, interfered with the physiological changes associated with meditation, and advised waiting for at least 2 hours after eating. More recent research, investigating the distribution of blood during meditation, supports Benson's view: Bricklin (1990) found that the blood flow to the brain during meditation increased dramatically, rising on average by 65% of its normal volume. It would not, therefore, be constructive to practise meditation at a time when other demands were being made on the vascular system.

7. The lotus position has been referred to as the posture traditionally adopted in the East. This posture, however, was never obligatory even in its country of origin. In the West it may be inadvisable for novices even to attempt it because of the excessive stretching of the joint structures which accompanies it. Sitting cross-legged on a cushion is no less conducive to meditation, and many people practise meditation sitting in a chair.

8. Some meditation may be disturbing if the stimulus object has unpleasant associations. A change of stimulus is therefore indicated.

9. The outcome should not be judged in terms of success or usefulness because these are rational dimensions. Progress is seen in terms of self-discovery rather than achievement (Fontana 1991).

10. Those who expect meditation to be a ready remedy for life's problems may become disillusioned. Meditation should be seen as a way of life, not as a panacea.

11. It is possible for an individual to experience euphoric states in which she believes she has made a profound spiritual discovery. Fontana (1992) advises a cautious approach to the interpretation of material from the inner self.

12. For those who have undergone psychoanalysis, the idea of ignoring their flow of thoughts may not come easily. Benson (1976) reminds us that psychoanalysis trains people to regard their

thoughts as a vital link with the inner self. People who have experienced this form of therapy may have some initial difficulty in learning meditation.

13. Because of individual variation, there will always be some people who gain very little from meditation.

Guidance should be sought from an experienced teacher by those wishing to pursue more advanced forms of meditation since they are beyond the scope of this book.

Further reading

Benson H 1976 The relaxation response. Collins, London

Chapter 22

Cognitive behavioural approaches

INTRODUCTION

Cognitive behaviour therapy (CBT) is an approach which uses a variety of modes of treatment. It seeks to address the client's difficulties from the client's point of view and to equip her with the information and confidence to become an active participant in the management of her condition (Marshall & Turnbull 1996). It thus lends itself to conditions such as anxiety, depression, psychotic disorders, eating disorders, chronic fatigue syndrome and chronic pain and is relevant in many other illnesses and dysfunctions.

DESCRIPTION AND RATIONALE

Its origins lie in cognitive and behaviour theories (Ch. 1). Cognitive theory states that our thoughts rule our feelings and so, they also rule our lives. Faulty patterns of thinking can lead to negative forms of behaviour which may need to be changed. This involves a restructuring of cognitions, i.e. a re-evaluation of the perception of vulnerability or danger, whether we are dealing with full-blown anxiety or day-by-day stress (Beck 1976, Greenberger & Padesky 1995). The cognitive view resembles psychodynamic explanations of behaviour in that irrational thoughts are seen to be interfering with healthy life (Donaghy 2003); their differences, however, are great: whereas psychodynamic theory sees thought processes as available only through unconscious determinants, cognitive theory views them as being readily available to the individual who can challenge them directly and if necessary, modify them (Roth & Fonagy 1996, Donaghy 2003). Cognitive therapy addresses problems in the context of the here-and-now, unlike psychodynamic therapies where life is seen as predetermined by past events which can only be accessed through some kind of analysis.

Cognitive theory views the individual as a self-determining agent in her own life, which means that, when receiving treatment, she needs to feel a degree of control in the management of her condition. This aspect makes the approach particularly applicable in the field of chronic disorder.

Behaviour theory, on the other hand, views human behaviour as a result of environmental conditioning, and when this behaviour is maladaptive, employs methods such as reinforcement, distraction and exposure to modify it. Positive reinforcement is a method for increasing the likelihood of a desired behaviour; negative reinforcement, of extinguishing it. Distraction, i.e. holding the attention elsewhere, can be a useful strategy particularly for people in chronic pain. Exposure, i.e. facing the anxiety-provoking situation itself, can be a useful tool for helping people who experience panic attacks or various forms of social anxiety.

The cognitive behavioural approach combines both theories. It sees thought processes as learned and maintained through reinforcement (Donaghy 2003); and by addressing the interrelationship of thoughts, feelings and behaviour, it creates a unifying philosophy with a strong psychosocial emphasis (Marshall & Turnbull 1996). In the therapy arising out of it, there is an attempt to foster more adaptive thoughts and emotions which, in turn, will influence the individual's behaviour to become more rewarding to that individual and so, help to promote a feeling of well-being.

A contract is drawn up between client and therapist at the outset whereby a limit is set on the duration of treatment and this is respected by both parties. Throughout therapy the relationship between therapist and client is one of collaboration with the client closely involved in drawing up the treatment programme and in the decision-making process. Thus the client is empowered to play a major role. Qualities of warmth, empathy and genuineness in the therapist (Rogers 1961)

will help to draw out the client's fears and heighten the effectiveness of the partnership.

CBT covers a range of therapeutic interventions and so, may be viewed as an approach rather than a treatment. Depending on the nature of the problem and the relevance of the technique, it may provide any of the following:

- education, i.e. advice on diet and exercise as well as information about the disorder and its treatment
- cognitive restructuring, i.e. identifying and challenging maladaptive thought patterns and making negative self-talk more positive
- goal-setting and pacing of activities
- motivational techniques such as diary-keeping
- reinforcing certain behaviours and discouraging others
- skills training to include social skills such as assertiveness
- problem-solving and other coping techniques
- relaxation training and imagery
- rehearsal of feared events and feedback
- graded exposure to feared events
- fitness training such as exercise or other physical activity
- strategies for maintenance of improvement and protection against relapse.

An example of the way in which selected items could form a treatment programme may be found in an article on pain relief (Harding & Watson 2000). The items selected were: education, goal-setting and pacing, fitness, relaxation, reducing pain behaviour, sleep management and relapse self-management.

EVIDENCE OF EFFECTIVENESS

CBT is now the most widely endorsed form of psychological therapy (Rachman 2003) and has wide application in both physical and mental health. Duncan (2003) points out that although cognitive behavioural approaches have featured in both occupational and physiotherapy treatment programmes, relatively few studies so far have been carried out. The research base is, however, growing. Donaghy & Durward (2000) report that systematic reviews have found these approaches to be an effective treatment for mild-to-moderate depression.

Other areas where the effectiveness of CBT has been investigated include social anxiety (Heimberg 2002), chronic fatigue syndrome (Prins et al 2001), psychotic disturbance (Chartered Society of Physiotherapy 1999), low back pain (Johnstone et al 2002) and chronic pain management (Harding & Watson 2000). Pain is an area which has attracted considerable interest: Sinclair et al (1998) demonstrated a significant improvement in terms of psychological well-being and personal coping resources in people experiencing chronic pain following a course of CBT, and Turner and Jensen (1993) found that pain intensity could be reduced by cognitive strategies. Relaxation techniques themselves were also shown to be effective but, as shown by Harkapaa (1991), best when combined with other cognitive behavioural strategies.

The perception of pain and its experience can be mediated by the feelings and beliefs that people hold; social and cultural factors will often determine how much pain an individual will feel or is prepared to tolerate (Bendelow & Williams 1995, Jones & Martin 2003). Research into the perception of pain suggests that too much sympathy can act as a reinforcer, intensifying the pain as experienced by the individual (Keefe 2003); and Tulkin et al (1996) found that perception of pain was reduced and mobility increased when people with musculoskeletal injuries were prevented from talking about their pain.

CBT has been compared with other approaches: Hassenbring et al (1999) found CBT more effective than electromyographic feedback in reducing pain and disability. Donaghy & Durward (2000) in their report found CBT more effective than psychoanalysis or counselling in generalized anxiety disorder; and Gould et al (1995) found that CBT with exposure provided more benefit than drugs treatment in panic disorder. Öst & Breitholtz (2000), on the other hand, comparing CBT with applied relaxation in a study of 36 outpatients with generalized anxiety disorder found no significant differences between the two methods, although both demonstrated large improvements.

Who should be using these techniques? Although CBT is a psychological specialty, many of its techniques are highly accessible to the health care professional, and since health care professionals have been asked to broaden their approach by taking account of psychosocial aspects of assessment and treatment, they will find in cognitive behavioural techniques a means of achieving this (Everett 2003, Johnstone et al 2002).

In summary, CBT helps people to challenge their beliefs and thoughts and to develop positive coping strategies. Insofar as the therapy contributes to a feeling of well-being, it can itself be seen as a relaxation technique: its effect, however, goes far beyond the strict bounds of relaxation.

Further reading

Duncan E A S 2003 Cognitive behavioural therapy in physiotherapy and occupational therapy. In: Everett T, Donaghy M, Feaver S (eds) Interventions for mental health. Butterworth-Heinemann, Oxford, Ch 10

Greenberger D, Padesky C A 1995 Mind over mood. Guilford Press, New York

Gregoris S 2002 Cognitive behaviour therapy. Brunner-Routledge, East Sussex

Hawton K, Salkovskis P, Kirk J, Clark D M (eds) 1996 Cognitive behaviour therapy for psychiatric problems: a practical guide. Oxford University Press, Oxford

SECTION 4

Miscellaneous topics

Chapter 23

'On-the-spot' techniques

CHAPTER CONTENTS

INTRODUCTION

The goal of most methods described in previous chapters has been the induction of deep relaxation: a slowly induced state which allows the individual to lose all tension. In order to achieve this, she must detach herself from environmental stimuli and focus all her attention on the method. This approach is appropriate where total relaxation is required and where the environment is making no current demands on her.

The individual may, however, be looking for a shorter technique which works fast: a strategy to lighten the effect of a stressor suddenly imposed upon her. The aim here is not to release all tension but to lose superfluous tension. Far from being detached from the environment, the individual wants to be fully alert to deal with its challenges. Instead of eliminating stressors, she wants to increase her tolerance of them. What she needs is a technique which can be implemented at a moment's notice, and still allow her to carry on with the task, whatever it might be.

Such an approach goes under a variety of names: instant, emergency, immediate, rapid, quick, all of which carry an appropriate hint of urgency. 'Brief', which sounds more neutral, is used by some practitioners. In the present work, the phrase 'on-the-spot' has been chosen, since, while acknowledging the need of the moment, it also conveys a sense of being equal to the occasion.

Shortened forms of techniques have already been referred to. The rapid relaxation of Öst (1987) is one example (Ch. 8, p. 73), where the individual recites a cue word on exhalation while scanning the body for tension. Mitchell's (1987) 'key movements', which are capable of unlocking the body from tense postures (Ch. 10, p. 88), are another example.

Although the aim of on-the-spot techniques is to lose excess tension, retaining only what is necessary for the task, these techniques are not the same as differential relaxation. Differential relaxation is a principle to be applied throughout the day, regardless of activity. By contrast, on-the-spot techniques are designed to exert a momentary effect in the face of sudden threat.

A variety of methods for inducing relaxation at short notice are presented in this chapter. They are derived from methods already described, being, for the most part, abbreviated versions of them. They work best in individuals who have given the parent method many hours of practice. It is practice that enables the individual to switch on the full effect at short notice. Thus, on-the-spot techniques are shorthand versions of lengthier methods previously learned.

CHARACTERISTICS OF ON-THE-SPOT TECHNIQUES

Lichstein (1988) lists the essentials of such techniques. They need to be:

- portable: short enough and convenient enough to be used in most situations
- unobtrusive: not attracting attention or interrupting ongoing work
- capable of inducing moderate levels of relaxation. The object is not to induce deep relaxation but to enable the individual to carry on with the task, in as relaxed a state as possible.

FACTORS AFFECTING THE SUCCESS OF ON-THE-SPOT TECHNIQUES

Not every strategy is going to succeed every time. A number of factors may influence the outcome.

1. *Situation.* The degree of inherent threat in a situation may vary. Situations of high threat tend to reduce the effectiveness of the technique.

2. *Sensitivity to internal cues.* A person's ability to recognize her own physiological

and psychological cues is important. As stress levels rise, the cues become more pronounced. The earlier she is able to pick them up, the more effective will be the relaxation device that she applies.

3. *Level of skill attained by previous practice.* The capacity to 'switch on' relaxation whenever the individual feels under stress depends to a great extent on the level of skill attained in any one technique. This in turn depends on the amount of home practice that has been carried out.

4. *Personal preference in choice of technique.* Individuals have preferences for some methods over others (Woolfolk & Lehrer 1984, Payne 1989). The method in which a person feels most at ease will be likely to induce greater relaxation than a method which feels alien to her.

5. *Diversionary content of the technique.* Diversion, such as the reciting of a mantra, is said to contribute to the effect of a relaxation device. The stronger the diversionary element, the greater the power of the technique (Lichstein 1988). It is a useful feature where all that is required is a reduction in stress levels, as in the condition of panic. Where successful coping relies on intellectual and verbal skills, distraction is less useful, and a technique which leaves the mind free to focus on the issue is more appropriate.

THE EXERCISES

A technique may be picked from any of the following approaches:

- physical actions
- scanning
- breathing
- cognitive strategies.

PHYSICAL ACTIONS

When under stress the individual tends to close up physically. It is an unconscious reaction to any kind of threat and has the effect of making her feel less exposed. Although the action may not be observable, the muscles involved may nevertheless be minutely contracting. To help release that tension, one of the following manoeuvres could be adopted:

1. key changes
2. posture
3. shaking a sleeve down
4. stretchings.

Key changes

Certain physical actions may serve as keys to unlock body patterns of tension (Mitchell 1987) (Ch. 10, p. 88). The individual may find her personal key in one of the following four actions.

1. Spreading the fingers. The order is:

> Fingers and thumbs long ... hold them there for a moment ... then stop ... let them recoil into a gently curved position.

2. Separating your teeth. The order is:

> Drag your jaw downwards ... feel your jaw hanging down inside your mouth ... then stop ... feel your throat slack, your tongue loose and your lips gently touching.

3. Pulling the shoulders towards the feet.

> Feel a distance growing between your shoulders and your ears ... and, stop pulling ... let your shoulders rest where they are.

4. Pushing the head back.

> With your shoulders pulled down, lift your head; carry it up and back, keeping your chin pointing towards your feet. Stop. The resulting position should feel comfortable.

Posture

A mental impression of being one's full height promotes a sense of ease and confidence. Reminders are contained in phrases such as:

- think 'tall'
- think 'up'.

The second item is drawn from the Alexander technique (Ch. 11, p. 94).

Shaking a sleeve down

This action loosens the muscles in the arm and shoulder and has the added advantage of appearing a quite natural thing to do.

Stretchings

Musculoskeletal benefit is derived from stretchings (Ch. 13). In the context of on-the-spot relaxation, they are aimed at structures which have been held in one position for some length of time, such as the spinal joints during long-distance motoring. A few examples appear below:

- trunk twisting (Fig. 13.14)
- back arching (Fig. 13.15)
- crouching (Fig. 13.16).

Other stretching exercises may be found in Chapter 13.

SCANNING

Scanning is a shortened version of passive relaxation. It involves a brief tour of the body during which the participant checks for unnecessary tension. Four approaches are described:

1. relaxation by recall with counting
2. behavioural relaxation checklist
3. sweeping the body
4. the ripple.

Relaxation by recall with counting

Bernstein & Borkovec (1973) condensed their progressive relaxation training programme into a release-only format for four groups of muscles: the arms, the head and neck, the trunk and the legs. In its most summarized form it consists of a counting procedure: two counts are allotted to each body part as attention is focused on it and tension released.

> One ... two, (arms relax) ... three ... four, (head and neck relax) ... five ... six, (trunk relax) ... seven ... eight, (legs relax) ... nine ... ten, (whole body relax) ...

Behavioural relaxation checklist

This is based on the assumption that if an individual looks relaxed, to some extent he will feel relaxed. A checklist (Table 9.1), which can be memorized, covers 10 postures characteristic of relaxation (Poppen 1988):

Feet ... resting with toes lying free
Hands ... fingers gently curled
Body ... without movement
Shoulders ... dropped and level
Head ... still, and facing forwards
Mouth ... teeth separated, lips unpursed
Throat ... loose
Breathing ... slow and gentle
Voice ... no sound
Eyes ... lightly closed behind smooth eyelids.

Sweeping the body

Kermani (1990) describes a routine used for releasing body tension. It involves sweeping the surface of the body with an imaginary large, soft paintbrush (Ch. 7, p. 65):

Starting at your feet, sweep the brush in your mind's eye, up your legs and the front of your body as far as your shoulders ... then down your arms to your fingertips ... then, a long sweep up the full length of the back ... continuing into the neck and scalp ... over the brow ... and down to the face and jaw.

The ripple

This is a single wave of relaxation which begins at the head and rolls down the body to the feet (Priest & Schott 1991) (Ch. 7, p. 62):

Starting at the top of your head, feel the relaxation rolling down your body in one continuous wave ... feel it releasing tension as it descends ... relaxing each part of your body in turn ... until it reaches the tips of your toes. Try synchronizing the ripple with a slow breath out.

BREATHING

Stress is associated with physiological arousal. This arousal is brought about by the action of the sympathetic nervous system, and includes an increase in the respiratory rate. Slowed breathing is associated with parasympathetic activity. Thus, by consciously slowing the breathing rate, it may be possible to counteract the effects of the sympathetic nervous system and generally check the symptoms of arousal.

Three techniques are described. Each one has a greater chance of success if it is introduced before the state of stress becomes established.

1. abdominal breathing
2. using words as cues
3. a breathing cycle.

Abdominal breathing

Since sudden stress is associated with apical (upper costal) respiratory movements, and relaxation with abdominal respiratory movements, breathing which is focused on the abdomen will tend to have a quietening effect (Ch. 15, p. 132).

Let your attention focus on your abdomen. Feel it swelling as you breathe in and sinking as you breathe out. Keep the breathing as gentle and as slow as you can.

Using words as cues (cue–controlled relaxation)

Repeated past associations of a word such as 'relax' with the relaxed state give the word the status of a cue. When subsequently recited on the outbreath, this word tends to bring about a state of relaxation (Öst 1987) (Ch. 8, p. 71).

Let your breathing be as natural as possible ... just before you begin to breathe out, think the word 'relax' ... slowly release the air as you focus on the word ... breathe in ... and, repeat the sequence ... keep the rhythm as gentle as you can ... avoid deliberately deepening the breaths ... continue for a few moments...

A short version might run:

In ... relax and out slowly ... in ... relax and out slowly...

or simply:

Relax.

A breathing cycle

Lichstein (1988) presents a breathing technique for helping to relieve stress in a crisis situation. It consists of a deeper than usual breath in, which is held for a few seconds before being slowly exhaled. Lichstein points out how each component of the exercise has value: the inbreath diverts attention from the distressing thoughts; the breath-retention raises the P_{CO_2} level, inducing mild lethargy, and the slow outbreath helps to reduce muscle tension. The cycle begins with an outbreath in the exercise below:

> Breathe out a little more fully than usual. Let the air flow in to fill your lungs. Hold it for 5 seconds. Then exhale slowly. As you let the air out, feel the tension going with it. Then, let your breathing recover its normal rhythm.

Since deep breathing can increase the possibility of hyperventilation, immediate repetition of this exercise is not recommended.

COGNITIVE STRATEGIES

These are methods which deal with stress by changing our thoughts. They include the following approaches:

1. self-talk
2. autogenic phrases
3. imagery
4. thinking of a smile
5. additional strategies
6. environmental markers.

Self–talk

Since thoughts influence feelings, positive thoughts will tend to generate positive feelings (Ellis 1962, Beck 1976). Phrases affirming the value of the self, repeated often, colour our view of ourselves, and in a positive direction (Ch. 18, p. 163). Feeling in control and feeling relaxed will tend to increase coping powers whatever the source of the stress.

Phrases tending to promote a sense of control over the situation include:

- I am competent
- I can deal with this
- I am in control
- My coping powers are good.

Phrases tending to induce a relaxed state of mind include:

- I feel at peace
- I am relaxed
- I am calm
- My thoughts are peaceful ones.

The above phrases provide examples of positive self-talk; however, the most effective phrases are those which the individual has composed for herself.

Autogenic phrases

Training in autogenics (Ch. 19) can result in relaxation occurring after recitation of a single phrase. It could be a heaviness phrase, a warmth phrase or one relating to feelings of peace. When recited it can act as a key to switch on autogenic effects.

Imagery

Both single images and transformations can promote relaxation. Two examples of the former are (Ch. 17, p. 154):

- the rag doll
- the piece of seaweed.

Identifying with the characteristics of an inert image can help to mitigate feelings of stress. Anger, panic and frustration may all respond to this kind of imagery.

Transformations refer to the mutation of one substance into another (Ch. 17, p. 155). The first substance is harsh, the second smooth and they are linked by some sensory quality as in the following items (Fanning 1988):

- sandpaper … to … silk
- chalk squeaking on the blackboard … to … high musical notes
- burnt toast fumes … to … baking bread
- fluorescent orange … to … soft peach
- sour gooseberries … to … sweet raspberries.

The individual focuses attention on the harsh image which she then resolves into the smooth one. The transformation becomes a metaphor for her own feelings which are thereby helped to undergo a change from negative to positive.

Thinking of a smile

Facial expression has been found to influence emotions. A positive expression tends to induce a positive feeling in that individual (Ch. 9, p. 75, Ch. 24, p. 215). Thus, if a person smiles, her feelings of stress will tend to be diminished. However, as it is not always appropriate to smile, it is enough to stay with the thought of it and simply to imagine the smile (L. H. Capel 1986, personal communication).

Additional strategies

The effect of stressors may be reduced by diverting the mind away from them. Techniques which can be used to distract the attention include images of strong light and memorized telephone numbers:

Strong light

Imagine an intensely bright light such as the rays from a powerful torch. Imagine it beamed into your eyes from a distance of 45 cm (18 in). Let it blot out all images.

Telephone number

Invent a telephone number. Make it a long one, so that you will have to concentrate hard. Hold it in your head for 1 to 3 minutes, depending on the situation.

The environmental marker

Several writers suggest marking appliances which are potential sources of stress (Öst 1987, Mitchell 1987) (Chs 8 and 10). Coloured dots stuck, for instance, on to the telephone, wrist-watch or steering wheel, serve to remind the individual to maintain low levels of tension. Öst suggests changing the colour of the markers frequently since their effect dwindles as the eye gets habituated to the dot.

Chapter 24

Other techniques

This chapter touches on a variety of relaxation techniques not so far mentioned and has been included in order to give the therapist a broader view of the field. Clients often ask about different approaches, so it is useful for the therapist to be able to answer these enquiries. The aim is not to provide a comprehensive list, but to include some of the best known relaxation techniques. Eleven methods are described here in summarized form. They are:

- massage
- aromatherapy
- biofeedback-assisted relaxation therapy
- body awareness therapy
- Feldenkrais relaxation
- functional relaxation
- yoga
- Eastern techniques
- reflex therapy
- shiatsu
- t'ai chi ch'uan
- smiling and laughter therapy.

MASSAGE

Massage is an ancient technique in which standard strokes and manipulations are applied to the soft tissues of the body. The techniques include effleurage which consists of long slow strokes, kneading (circular movements with compression), skin rolling, frictions, percussive movements and vibrations. It is claimed that circulatory benefits in the form of improved venous and lymphatic drainage are gained from these procedures together with a decrease in pain, muscular tension and psychological stress (Kerr 2000, Ernst 2003).

Early attempts to measure its effectiveness tended to suffer from methodological flaw but some of this stems from research difficulties such as finding an acceptable placebo. It is, however, interesting to look at some of the research that has been carried out and subsequently reviewed by Kerr (2000). Several studies have investigated the effects of massage on elderly people. For example, Fraser & Kerr (1993) studied the effects of 5 minutes of slow rhythmical back massage on 21 residents of a care institution and found that electromyographic and anxiety scores in the groups receiving massage were significantly lower than in the control group 10 minutes following intervention.

Other studies have demonstrated considerable effects on physiological parameters following massage. For example, Fakouri & Jones (1987) measured heart rate, blood pressure and skin temperature in 18 elderly clients after 3 minutes of slow stroke back massage. Following treatment, heart rate and systolic blood pressure were significantly lower than before treatment while skin temperature was significantly higher, indicating an overall benefit. Where people have been diagnosed with hypertension, researchers find that massage may be effective in reducing diastolic blood pressure and in ameliorating the symptoms associated with hypertension (Hernandez-Reif et al 2000).

Massage has been found effective in the context of cancer. Meek (1993) studied the physiological effects of 3 minutes of slow stroke back massage in 30 terminally ill hospice patients and obtained significant findings for heart rate, blood pressure and skin temperature. Ferrell-Torry & Glink (1993), investigating the psychological effects of massage in nine male inpatients suffering cancer pain, found significant reductions in both pain and anxiety. Such results persuaded the Oncology Department of the Hammersmith Hospital to introduce massage as a standard component of treatment, seeing it as offering benefit in terms of quality of life without the negative consequences of other forms of treatment (Burke et al 1994).

In the area of back pain, massage has been shown to be more effective than placebo, muscular relaxation and acupuncture, but less effective than shiatsu, transcutaneous electrical stimulation and manipulation, while it was found equal to exercise and therapeutic corsets (Furlan et al 2000, Ernst 2003).

Normal healthy adults have also been studied, where it was shown that massage can provide relaxation, thus lending itself to the treatment of workplace stress (Cady & Jones 1997). Massage also offers immunological benefits. Lovas et al (2002) demonstrated a significant increase in the proliferative response of T and B lymphocytes, and also in the levels of serum IgG during full-body Swedish massage on healthy females.

What is the mechanism behind these effects? Is it the pressure of the massage? Or the rhythm of the stroking? It has been suggested that massaging particular segments of skin can have specific effects (Kurosawa et al 1995) and this notion might help to explain why results are not always consistent (Kerr 2000).

Most people seem to find massage a pleasant experience. Research shows that when performed slowly it increases feelings of relaxation (Kerr 2000). It does this at relatively little financial cost and without side effects or negative interactions.

AROMATHERAPY

Loosely connected with massage is aromatherapy. Here, concentrated essential oils from aromatic plant extracts are applied to the body. These oils are generally conveyed through massage or sometimes by steam infusion, while the massage itself may cover the whole body or focus on a part of it, for example, the foot. Of the very few published trials that exist, Cooke & Ernst (2000) have reviewed six. They all had similar designs in that massage with essential oil was compared to massage without essential oil and the participants were all suffering from anxiety. Results showed that, on the whole, aromatherapy massage was slightly more effective than massage on its own, although the benefits were short-lived. The reviewers concluded that aromatherapy has a mild and transient anxiolytic effect.

Regarding the mechanisms of action, Cooke & Ernst find they are unclear and propose that future investigations should attempt to separate the effects of transdermal absorption from the effects of smell.

The popularity of aromatherapy as a relaxation technique is undeniable and has led to a growing use of it in the fields of midwifery and cancer care.

BIOFEEDBACK–ASSISTED RELAXATION THERAPY

Biofeedback (BFB) is 'a descriptive term for the process of providing an organism with information about its biological functions' (Reber & Reber 2001). In one sense, such information is relayed to us every day by the sensory systems in the body. It is illustrated by, for example, the way joint proprioceptors inform the individual about the position of her hands when she cannot see them, i.e. when they are clasped behind her back. The benefit of the information is that adjustments can be made to the movements in her arms.

In the case of the workings of the internal body organs this information is normally unavailable. However, it can become available with the help of an instrument capable of converting the inner workings of the body into visual or auditory signals. It is claimed that an individual who is provided with signals from a particular organ can modify the functioning of that organ. The instrument picks up stress responses such as muscle tension, high blood pressure, raised heart rate or sweat gland activity. The client then reads the signal. If the stress indicator is high she practises a relaxation technique and observes the result. This tells her how effective her attempts have been. Such feedback gives her clear evidence of the result of her efforts and any success she achieves serves to increase her motivation (Stoyva & Anderson 1982). In this way she learns how to reduce the effects of stress on her internal organs.

There is a substantial body of evidence relating to biofeedback-assisted relaxation therapy. Not all of it is favourable. However, a proportion of studies have found the method effective in reducing the stress response and promoting a state of mental tranquillity. Chandler et al (2001) found the technique successful with counsellor trainees as did Fehmi (1974) with middle management executives.

Patient populations have also benefited, particularly those suffering from psychosomatic disorders. Duckro & Cantwell-Simmons (1989) reviewed studies investigating biofeedback-assisted relaxation in the management of paediatric headache and found good support for its use as a stress-reducing technique.

Research comparing BFB with other relaxation techniques has so far been unable to show that BFB is more effective than other methods of inducing relaxation (Brannon & Feist 1992).

BODY AWARENESS THERAPY

Body awareness therapy is based on the notion that human movement has a psychological dimension, i.e. that it means something in emotional terms (Piret & Beziers 1979). For example, each movement has a purpose; each movement creates a subjective experience; each movement expresses some aspect of the individual's life (Roxendal 1990). Movements carried out by the body are recognized as part of the self and are therefore part of a person's identity. The aim of treatment is to integrate the body in the total experience of identity and by way of achieving this, emphasis is placed on sensory awareness at a conscious level (Roxendal 1990).

Gjertrud Roxendal, a Swedish physiotherapist, presents two aspects of the approach: basic and expressive. Basic refers to general movement functions, such as posture and gait, and it consists of structured exercises covering concepts such as the body's relation with the ground, its contact with the supporting surface, posture, balance, free breathing and muscle relaxation. Boundaries of the body in different contexts are discussed; for example, the experience of holding hands in formal dances.

The expressive aspect refers to a person's experience of the movements she makes and to her uniqueness as an individual. The exercises are related to personal style as expressed in gait, voice, degree of eye contact, way of interacting with other people and how comfortable she is with her mirror image and the sound of her name. Partner exercises form a context for exploring the need for human contact and the sense of security or insecurity attaching to it.

Progress is measured on the Body Awareness Scale which contains an assessment of movement, together with a structured interview on body image and attitudes to movement. The Scale has been tested for validity by Gyllesten et al (1999).

Clients seem to find the approach helpful. Irritable bowel syndrome is one area where it has been found effective (Eriksson et al 2002). Another is sexual abuse where Mattsson et al (1998) studied seven women over 20 months. An improvement in body image and self-image occurred in the majority of the women and their symptoms were reduced by half. Anorexia, schizophrenia, and chronic pain are other conditions which have benefited from it.

Body awareness therapy is not primarily a relaxation technique but in promoting a sense of well-being, it induces a feeling of serenity.

FELDENKRAIS RELAXATION

Moshe Feldenkrais was a physicist who began to study human movement following an injury to his knee. He developed an approach whose aim was to improve function by teaching the individual to move with greater ease and efficiency (Kolt & McConville 2000). His method consists of training the client to be more aware of the body in order to enhance sensitivity to existing movement patterns. These can then be replaced by more efficient new ones. In addition to improving neuromuscular function, the method also claims to influence the way an individual thinks and feels. Thus it has psychological benefit and can be said to promote a sense of well-being.

The Feldenkrais method covers two training systems: awareness-through-movement and functional integration. The first consists of verbally directed movements designed to increase sensorimotor awareness and leading to improved coordination (Malmgren-Olssen et al 2001). Treatment starts with a simple exercise; it is repeated, then developed into a more complex movement with a coordinated pattern which involves the whole body. The emphasis throughout is on awareness of the movement.

The second, functional integration, focuses on individual functional problems and uses guiding techniques, such as touch and manipulation, tailored to the individual's need. Treatment is intensive and one-to-one and designed to 'communicate new possibilities of body organization' (Kerr et al 2002).

Feldenkrais relaxation (FeldR) has been compared to the Alexander technique by Fulden (1989) who points out that whereas FeldR promotes awareness of the body while it is in motion, the Alexander technique concentrates on the body in space. In general, however, Fulden sees FeldR as a fusion of the Alexander technique and Oriental body training.

Malmgren-Olssen et al (2001) compared FeldR with body awareness therapy and conventional physiotherapy in patients suffering from musculoskeletal disorders. There were few differences in outcome among the groups, but significant positive changes occurred before and after treatment with respect to distress, pain and negative self-image in all three groups. This led the researchers to suggest that psychological aspects be addressed in the management of all musculoskeletal injuries.

Evidence of the efficacy of awareness-through-movement in reducing anxiety was demonstrated by Kolt & McConville (2000). Of the 35 female and 19 male undergraduate participants in their study, the female ones reported significantly lower anxiety scores following treatment.

FeldR is steadily gaining in popularity and is used in the management of a range of disorders, such as cerebral palsy and multiple sclerosis, where its holistic approach is found particularly helpful.

FUNCTIONAL RELAXATION

Devised by a German physiotherapist, Marianne Fuchs, functional relaxation (FunctR) consists of small movements of the jaw, neck, spine and shoulders. These are performed smoothly in a snake-like fashion while breathing out. The participant focuses her attention on the movements themselves and on the body feelings elicited by the movements, thus intensifying her perception of them and enhancing body awareness. It is said that, as a result, a spontaneous physical relaxation occurs.

This is a relaxation technique which can be readily integrated into the lives of people suffering from disorders, such as tension headache and asthma, where its effectiveness has been tested by Loew and colleagues (2000). These researchers showed significant differences between measurements before and after treatment with FunctR in total headache hours and intensity of pain. These results support the view that FunctR may have a use in the relief of tension headache, both as an adjunct to pharmacological treatment and as a prophylactic.

Loew et al (2001) have also explored the effect of FunctR in the context of asthma. Twenty-one asthma sufferers were randomly assigned to three groups: FunctR, the drug terbutaline and placebo. Results showed that FunctR was significantly more effective in decreasing airway resistance than the placebo, although FunctR was not as effective as terbutaline. In their conclusion the researchers suggested that FunctR had potential as a supplementary therapy in cases of asthma.

FunctR is easy to learn and, on account of its unobtrusive nature, can be practised in any situation. Although 20 1-hour sessions are needed to acquire full proficiency, small benefits can be gained in considerably less time.

YOGA

Yoga is a discipline with a long history in Hindu philosophy. As a method, it integrates physical, psychological and spiritual aspects of life. Physical postures and breathing-control prepare the body and mind for the rigours of meditation which, in turn, lead to a state of harmony in which the soul is able to reach a higher level, communicating with the Universal Spirit (Gilbert 1999).

Within this general concept there are different schools, each with its own emphasis. Hatha yoga or 'the yoga of health' is the one most frequently practised in the West. Its focal elements are postures, breath control and simple meditation in the form of chantings or candle-gazing. It attracts people for a variety of reasons, such as relief from stress, healing after body injury, or simply, the wish to increase one's joint flexibility.

Kerr (2000) has found evidence of its effectiveness in her review of relaxation techniques. In one study, 40 male physical education teachers attending a residential camp were trained in yogic procedures. After 3 months significant reductions in autonomic arousal and increased psychophysiological relaxation were demonstrated (Telles et al 1993). In 2000 these researchers turned their attention to a notion referred to in ancient yoga texts, i.e. the effect of combining stimulating and calming yogic procedures in the same session. Their results supported the notion that a greater reduction in autonomic arousal followed the combined procedures than that which followed the relaxing procedures on their own (Telles et al 2000).

Yoga has been shown to provide benefit in a variety of medical conditions, one of which is asthma. Khanam et al (1996) demonstrated a significant decrease in sympathetic activity in nine participants following a 7-day course.

Psychological benefit has been demonstrated in the work of Schell et al (1994). Twenty-five young, healthy females were instructed in yogic procedures in the form of spinal stretches, breathing and meditation and tested along a variety of dimensions including life satisfaction, mood and coping with stress. Results were compared with those of a control situation consisting of quiet reading. A significant difference was demonstrated in favour of the yoga-practising group.

Despite its popularity, yoga should not be seen as an easy remedy. On the contrary, it requires infinite patience. Neither should it be seen as a test of pain endurance (some of the postures can be uncomfortable for the novice); rather, it may be seen as a test of self-discipline where progress is viewed in terms of process, not end-result (Gilbert 1999).

EASTERN TECHNIQUES

These are based on the Taoist principles of yin and yang, which are themselves a product of the Ultimate Source of Being. Yin and yang are opposing principles in Chinese philosophy but they are not in conflict; rather, they complement one another, and when they are balanced, a state of harmony is said to exist. Yin and yang, which are present in all living things, interact with each other to produce the vital energy force, called ki or chi, which flows through the meridians to all the organs and parts of the body. In health its flow is unimpeded. However, if there is imbalance between yin and yang the flow can get blocked and disease may develop. Treatment, which is aimed at releasing the blocked energy and restoring equilibrium, addresses the mind and body as an integrated whole. In this way it helps to promote relaxation. A few of the Eastern methods are described here: reflex therapy, shiatsu and t'ai chi ch'uan.

REFLEX THERAPY

Reflex therapy owes its name to the belief that the sole of the foot carries a representation of the entire body. It is claimed that treatment of these reflected areas can influence healing in related parts of the body. The approach has a long history in the East where its practice is linked to the principles of Chinese medicine, i.e. locating imbalances in the body and restoring harmony of body and mind. Today its use is growing in the West where many people are looking for the kind of holistic approach it offers with its acknowledgement of the anxiety that accompanies physical disease.

Reflex therapy is a gentle manual technique consisting of pressure massage of the foot. This massage covers the whole foot but focuses on points relating to organs where symptoms of trauma have been detected. In addition to regulating imbalances, one of the aims is to stimulate self-healing powers (Association of Chartered Physiotherapists in Reflex Therapy (ACPIRT) 2001).

The rationale in Chinese terms concerns the free flow of chi which is promoted by the massage. In scientific terms its rationale is not known, but one possible explanation is that stimulation or sedation of certain points in the foot releases endorphins which relieve pain. This induces relaxation. The relaxation may, in its turn, result in a freer-flowing circulation and improved nourishment, both of which promote healing.

Diagnosis may lie outside the therapist's domain and acute pain and fever should always receive medical attention. However, once the diagnosis is established, reflex therapy may help in a wide range of disorders. Some of the areas in which its

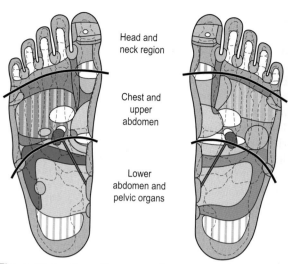

Figure 24.1 The reflex zones of the feet. With acknowledgement to the Association of Chartered Physiotherapists in Reflex Therapy (ACPIRT).

benefits have been measured are cancer, sinusitis, menopause, childbirth and mental health. With regard to cancer, substantial reductions in pain, nausea and anxiety have occurred after reflex therapy, leading some researchers to suggest that the approach should feature in all cancer units (Grealish et al 2000, Stephenson et al 2000).

In the mental health field, significant improvement in general emotional state has occurred in individuals receiving reflex therapy in a drop-in and day centre in Worthing. The data were qualitative but indicated a marked increase in confidence and self-esteem levels (Trousdale et al 1997). This service was reassessed in 2000 when it was found that 74% of respondents reported improvement in their physical health in addition to the psychological benefits. Chronic sinusitis also appears to benefit from reflexology as Heatley et al (2000) demonstrated when they found its effect equalled that of nasal irrigation.

These results suggest that reflex therapy has much to offer. However, some studies have compared the approach with standard foot massage and found no discernible difference in effectiveness. Cornbleet (2001) has reported this in the field of palliative care, and Williamson et al (2002) in the field of menopause where, following treatment, scores for negative mood fell in equal measure, whether the group were receiving reflex therapy or non-specific foot massage.

This might suggest that the benefits of reflex therapy are mainly a function of manual contact; and yet, many other studies have shown the approach to be effective in a variety of settings. Like massage, it is also non-invasive and, since it does not rely on special equipment, is relatively low-cost. As with other complementary approaches, however, scientific measurement of its effectiveness has only recently begun, so that no established body of research yet exists.

SHIATSU

As a branch of Oriental medicine, shiatsu looks at the whole person, checking the meridians, diagnosing weak points and applying a range of manual techniques, such as palpations, stretchings and pressure. The pressure is applied inwards, which distinguishes it from most other massage techniques where strokes and circular movements predominate. The therapist generally uses her fingers to apply the pressures but her thumbs, palms, elbows and even knees and feet may play a part.

Psychosomatic and musculoskeletal disorders particularly respond to this approach but, since a shiatsu treatment covers the whole body, it can be applied in a wide range of conditions (Beresford-Cooke 1996).

Stevenson (1995) investigated the effects of shiatsu as a palliative procedure in a single case study of a patient diagnosed with lymphoma of the lung. Results were favourable as registered by the patient's self-report and the physician's observation. No statistical analysis was reported.

T'AI CHI CH'UAN

A non-aggressive form of the martial arts, t'ai chi ch'uan consists of a series of slow, circular and deliberate movements which flow from one into another. Their slowness tends to be reflected throughout the body organs, including the respiratory system where the breathing rate falls. T'ai chi ch'uan thus appears to induce the relaxation response and, as this influences the mind also, the method helps to promote a sense of personal harmony and inner calm (Mack 1980, Fasko & Grueninger 2001). The gentle character of the exercises makes the approach particularly suitable for older age groups where, as the muscles become stronger and the balance improves, the tendency for falls to occur is reduced (Luskin et al 2000).

Practice periods last about 15 minutes and are carried out twice a day, singly or in groups. During the movements the practitioner focuses her attention on them and on her breathing which should be slow and even. The emphasis placed on concentration has earned the method the name of 'meditation-in-motion'.

Fasko & Grueninger (2001) have reviewed studies investigating the effectiveness of t'ai chi; these researchers conclude that benefit is to be gained from the practice of t'ai chi along all dimensions of health: physical, physiological, cognitive and emotional.

SMILING AND LAUGHTER THERAPY

William James (1890/1950) remarked over a century ago that the way to cheerfulness is to act and speak as if cheerfulness were already there. In other words, smiling makes us feel happy (Ch. 23, p. 208). This idea has given rise to the facial and postural feedback hypotheses (Ch. 9, p. 75) which state that feedback from facial expression and posture induces the emotion associated with that expression and posture (Izard 1977, Duclos et al 1989, Hatfield et al 1992).

Humour and laughter are related to positive moods, and few would deny that laughter releases tension. Ekman (1984) has posited the existence of neural connections between the facial muscles and the autonomic system; an idea which has been supported by research (Berk et al 1988). It has been shown that levels of hormones related to sympathetic activity are reduced by humour and mirthful laughter, thus suggesting an association between laughter and parasympathetic activity. In this light, laughter can be seen as a natural tranquillizer (Hodgkinson 1987).

Smiling and laughter have been referred to as overlapping but distinct domains, the one of friendliness, the other of amusement (Van Hooff 1972). Both can be effective stress-relievers.

Further reading

Massage

Holey E A, Cook E M 2003 Evidence-based therapeutic massage, 2nd edn. Churchill Livingstone, Edinburgh

Rosser M 2004 Body massage: therapy basics. Hodder & Stoughton, Abingdon

Yoga

Meaux K 2002 Dynamic yoga. Dorling Kindersley, London

Reflexology

Gillanders A 1995 Reflexology: a step-by-step guide. Gaia Books, London

Chapter 25

Relaxation in pregnancy and childbirth

RATIONALE

This chapter differs from the rest of this book in that it focuses on a condition for which relaxation training is offered, rather than the description of a particular technique. It has been included because of the widespread use of relaxation in the field of obstetrics, where the aim has been to achieve an altered response to physical pain through acquired skills (Culverwell & McKenna 1988).

Relaxation has been taught antenatally since the 1930s when Grantly Dick-Read saw it as a means of breaking the cycle of pain–fear–tension–pain in childbirth. His particular concern was to reduce the fear many women have of labour (Dick-Read 1942). Others followed, teaching a variety of methods, most of which were concerned in different ways with the control of breathing. The purpose of these methods was to provide a distraction from the discomfort of strong uterine contractions (Noble 1988), and also to ensure that the fetus received an adequate supply of oxygen.

BREATHING AND ANTENATAL TRAINING

Techniques using contrived forms of breathing have lost credibility over the years. Research has shown that a pregnant or labouring mother whose natural breathing is artificially augmented is more likely to suffer from the ill-effects of lowered carbon dioxide levels than to gain from increased levels of oxygen (Buxton 1973). Buxton's study included a group who had been taught controlled breathing. It was found that this group, compared with participants who had been given other forms of antenatal training, exhibited marked hyperventilation with resulting adverse effects (Ch. 15, p. 134). Stradling (1983) has since re-emphasized the dangers of overbreathing during labour.

Some hyperventilation may occur physiologically in labour without affecting the normal fetus (Polden & Mantle 1990). It is not, however, in the interests of the fetus to increase the degree of hyperventilation, because the resulting low carbon dioxide levels could theoretically lead to both vasoconstriction of uterine blood vessels, and interference in the transfer of oxygen to the tissues and fetus (Ch. 15, p. 135). Moreover, hyperventilation can be followed by apnoea (temporary cessation of breathing) which could also reduce the availability of oxygen. A fetus which was already compromised would be more vulnerable to these effects than a normal one (Mantle et al 2004).

In the light of such findings, antenatal teachers no longer use controlled breathing exercises but instead encourage women to breathe freely, naturally and easily, seeing the interests of the fetus best served by breathing rates and rhythms determined by the mother's own physiology (Stradling 1983, Noble 1988). Breathing exercises, in their original sense, are no longer a feature. *Awareness* of breathing, however, is widely taught. It is seen as a means of helping the mother to understand her body.

AWARENESS OF BREATHING

While emphasizing that breathing should be effortless, mothers are invited to explore the different aspects of the expanding chest (Schott & Priest 2002). (Plenty of time should be allowed for this exercise.)

Sit quietly. Allow your breathing to settle to a resting rhythm. Place your hands over your lower ribs (fingers almost touching), and become aware of the movements that occur underneath them. Think of the air gently flowing in and down towards your hands ... and then flowing out along the same

route ... make sure the rate is a natural one and that you don't overbreathe. Let your body tell you when to breathe in and out ... Move your hands down a bit lower and feel the whole abdomen gently rising and falling in synchrony with your breaths.

Take a little rest, then lean forwards with your arms resting on a table. This position gives full play to chest movement in the back. Perhaps you have the sensation of your ribs expanding backwards. Don't be in a hurry. It's important to keep the breathing natural ...

Finally, sit back and lay one hand over your upper abdomen and the other over your chest just below your collar bones. Take plenty of time. Notice movement taking place under both hands. Perhaps you also notice that the more relaxed you feel, the more movement there is under your lower hand. Conversely, a slow, abdominal breathing rhythm helps to induce relaxation. It is useful to remember this in moments of emotional unease, since slowing the breathing can help to calm the feelings. Otherwise, your body takes care of your respirations, giving you more air when you need it and reducing the supply when you don't.

The connection between respiration and the experiences of exertion, pain and emotion can be made by asking the women to consider what happens to their breathing when they run for a bus, bang their shin or get angry. The women will understand how effort, discomfort and emotion can temporarily disrupt the breathing pattern (Schott & Priest 2002). Since disrupted breathing can take the form of increased ventilation, this is an opportunity for discussing hyperventilation: its causes, how to recognize it, and how to relieve its symptoms (Ch. 15).

Breathing awareness exercises for inducing relaxation

Many women find breathing awareness exercises have a relaxing effect. Two examples follow.

1. Sit, lie or stand comfortably. Turn your thoughts towards your breathing and watch it settling down to a resting pattern. Become aware of the movement occurring in your upper abdomen and lower chest. Without doing anything to change the

rhythm, focus your attention on these areas. Perhaps your breathing is also getting slower. Above all it is gentle. Notice how calm you feel, breathing in this way. Feel the soothing nature of this quiet breathing.

2. Settle down in any position you find comfortable. Let your body decide when to breathe in and out. Enjoy the feeling of being in tune with your body's needs. Notice how the rate slows down, reflecting your resting state. Notice also, the gentle rhythm. Next time you breathe out, let the breath carry your tensions away. Next time you breathe in, let the breath bring calmness... breathe out tension... breathe in calm...

OTHER FORMS OF RELAXATION

Other forms of relaxation as well as breathing awareness are widely taught in pregnancy, their object being to help the mother through the birth experience. Three are mentioned here:

- muscle relaxation
- massage
- visualizations.

MUSCLE RELAXATION

Muscle relaxation is a well-known method of reducing tension for labouring mothers. In its early days it was presented as a series of tense–release procedures deriving from Jacobson's work. In recent decades, however, this approach has given way to Mitchell's method (Ch. 10) whose advantages include the following points:

1. Mitchell's method avoids activating the muscles typically associated with tension, i.e. the clenching and hunching muscles as this might interfere with uterine contractions. Instead, by a simple change of joint position, it creates a reciprocal state of ease and comfort.
2. Joint change, when applied to a 'key' area in a trained individual, can relax the whole body in the space of a few seconds. Thus, Mitchell's method can have a general and immediate effect.
3. Mitchell discourages any kind of interference with the natural breathing pattern.

MASSAGE

Kitzinger (1987) advocates massage and suggests a form in which gentle stroking movements from the centre to the periphery are carried out. As the hand moves down the extremity, the woman can imagine her tensions flowing out.

VISUALIZATION

Imagery can be used to enhance relaxation during both pregnancy and labour since by its capacity to hold the attention, it may help to block pain pathways to the brain (McKenna 1988).

Getting in touch with the baby

The following script is based on a passage by Priest & Schott (1991).

> Let your thoughts focus on the baby growing inside your uterus. Imagine him or her lying safe and warm and comfortable, lulled by your heartbeat and rocked by your movements. Your baby can move his or her limbs, can swallow and can hear sounds. He or she is familiar with your voice and the voice of the father and will recognize them after birth. Think of your baby growing inside you, getting ready to be born, while you are waiting to receive him or her...
>
> Slowly, in your own time, bring your attention back to the room, but do not be in a hurry to get up.

Some women like to sing to their unborn baby, soothing it and welcoming it into the family.

Comparing labour to the sea

Polden & Mantle (1990) offer several examples of imagery for use during the first stage of labour. Ocean waves and mountain peaks are used as metaphors, to help women withstand the intensity of the contractions. The following is adapted from one of their suggested pieces:

> Imagine a beautiful day out at sea... with blue sky, still air and calm water. As the day wears on, perhaps the surface of the water begins to show the odd ripple. These ripples may be small so that at first you hardly notice them. Gradually, the tiny ripples turn into small waves; waves which you feel you can ride quite easily. After a while, the waves may get higher, and as they get higher, perhaps

they also get closer together. You find you continue to ride them. Still higher and closer together ... the waves seem almost to overwhelm you, but as they dip, you notice they are carrying you nearer to the shore ... nearer to the shore where your baby will be born.

FOR RELAXING DURING DISCOMFORT

Some teachers prepare women for the birth by simulating the discomfort of a contraction. They do this by getting the woman's partner or another member of the group to apply an uncomfortable pinch or squeeze to her arm or thigh. The woman is asked to relax towards the pressure in an effort to reduce the sensation. The aim is to help the woman feel she can raise her pain threshold. The pinch or squeeze should last about a minute. It starts with a light touch and gradually builds up in intensity over the first 30 seconds; in the second half-minute it is gradually released. Slow, gentle breathing should accompany the exercise (Polden & Mantle 1990).

HOME PRACTICE

Relaxation is a skill, and like any skill it requires practice for proficiency. This practice can be done in any position which the mother chooses: lying, sitting, kneeling on all fours, kneeling with arms supported on a chair seat, standing with raised arms resting on the wall or any other position which the woman finds comfortable. She can try out different ones to find the one that suits her best.

EVIDENCE OF EFFECTIVENESS

A number of studies have been carried out in the area of childbirth and relaxation, for example the controlled investigation of Rees (1995). This author examined the effect of relaxation training on levels of anxiety, depression and self-esteem in primiparas. Sixty participants were randomly assigned to experimental and control groups. The experimental group received 15 minutes of taped relaxation which included muscle routines, breathing awareness, meditation and imagery, while the control group listened to tape-recorded music for the same length of time. Results showed the experimental group to have significantly lower scores on anxiety and depression than the control, and significantly higher scores on self-esteem than the control. Thus, it is suggested that relaxation techniques can contribute to the psychological well-being of women giving birth to their first child.

Before using the techniques contained in this chapter, the pitfalls relating to each should be read in the corresponding sections of the book. The chapters on breathing (Ch. 15) and visualization (Ch. 18) both contain lists of relevant pitfalls (p. 138 and p. 170 respectively).

This chapter does not cover all the relaxation strategies for helping women through labour. For further information in this highly specialized field, readers are referred to the Further reading section below.

Further reading

Mantle J, Haslam J, Polden M 2004 Physiotherapy in obstetrics and gynaecology, 2nd edn. Butterworth-Heinemann, Oxford

Schott J, Priest J 2002 Leading antenatal classes: a practical guide, 2nd edn. Books for Midwives, Oxford

Chapter 26

Measurement: patient assessment and clinical audit

This chapter is devoted to the topic of measurement and includes a discussion of patient assessment and clinical audit. The first is considered at length; the second is touched on and the reader referred to other works as the topic justifies a separate study. Both patient assessment and clinical audit call for careful record-keeping and, although their common goal is to serve the patient's interests, they may have different approaches to it.

PATIENT ASSESSMENT

Assessment means 'estimating' or 'judging' (Chambers 20th century dictionary 1983); in this case estimating the degree of stress or relaxation present in an individual. With regard to relaxation training, assessment is needed for the following reasons.

1. To obtain a profile of the individual's problems. It is likely that the relaxation training will be part of a wider programme of anxiety management, in which case the activities of the professionals concerned will need to be integrated.

2. To measure existing tension levels. Such a measure provides a baseline when evaluating progress. It should be carried out after a short period of rest to allow for the relaxation effects which occur, in the absence of any relaxation technique, as part of the process of adapting to a restful environment (Lichstein et al 1981).

3. To choose the most appropriate method of relaxation. The results of the first assessment may

reveal information which suggests that a particular approach is indicated.

4. To measure the benefit from the relaxation training in terms of reduced tension levels. Alternatively, assessment may focus on symptoms, such as tension headache or hypertension, and the degree to which these have been relieved by the relaxation training.

5. To provide feedback for the participant. Positive feedback acts as a reinforcer, negative feedback indicates the need for corrective action.

6. To collect quantifiable data for research. Therapy can be designed in a way which lends itself to the development of a research project. Research methods themselves, however, are not covered in this book.

Thus patient assessment covers questions such as :

- What is the problem?
- What is the best way of approaching it, i.e. which relaxation method or methods are indicated?
- Is the selected method based on sound evidence?
- How tense is the individual before training?
- How relaxed is the individual as a result of the relaxation training?
- Is her tension headache/hypertension relieved?
- Is she aware of her progress?
- Can this work contribute to research?

Although patient assessment is time-consuming, its benefits are clear and every effort should be made to carry it out in some form.

WAYS OF MEASURING RELAXATION

Relaxation has psychological, physiological and behavioural components, so a test which is restricted to only one of these cannot claim to be comprehensive. To give an accurate measure of the degree of relaxation present, assessment should cover all three components. Only an assessment which takes account of these multiple dimensions can reflect the complexity of the relaxation state.

Since there is no test which covers all three, the components must be measured separately. Possible forms of measurement include the following:

1. questionnaires
2. self-rating

3. physiological measurement
4. observation
5. counting the training sessions.

QUESTIONNAIRES

A questionnaire is a list of questions requiring 'yes/no' or similar answers, which can be converted into numerical scores. Its purpose is to obtain information about a specific topic. A standardized questionnaire is the instrument of choice as it will have been tested on different groups of people and average scores will have been established, against which the individual's scores can be compared. This kind of questionnaire is the only kind that can be used for quantitative assessment and research. In the case of relaxation, such a questionnaire could be used to obtain information both at the start and at the end of a course of treatment, in order to see how people progress and to compare them with groups diagnosed as 'anxious' or 'normal', for example.

The advantages of questionnaires are that they are quick, cheap and easy to complete. It is also easy to collate the results. Their disadvantages include the possibility of inaccuracy if the questions are misunderstood, or of missing out information, if forcing responses into yes/no categories should fail to express the complexity of a person's position.

The interview schedule

An alternative and more sensitive approach is to use an interview schedule. Here, the interviewer guides the individual through a list of questions, making sure those questions have been understood and drawing fuller answers than are possible in a questionnaire. Thus, the interview schedule provides more detailed and more complete information than the questionnaire. Quantifying the results, however, is more difficult and the interview schedule is subject to variability between interviewers, each of whom may have different ways of interviewing people.

Examples of questionnaires

There is available a wide range of standardized questionnaires, each designed to measure a particular aspect of mental distress. The following are examples.

The Hospital Anxiety and Depression Scale (HAD) (Zigmond & Snaith 1983). This contains 14 items, seven relating to anxiety and seven to depression. The score gives an indication of the degree to which the individual is suffering from either condition. The scale is also able to pick up alterations over time.

The General Health Questionnaire (Goldberg & Williams 1988). This consists of 12 items and is designed to detect feelings of distress in the individual. As a simple screening device it is used for much the same purposes as the HAD.

The Beck Depression Inventory (Beck et al 1961, Beck 1988). Measures of the level of depression can be obtained from this questionnaire which can be used at different stages of illness and recovery.

The Cognitive Anxiety Questionnaire (Lindsay & Hood 1982). This contains 12 items and reflects some of the commonest thoughts associated with anxiety. The scale measures the tendency of the individual to engage in such thoughts.

These are all simple screening devices for use with individuals. The results, when obtained at the beginning and at the end of a training course, give an indication of change over time in the individual concerned.

The results can also be used to assess the effectiveness of relaxation training on groups of people. In this case, means and standard deviation are calculated so that the data can be used for statistical purposes and employed, for instance, in building a case for funding.

The Hospital Anxiety and Depression Scale is shown in Figure 26.1. It has been picked as an example because of its widespread use and general applicability. Questions 1, 4, 5, 8, 9, 12 and 13 relate to anxiety, and questions 2, 3, 6, 7, 10, 11 and 14 relate to depression. Scoring instructions are attached to the assessment sheet but not included here. A score of 8–10 in either section indicates a mild degree of the condition, while a score of 11 or above suggests the advisability of referral to a specialist agency. Although the scale is seen as a screening tool, it is, in the present context, used primarily to measure tendencies to mental distress

which may change over the period in which relaxation is practised. Any resulting change should not, however, be totally attributed to relaxation, since other factors such as changing environmental circumstances may be contributing to alterations in scores.

Tests show that the HAD possesses a considerable degree of validity and reliability although, as with most scales, further testing is required before confident judgements on its performance can be made. Its ability to detect minor degrees of psychiatric disorder has been shown and it has been found responsive to changes in individuals with neurotic disorders. The scale is also easy to understand and has been found acceptable to patients, taking only 5 minutes to complete (Bowling 1997).

A fuller list of self-administered questionnaires appears in Appendix 2. It relates particularly to the condition of depression.

Specific questions for participants

To make the assessment information more specific to the group whose problems are being measured, additional questions could be put to the participants, for example:

- In the case of a smoking cessation group, 'How many cigarettes are you now smoking a day?'.
- In the case of a person suffering from agoraphobia, 'How many times have you been out of the house in the past week?'.

Each person could select two or three personally meaningful targets like these and keep a record of their progress in relation to them. Precise targets, such as the above examples, are measurable and therefore preferable to vague aspirations such as 'I'd like to feel better'.

SELF-RATING

Related to the questionnaire is the self-rating scale, i.e. the rating an individual gives herself. It often takes the form of a visual analogue. Though it is a highly subjective assessment, it nevertheless has value since relaxation is an internal state with a strong subjective component. The self-rating scale is particularly useful for recording levels of pain and anxiety.

SECTION 1

NAME:

DATE:

AGE:

This section is designed to help identify how you feel. Read each item and place a tick in the box opposite the reply which comes closest to how you have been feeling in the past few weeks. Don't take too long over your replies: your immediate reaction to each item will probably be more accurate than a long thought out response.

Tick only one box in each section

(1) I feel tense or 'wound up':
Most of the time
A lot of the time
Time to time. Occasionally
Not at all

(2) I feel as if I am slowed down:
Nearly all the time
Very often
Sometimes
Not at all

(3) I still enjoy the things I used to enjoy:
Definitely as much
Not quite so much
Only a little
Hardly at all

(4) I get a sort of frightened feeling like 'butterflies' in the stomach:
Not at all
Occasionally
Quite often
Very often

(5) I get a sort of frightened feeling as if something awful is about to happen:
Very definitely and quite badly
Yes, but not too badly
A little, but it doesn't worry me
Not at all

(6) I have lost interest in my appearance:
Definitely
I don't take so much care as I should
I may not take quite as much care
I take just as much as ever

(7) I can laugh and see the funny side of things:
As much as I always could
Not quite so much now
Definitely not so much now
Not at all

(8) I feel restless as if I have to be on the move:
Very much indeed
Quite a lot
Not very much
Not at all

(9) Worrying thoughts go through my mind:
A great deal of the time
A lot of the time
From time to time but not too often
Only occasionally

(10) I look forward with enjoyment to things:
As much as ever I did
Rather less than I used to
Definitely less than I used to
Hardly at all

(11) I feel cheerful:
Not at all
Not often
Sometimes
Most of the time

(12) I get sudden feelings of panic:
Very often indeed
Quite often
Not very often
Not at all

(13) I can sit at ease and feel relaxed:
Definitely
Usually
Not often
Not at all

(14) I can enjoy a good book or radio or TV programme:
Often
Sometimes
Not often
Very seldom

Figure 26.1 The Hospital Anxiety and Depression Scale. (Adapted from Zigmond & Snaith 1983 Acta Psychiatrica Scandinavica 67: 361–370 with permission from Munksgaard, Copenhagen, and reproduced from Anxiety and Stress Management by Powell & Enright 1990 with permission from Routledge, London.)

Self-rating may take different forms:

- A rating scale in the form of a line calibrated from 0 to 10 where 0 represents total relaxation, and 10 maximum tension. The intervening numbers refer to intermediate states. The trainee rings the appropriate number.
- A rating scale which consists of numbered descriptors signifying different degrees of relaxation and tension, as in Poppen's (1988) self-rating scale (Ch. 9, pp 80–81). Again, the trainee rings the appropriate number.

These may be used before and after the relaxation session. Marking scales in this way gives a measure of the effect of the treatment.

During the homework periods a form such as the one illustrated in Figure 8.3 (p. 71) may be completed. This helps to ensure that practice is carried out as well as providing an indication of the degree of benefit obtained. A diary, when used to record instances of high stress, is another form of self-report; so is the record sheet (Fig. 8.2, p. 69) in which the occurrence and intensity of anxious feelings are recorded on a numbered scale together with details of the particular coping strategy adopted.

The advantages of the self-report method are that it is quick, easy, cheap and non-threatening to the trainee. It does, however, have limitations:

1. Responses may be influenced by social concerns which enter into the individual's judgement, for example:
    a. people tend to say what they feel is expected of them
    b. they may say what they think the trainer wants to hear
    c. they may present a view which shows them in a favourable light.
2. A placebo effect may be operating, whereby belief in the approach leads some people to report more benefit than has in fact occurred (see below, p. 226).

These factors result in a tendency for the responses to be unduly positive.

In his discussion of the verbal aspects of multimodal assessment, Poppen (1988) suggests remedies for this tendency. The participant can be reminded that questions of any sort tend to be answered differently, depending on who is asking the question: whether, for instance, it is a friend, a newspaper reporter or a doctor. This highlights the fact that there are many ways in which a question may be answered. The participant can then be asked to distinguish between the answer she feels is expected of her and the answer that reflects what she really feels. The second interpretation is, of course, the one that is required.

Self-rating can only provide a rough guide as to the effects of training. Its value lies particularly on an intrapersonal level, that is, where measurements are taken in the same individual before and after training sessions. Interpersonally, i.e. when comparing one individual with another, self-rating is less useful because of the varying standards of the reporters (Lichstein 1988).

A range of self-report measures can be found in Johnstone et al (1995).

PHYSIOLOGICAL MEASUREMENT

Assessing the effect of relaxation training on body systems provides an objective measurement. A variety of indicators are in current use, including pulse rate, blood pressure, respiratory rate, muscle tension, peripheral blood flow, palmar sweating, and electrical activity in the brain. Most of these can easily be measured, and machines are available for the purpose. The results indicate the level of physiological arousal in an individual, and the test or tests are carried out before and after relaxation sessions. The baseline is established before training begins and, in common with all pre-treatment measures, should be recorded after a short period of rest (see above).

It might be supposed that this approach offered the perfect solution. The field of physiological assessment, however, is not as straightforward as it appears. Keable (1997) discusses certain points:

- Physiological measures can be distorted by circumstances. The individual may, prior to a relaxation session, have eaten, which would result in artificially low arousal scores; she may have taken exercise immediately before, which would raise her scores; emotional distress would also raise them and drugs could distort them. Tests therefore need to be conducted under controlled conditions.

- Since the physiological response of individuals is to some extent idiosyncratic, a single measure may not include relevant information. To gain an accurate picture, therefore, a system which provides multiple measurements is needed.

Poppen (1988) adds the following point.

- Even in the case of specific symptoms, it is not always clear how their measurement should be approached. In tension headache, for example, it might be thought that electromyography of the surrounding muscles would be appropriate; however, exactly which muscles should be measured is less clear. Or again, instead of measuring the electrical activity, it might be more constructive to measure the bloodflow through the surrounding muscles (Olton & Noonberg 1980). Researchers hold different views.

Furthermore, while measurement of the pulse and breathing rate are simple procedures, most other physiological measures require equipment and expertise, neither of which may be available.

In spite of these difficulties, however, physiological measurement is an important aspect of general assessment.

OBSERVATION

Informal unstructured observation is practised by most trainers and used to corroborate information collected from other sources. A structured form of observation, such as role play, may also be employed. However, since the presence of the observer tends to affect the outcome, it is sometimes carried out in her physical absence but with the use of videos, tape recorders and two-way mirrors. (Ethical considerations demand that the individual's consent must first be obtained.)

It was in an attempt to structure the observation process that Schilling & Poppen (1983) devised the Behavioural Relaxation Scale as an assessment tool (Ch. 9, p. 79). As mentioned in Chapter 9, the scale provides a quantified measure of the motor component of relaxation (Poppen 1988).

COUNTING THE TRAINING SESSIONS

In the absence of an easy and accurate method of measuring the effects of relaxation training, some clinicians may resort to counting the sessions attended on the assumption that a fixed number of sessions will create a predictable level of relaxation skill. This method can never be more than a rough guide of progress, since there is known to be a mismatch between the amount of teaching and the amount of learning that occurs in any lesson (Poppen 1988).

A PRACTICAL APPROACH TO ASSESSMENT

Because none of the above measures alone offers the perfect solution, and because relaxation is a multimodal state, assessment ideally includes a variety of measures, each reflecting a different dimension of relaxation. Time-consuming as it is, careful assessment is important. Its value cannot be overemphasized if clinical methods are to have credibility.

However, it is acknowledged that overworked health care professionals may find it difficult to meet the above requirements, particularly if their groups are large. In this event, the following procedure could be set up:

- Participants are asked to state (verbally or in writing) what they hope to gain from the course. They can be asked to list three targets as described above.

While the course is in progress:

- Some kind of self-rating is carried out regularly.
- Some kind of physiological assessment is carried out regularly (pulse or breathing rate).
- The attendance rate is noted.
- Home practice is monitored (Fig. 8.3).

At the end of the course:

- Participants are asked if the course satisfied the three targets they listed in the beginning.

It should be noted that this kind of assessment is minimal. A system which provides fuller information is desirable for clinical purposes, and essential for research purposes.

THE PLACEBO EFFECT

Any measurement of relaxation is likely to be influenced to some extent by the placebo response.

This is the benefit derived by the individual as a result of her belief in the efficacy of the procedure, and it is separate from the procedure's intrinsic value. Simply believing in the treatment creates benefit, and this contributes to the total effect. The placebo response, however, is not the same as spontaneous improvement. It may produce the same result, but whereas spontaneous improvement is unrelated to treatment, the placebo response is an intrinsic feature of treatment. The placebo effect should be borne in mind in clinical work, while in research it must be controlled for.

CLINICAL AUDIT

Clinical audit consists of the systematic analysis of procedures used for diagnosis, care and treatment (Department of Health 1994). It poses questions such as:

- To what extent do these procedures benefit the patient?
- Do these procedures make the best use of resources?
- Can this service be improved?

Audit assesses the effectiveness of a particular intervention in a particular context or location and acts as a guide in the planning of services. As well as measuring the effects of clinical practice, it is concerned with issues such as resource allocation and may be used to highlight a need for departmental funding. This distinguishes it from research whose aim is to generate new knowledge or to test old knowledge and methods of treatment, seeking to identify the most effective intervention. Put another way, audit examines existing practice while research defines best practice (Sealey 1999). However, there is an interaction between audit and research in that the standards by which clinical practice is measured are established mainly from the research literature (Barnard & Hartigan 1998, Bury & Mead 1998). This relationship underlies the principles of evidence-based practice.

OUTCOME MEASUREMENT

All measuring procedures produce an outcome, which has been defined as 'that part of the output

of a process which can be attributed to the process' (Long et al 1993). In the context of health care, outcome can be seen as change in the health of an individual which is likely to be due to the therapeutic intervention.

Outcome is measured by an instrument which might be a questionnaire or other measuring tool and the results then undergo analysis in order to determine the degree to which the intervention was responsible for any change in the health status of the individual.

Outcome measures can be objective or subjective. Objective measures include quantifiable factors such as arterial blood gas levels; subjective measures include on the one hand, the level of pain experienced by the patient, and on the other, observational judgements made by the therapist (Barnard & Hartigan 1998).

Tools for measuring outcome are designed for different purposes, such as goal attainment, functional status, pain levels or patient satisfaction (Romain 1995). They may also vary in their range of concern, i.e. be multidimensional or condition-specific. An example of a multidimensional outcome measure is the Short Form 36 (Ware & Sherbourne 1992) which assesses physical and mental components of health, giving an indication of quality of life; an example of a condition-specific outcome measure is the Self-esteem Inventory (Rosenberg 1965) which focuses on one particular area of mental health. Since a treatment outcome can have several aspects, the question can be answered more fully if a variety of measures are used. Some examples of standardized devices for measuring therapeutic outcome may be found in Appendix 2.

It can be seen that the same devices may be used for assessing the patient's progress as for auditing the service or conducting research. For example, an instrument such as the Beck Depression Inventory can be useful in all contexts. To make outcome measurement as accurate as possible, certain criteria must be fulfilled (Donaghy 2001). The measuring device should be:

1. appropriate, i.e. suitable for the purpose and contain relevant items
2. valid, i.e. shown to be measuring what it claims to measure

3. reliable, i.e. capable of providing the same answer when the test is repeated by other therapists or by the same therapist on different occasions

4. responsive, i.e. sensitive to change, able to detect small variations over time and sensitive to individual differences

5. specific, i.e. able to isolate particular characteristics, for example, to focus on depressive symptoms as opposed to general symptoms of ill-health

6. acceptable, i.e. presented in such a way that the clients feel comfortable with the questions and fully understand what is being asked

7. feasible, in the sense of the equipment being available and within budget costs.

Clinical audit is thus concerned with the ability to demonstrate effectiveness, which, together with efficiency, form the twin pillars of Cochrane's

---

Box 26.1 Sources of information regarding outcome

1. National Centre for Health Outcomes Development: http://phi.uhce.ox.ac.uk
2. National Institute for Clinical Excellence: http://www.nice.org.uk

---

philosophy (Cochrane 1972). Its essential feature is measurement, as it is in patient assessment. However, in seeking to make therapeutic care more effective for all clients, audit goes beyond the treatment outcome of the individual patient to encompass wider issues.

Further discussion of audit is beyond the scope of this book but the interested reader is referred to the works of Bury & Mead (1998) and Barnard & Hartigan (1998).

Further reading

For assessment and research

Barnard S, Hartigan G 1998 Clinical audit in physiotherapy: from theory into practice. Butterworth-Heinemann, Oxford

Bowling A 1997 Measuring health: a review of quality of life measurement scales. Open University Press, Buckingham

Bowling A 2001 Measuring disease: a review of disease-specific quality of life measurement scales, 2nd edn. Open University Press, Buckingham

Bury T J, Mead J M (eds) 1998 Evidence-based health care: a practical guide for therapists. Butterworth-Heinemann, Oxford

Tansella M, Thornicroft G (eds) 2001 Mental health outcome measures. Gaskell, London

Acknowledgement

The author is indebted to Ian Hughes for his advice on this chapter.

Chapter 27

Evidence from research suggesting choice of technique for particular conditions

INTRODUCTION

There is a pressing need for therapists to demonstrate the effectiveness of their treatments, not only to serve the client in the best way but also to validate their work. Carefully designed and rigorously executed studies, repeated many times, help to build a robust foundation of effective treatments which contribute to the current best practice.

Much work has been done to measure the effect of different methods or to weigh up relaxation training against other approaches such as cognitive treatment, exercise or pharmacology. The results are, however, beset by methodological shortcomings; moreover, the diversity of methodologies makes it difficult to compare one study with another (Donaghy & Morss 2000). Kerr (2000) reports that all techniques have the potential to reduce indicators of stress, whether physiological or psychological, thereby suggesting benefit; however, regarding the superiority of one technique over another, no clear picture emerges. In her review, Kerr (2000) lists some of the reasons for this: variations in sample size, varied durations of the intervention and different outcome measures. Only further research can resolve these matters.

While assessment measures the relaxation achieved in the individual, research tests the general value of the relaxation method. Among the questions asked by the researcher are:

- Is method X useful in condition A?
- Is it more effective than method Y?

- Does it provide more benefit in one setting than another?

This chapter draws on existing research into the effectiveness of relaxation techniques in the context of specified conditions. The range of conditions discussed is by no means comprehensive. Many other conditions have been investigated which are not included. The chapter simply offers a selection to give the reader a glimpse of the kind of work that is being carried out in the field of relaxation training. A table suggesting appropriate techniques for particular conditions may be found in Appendix 3. Although the choice of technique is based on information from research, it is intended only as a guide.

WHAT IS THE EVIDENCE?

Mandle et al (1996) conducted a review of 37 studies exploring the efficacy of relaxation training in different diagnostic categories and clinical settings and found conflicting evidence of its value. In their conclusions they report that the most consistent positive results were found in patients with mild to moderate hypertension while other conditions where benefit was demonstrated were headache, insomnia, anxiety and pain. On the whole, improvement was more marked in the medical than in the surgical field.

Of the areas which attract research interest, the following are discussed in this chapter:

- anxiety
- panic disorder
- depression
- headache and migraine
- asthma
- insomnia
- hypertension and cardiac rehabilitation
- pain
- cancer
- pre- and post-surgery
- alcohol misuse
- menopause
- epilepsy
- learning disabilities
- athletic injuries
- chronic fatigue syndrome and fibromyalgia

- HIV/AIDS
- occupational stress.

Many of the studies reported are of sound quality (Kerr 2000); some may be deeply flawed, but in the way in which they are presented in this work they should not be seen as having undergone the critical scrutiny required for a scientific review. Such a work is beyond the scope of this book. Rather, the chapter is written to inspire the reader's interest and the author has hoped to do this by sharing a few reflections in the context of recent investigations. For critical appraisal of the individual studies, the reader is urged to look elsewhere.

ANXIETY

Most diseases and conditions are accompanied by some degree of anxiety: fear of pain, fear of deterioration and doubts about recovery. The notion of relaxation training as a useful intervention would, therefore, seem to be a logical one. Anxiety conditions themselves have been found to respond to this training. One of these is social anxiety disorder. This has been shown to benefit from cognitive behaviour therapy (of which relaxation training is a component) in a number of investigations (Heimberg 2002). Heimberg discusses the common clinical practice of combining cognitive behaviour therapy with pharmacological treatment and points to a need for further study of this dual approach which he feels does not yet stand on firm empirical ground.

The effects of relaxation training itself on anxiety have been studied in both healthy and clinical populations with positive results. Many of the non-clinical populations have been student groups, as for example in the study of Rasid and Parish (1998). These researchers studied the relative effects of behavioural relaxation training and progressive relaxation on American male and female high school students. Results showed state anxiety scores of both treatment groups to be significantly lower than those of control group participants who received no such training.

Stephens (1992) looked at the effects of imagery and progressive relaxation on first year nursing students and found that training in either was associated with significantly lower state anxiety scores than no training. Students in the treatment groups also reported additional benefits such as greater energy, more self-confidence, increased ability to sleep and improved sense of well-being.

With regard to clinical populations, Weber (1996) gave 39 inpatients in a general psychiatric unit a course of relaxation training consisting of progressive muscle relaxation, meditation, breathing, guided imagery and soft music. Results showed a significant reduction in anxiety levels from pre- to post-test, although methodological deficiencies in the form of non-random sampling and absence of control necessarily diminish the value of the findings. However, the author draws attention to the low cost of the relaxation techniques employed.

It is often said that research findings might have been different if the period of training in the technique had been longer or the participants had spent more time practising it. One study which bears out both these points is the randomized and controlled trial of Borkovec & Mathews (1988). These researchers compared the anxiety levels of individuals trained in progressive relaxation training with the levels of those untrained and found that the reduction in anxiety demonstrated in the trained group became still more pronounced as practice of the technique increased.

PANIC DISORDER

Both psychological and pharmacological approaches are conventionally employed in the treatment of panic disorder. Clum and colleagues (1993) looked at their relative value in meta-analysis, which revealed that treatments involving relaxation training, cognitive restructuring and exposure appeared to be the most effective strategies. Pharmacological treatments seemed to be less useful.

The benefit of psychological treatments was again demonstrated in a study by Penava and colleagues (1998) in which, following 12 sessions of treatment, a significant reduction in symptoms was found, with the greatest effect occurring in the first 4 weeks. The authors discuss the benefit of giving the clients information about predicted rates of improvement since such information helps them to form accurate expectations, which in turn may influence their motivation.

DEPRESSION

Depression is characterized by a lack of interest and loss of pleasure in usual concerns. It is described as clinical when symptoms become marked enough to interfere with normal activities and to persist for 2 weeks or longer (Peveler et al 2002). Depression can be a primary disorder, as in the case of major depression, or it may be secondary to the experience of an already existing disorder, such as cancer (Craft & Landers 1998).

Donaghy & Durward (2000) find some evidence to suggest that relaxation training may be beneficial (particularly for women) in relieving symptoms of mild-to-moderate depression, adding however, that the evidence is tentative. Cognitive behaviour therapy, drugs and psychotherapy are currently seen as having more to offer.

Since anxiety and depression so often occur together, they are increasingly being viewed as a single condition (Sloman 2002).

HEADACHE AND MIGRAINE

Headache is an area in which psychological treatments are widely used in a variety of populations including children, adolescents, young women and the elderly. The review by Reid & McGrath (1996) examined the effects of such treatments on migraine, and indicated that considerable benefit could be derived from biofeedback (Ch. 24, p. 211), relaxation training and stress-coping training. The authors concluded that for most people relaxation is an effective treatment, producing benefit which is maintained for at least a year. Marcus et al (1998) support this view and consider relaxation training with thermal biofeedback to be the treatment of choice for this condition.

Anxiety-related headaches are common in children preparing for exams. Relaxation techniques are frequently offered with the object of reducing anxiety to normal levels. In their review of school-based programmes, most of which delivered a modified version of progressive relaxation training, King and colleagues (1998) concluded that the benefits of such treatment on its own are modest. They suggest its impact would be greater if relaxation training were incorporated into more comprehensive packages.

Since this review, Sartory and colleagues (1998) have published a study involving 43 children, aged 8–16 years, with migraine, in which three different strategies for reducing the frequency, intensity and duration of children's headaches were tested. Of the three strategies, the most successful one was found to be relaxation training, followed by cephalic vasomotor feedback, with beta-blockers taking third place.

ASTHMA

A number of non-pharmacological treatments are offered to asthma sufferers. These include relaxation therapy, biofeedback, educational self-management and family therapy. In their review of scientific work in the area, Lehrer and colleagues (1992) found that relaxation therapy occasionally produced some significant effects, in particular with the use of progressive relaxation. While not all results reached levels of statistical significance, they did consistently lie in that direction, which led the reviewers to suggest that relaxation therapy be seen as a useful adjunct to medical management of the condition. A recent systematic review (Huntley et al 2002) drew similar conclusions and singled out muscular relaxation as conferring more benefit than other forms of relaxation training. In general, however, the evidence in favour of relaxation training in the management of asthma was not strong. Reviewers point to the poor quality of many of the studies and the problems inherent in this field of study – factors which make it difficult to draw firm conclusions.

It is possible that some asthma sufferers are more responsive to relaxation training than others. This might suggest that stress plays a part of varying importance as a trigger of attacks. To test this hypothesis, Vazquez & Buceta (1993) highlighted a sub-group of people whose attacks were triggered by emotional factors. Focusing on children with light to moderate degrees of asthma, these researchers found that participants who displayed emotionally triggered attacks, and who were treated with progressive relaxation training, experienced significantly shorter durations of attack and significantly greater increases in peak expiratory flow rate than those who displayed emotionally triggered attacks and received

pharmacological treatment. Thus, a stress-relieving technique was shown to be effective in this sub-group, leading the authors to conclude that progressive relaxation training could be a useful intervention for people whose asthma was associated with stress. They further suggested that, before treatment programmes were drawn up, it might be useful to identify those asthma sufferers whose attacks were triggered by emotional factors.

Evidence regarding the effectiveness of relaxation training in adult asthma is presented in a paper by Ritz (2001, p. 659) in which he discusses possible mechanisms. In the case of progressive relaxation training, he suggests that it might be the tensing component rather than the release component which is useful in relieving asthma since tensing is associated with excitation of the sympathetic nervous system, one of whose functions is to open the airways. By contrast, the release component is associated with parasympathetic influence and a restriction of airflow.

INSOMNIA

Interventions for the relief of insomnia have typically been pharmacological. However, a wide range of non-pharmacological treatments exist in the form of sleep hygiene techniques, stimulus control instruction, sleep restriction, chronotherapy, relaxation therapy, biofeedback, paradoxical intention and cognitive therapy. These approaches are popular with people who fear the possibility of drug side effects and dependency, which can occur with many pharmacological remedies.

In their review of the relevant literature, Bootzin & Perlis (1992) indicated the particular benefit of stimulus control, an approach which is concerned with the setting up of sleep/wake patterns such as using the bedroom exclusively for sleep, rising at the same time every day and avoiding a daytime nap. Relaxation training was also shown to have value, and the same reviewers referred to one of the better designed studies in which the effectiveness of progressive relaxation training as a sleep-inducing technique was demonstrated.

Other reviewers (Richmond et al 1996) weighing the evidence in respect of insomnia report that, although relaxation training can be effective, its benefits seem to be confined to certain aspects of sleep. In their opinion, meditation produces good results, which are sometimes better than those produced by muscular methods. Overall, however, they agree with Bootzin & Perlis (1992) that stimulus control is a highly effective non-pharmacological treatment for insomnia.

HYPERTENSION AND CARDIAC REHABILITATION

Relaxation training has been extensively studied with respect to its effectiveness in reducing blood pressure. This literature was reviewed by Eisenberg and colleagues in 1993. From a pool of 800 published works, 26 met the strict criteria of the authors, and these 26 covered such approaches as meditation, muscle relaxation and biofeedback. Meta-analysis revealed that these interventions were more effective than no therapy, but not more effective than credible sham techniques. This suggested that the effect of relaxation training was primarily that of placebo. Thus it seemed that the benefits of relaxation training for reducing blood pressure were, at best, modest, and the authors concluded that anti-hypertensive pharmacotherapy had more to offer.

By contrast, the findings of a large study conducted in Taiwan were more supportive of the claims made for relaxation training. In a trial consisting of 590 hypertensive people, Yen and colleagues (1996) found progressive relaxation and meditation to be more effective than either regular blood pressure monitoring or self-learning packages, although all interventions significantly reduced systolic blood pressure. Further support has come from the findings of a study which set out to explore the relative effectiveness of two relaxation techniques. Salt & Kerr (1997) found that both progressive relaxation and the Mitchell method were significantly more effective than supine lying at reducing systolic blood pressure (Ch. 10, p. 90).

Biofeedback-assisted relaxation training is another approach which has resulted in significant reductions of systolic and diastolic blood pressure as was demonstrated in a meta-analysis of randomized controlled clinical trials on adults

(Yucha 2001). These reviewers concluded by urging health care professionals to offer relaxation techniques as a treatment adjunct to their hypertensive clients.

In the management of essential hypertension it has been shown that the risk factor with the strongest and most consistent correlation (apart from age) with blood pressure is weight (Anand 1999). A cognitive behavioural approach with relaxation component would seem an appropriate way to address this problem.

Relaxation training has also been studied with regard to its usefulness following myocardial infarction. In a study involving 156 patients, post-infarction hospitalizations were shown to be reduced by 31% following a relaxation programme (Van Dixhoorn 1997). The authors suggest that the addition of such procedures to cardiac rehabilitation might favourably influence the course of the underlying disease.

King et al (2002) reviewed the research on transcendental meditation in the treatment and prevention of coronary heart disease. In their conclusions they found a measurable association between transcendental meditation and decreased hypertension together with indications that the approach had potential as a preventive strategy for coronary heart disease.

People with cardiovascular problems can benefit from interventions which modify their autonomic changes. Studying ways of reducing the intensity of sympathetic responses to environmental stimuli, Lucini and colleagues (1997) compared a combination of muscle relaxation and breathing awareness with beta-adrenergic blockade and found them equally effective, and significantly more effective than sham training. This apparent capacity of relaxation techniques to blunt excitatory autonomic responses has implications for behaviour in all situations which the individual finds challenging.

PAIN

A widely adopted view sees the perception of pain as governed by a neural 'gate' in the spinal cord (Melzack & Wall 1965). When this gate is open it allows signals from the pain receptors on the skin to pass to the brain, exposing the individual to the full experience of the pain; however, signals sent down from the cortex can close the gate, thereby reducing the perceived intensity of the pain. For example, if you are enjoying a film, you will be less inclined to notice bodily irritations that might otherwise claim your attention. Most non-pharmacological pain relief can be explained by the gate theory.

Seers & Carroll (1998) singled out the effects of relaxation training in a review of the literature in the context of acute pain, i.e. pain experienced following surgery or during procedures. They examined seven randomized controlled trials where relaxation was the only intervention and found that three of them showed a significant reduction of pain sensation and pain distress while the other four demonstrated no difference. The reviewers concluded that while there is some evidence to support the use of relaxation techniques in acute pain, that evidence is not strong and, in the present state of knowledge, relaxation training should therefore be seen as an adjunct rather than a principal form of treatment in the management of acute pain. However, many patients are reluctant to rely too heavily on analgesics, and for them it could be a useful alternative.

It was not possible to compare the various techniques for effectiveness because in most of the studies they were used in combinations.

A second review was conducted by the same two researchers, with the focus of interest this time on chronic pain (Carroll & Seers 1998). The studies covered a range of conditions but all used relaxation training (in different forms) as the sole intervention. Nine randomized controlled trials met the inclusion criteria. Chronic pain levels, which in most cases were measured on the McGill Pain Questionnaire (Melzack 1975), were lowered following training and, in four of the studies, showed a significant difference between pre- and post-test scores. Three studies comparing relaxation with other treatments reported significant findings in favour of relaxation training.

Some studies showed relaxation training to be particularly effective in certain conditions, for instance in rheumatoid arthritis where subjective ratings of pain were significantly lower following training in the relaxation group than in the routine-treatment control group; and in ulcerative colitis where as many as six out of seven pain outcome measures showed relaxation training to be significantly more effective than being in a waiting-list control group. (In this study, progressive relaxation was the technique used.) One cancer pain study showed a significant reduction in pain sensation scores where relaxation was taught by the nurses on the ward.

Carroll & Seers conclude that there is not enough evidence to state that relaxation can, by itself, reduce chronic pain; however, it does seem to be a useful component of treatment when used in combination with other cognitive behavioural strategies (Carroll & Seers 1998, Johnstone et al 2002).

Chronic pain featured as a topic of discussion among the 12 members of a panel set up to consider the merits of behavioural and relaxation approaches (Richmond et al 1996) (see section on insomnia). The members represented different fields of medicine. In their conclusion relating to chronic pain, the panel indicated the clear benefit of relaxation training over a wide spectrum of medical conditions where, in many instances, the evidence was judged to be quite strong. They also found relaxation approaches to be more effective than other cognitive behavioural methods and biofeedback. Regarding the choice of technique, there was no indication that any one method was more successful than another for reducing pain in a given condition.

Thus, it would seem that relaxation techniques in general have a place, if a modest one, in the management of chronic pain.

CANCER

There is a large body of research focusing on the pain and distress associated with different forms of cancer. Wallace (1997) examined the effect of relaxation and imagery within this context. In her review of studies, which included a variety of techniques and combinations, she could find few that were without methodological flaw. However, in spite of such weaknesses, a trend of benefit emerged in the sense that relaxation and imagery seemed to reduce the sensory experience of pain. More recently, Ernst et al (2001) referred to the complementary therapies as having some potential for benefit in palliative cancer care and Sloman (2002) found significantly positive changes in quality of life resulting from such therapies.

Some authors have explored ways of relieving the distress following chemotherapy. One such study (Vasterling et al 1993) examined the relative values of cognitive distraction (video games) and relaxation training (progressive relaxation and guided imagery) in this context. Both interventions resulted in less nausea and showed lower systolic blood pressures than the control (no intervention), while the relaxation group exhibited reduced diastolic blood pressures in addition. Although significance was not always achieved, the authors suggest that relaxation may have a useful adjunctive role to play in the relief of distress caused by chemotherapy.

Relaxation training with imagery has been associated with increases in survival duration. Spiegel & Moore (1997) followed up 86 women from a previous randomized trial and found that group therapy over the period of a year was not only supportive, as described by the participants, but was related to significant increases in length of survival time. The groups, which met at weekly intervals, received various forms of relaxation training together with healing imagery.

PRE- AND POST-SURGERY

Relaxation training can help people manage the distress they experience before and after surgery. Petry (2000), in her review of complementary therapies, indicates the benefit of such strategies for the well-being of the client. She also points to the advantage of such interventions in reducing the need for pain-relieving medication. It is further suggested that immune function, stress hormone levels and wound healing may also benefit from the effects of relaxation strategies. Among the techniques considered in Petry's article are muscular routines and imagery.

Some researchers have suggested that music might help provide pain relief. Good et al (2001) tested this hypothesis during the first 2 days following surgery. Four hundred and sixty-eight participants were divided into four groups: relaxation, music, their combination and a control. Results showed significant effects in all three intervention groups but very little difference between them.

In the field of cardiac surgery, Halpin et al (2002) showed that patients treated with guided imagery before and after surgery had a shorter length of stay in hospital and a reduced level of pain medication, while high overall patient satisfaction was maintained.

ALCOHOL MISUSE

Problem drinking is a condition that seems to respond better to exercise than to relaxation training (Donaghy et al 1991). However, relaxation training may have a place in helping to alter the individual's locus of control. This refers to the degree to which events are viewed as being within the individual's control: an internal locus implies a strong sense of personal control; an external locus implies a tendency to believe that events are controlled by factors outside the individual. The alcohol misuser is inclined to be more external in her locus of control than others; therefore, a treatment which could increase her sense of personal control might be helpful to her.

This topic interested Sharp and colleagues (1997) while they were working with young residents in North American treatment centres. Using autogenic training with biofeedback, these authors showed that relaxation techniques could increase the individual's sense of internal locus. They concluded that autogenic therapy might be a useful component of the total treatment package for young misusers of alcohol.

Relaxation training has also been shown to help alcohol misusers through periods of insomnia. In their study of 22 adults, Greeff & Conradie (1998) demonstrated significant improvements in sleeping patterns and in the quality of sleep following a programme of progressive relaxation training.

MENOPAUSE

The efficacy of relaxation training has also been investigated in conditions relating to women's health. One of these is the menopause. Irvin and colleagues (1996) studied the effects of instruction in Benson's method on a volunteer sample of women aged 44–66 years who were not using hormone replacement therapy.

Results showed a significant reduction in hot flush intensity, tension–anxiety and depression in the group receiving relaxation training, while a control group with whom they were compared showed no reduction. In their conclusion, the authors suggested that daily practice of Benson's method might help to reduce symptoms of the menopause and could be particularly useful for women who do not wish to use hormone replacement or whose health status precludes its administration.

EPILEPSY

Seizure reduction has been associated with regular practice of relaxation techniques, as in the controlled study of Puskarich et al (1992). Progressive relaxation training was the method employed. Of the 13 participants who received the intervention, 11 experienced a reduction in seizure frequency, while only 7 out of 11 in the control group of quiet sitting showed a decreased frequency. This suggests that the technique might be a useful adjunctive procedure for some people with epilepsy. Moreover, it is non-invasive, inexpensive and gives the client a sense of being in control.

In discussing the mechanism by which seizure frequency is reduced in this study, the authors propose that relaxation acts as a mediating factor, diminishing the impact of the stressor.

LEARNING DISABILITIES

(See Ch. 9, p. 81)

ATHLETIC INJURY

Athletic injury carries with it a number of stresses. In addition to the fear of pain and the fear of non-recovery there is the fear of re-injury when play is resumed. Cupal & Brewer (2001) studied the effects of relaxation and guided imagery in 30 participants undergoing rehabilitation following anterior cruciate ligament reconstruction. Among the positive effects demonstrated at 6-month follow-up was a significantly reduced level of re-injury anxiety and pain.

Long-term injuries are known to lower the mood of injured athletes. In an attempt to find a way of raising that mood level, Johnson (2000) studied the effect of different short-term interventions such as stress management, goal-setting skills and relaxation training with guided imagery. Of the three interventions, the only one to show statistical differences was relaxation training with guided imagery.

Imagery is widely used in sport, and particularly by athletes in training and competition. Both cognitive and motivational forms of imagery are practised (Ch. 18, p. 169). When athletes are injured they also use healing imagery which has been found to be associated with reduced pain, anxiety and distress, with accelerated healing and improved immune responses (Sordoni et al 2002).

CHRONIC FATIGUE SYNDROME AND FIBROMYALGIA

Chronic fatigue syndrome (otherwise known as myalgic encephalomyelitis) is a condition in which the predominating symptom is tiredness in the absence of previous exertion. Price & Couper (2000) conducted a systematic review of studies with adults which provided evidence of the benefit of cognitive behaviour therapy in this condition. In three of the trials greater benefit was demonstrated from this method of treatment than from orthodox medical management or from relaxation. Other researchers, for example Fulcher & White (1998), report that graded exercise and physical activity are effective approaches. The conclusion reached by Everett (2003, p. 257) is that both cognitive behaviour therapy and graded exercise can be useful approaches in the treatment of chronic fatigue syndrome.

Fibromyalgia is a chronic disorder characterized by a variety of symptoms which include aching muscles, general fatigue, sleep disturbances, anxiety and bowel problems. Many of these symptoms resemble those of chronic fatigue syndrome with which the condition is sometimes confused. Research into fibromyalgia syndrome has been systematically reviewed by Sim (2002). It indicates an absence of strong evidence for any single non-pharmacological intervention in the treatment of this condition, although there was some preliminary support for aerobic exercise. A systematic review in the preceding year (Oliver et al 2001) found cognitive behaviour therapy effective.

HIV/AIDS

It has been shown that cognitive behavioural programmes which include relaxation techniques can have favourable results, both psychological and physical, in HIV disease. Such outcomes represent an improved quality of survival time in individuals found to be HIV-positive. Several randomized controlled trials have shown significant reductions in anxiety and distress, while at the same time improving mood and self-esteem (Taylor 1995, Lutgendorf et al 1997). A decrease in the severity of physical symptoms was also reported by these authors, who demonstrated significantly lowered herpes simplex virus type 2 antibody titres (Lutgendorf et al 1997) and significantly raised T-cell counts (Taylor 1995) resulting from such programmes.

In the case of Lutgendorf et al's participants, the more consistently they practised the relaxation technique, the more their distress was relieved. The study ran for 10 weeks. Taylor's participants, who had trained for 20 weeks using progressive relaxation, meditation, biofeedback and hypnosis, demonstrated significant improvement which was maintained at follow-up 1 month later.

These researchers suggest that relaxation is a useful component of treatment for people diagnosed as HIV-positive.

OCCUPATIONAL STRESS

The Health and Safety Executive report that half a million people every year suffer from the effects of stress at work (Frontline 1999). From a large number of published studies on the subject of occupational health, the most successful programmes seem to be those which not only involve the entire organization and have the full support of management, but also engage the cooperation of the workforce during the planning stage (Van der Hek & Plomp 1997).

Several studies have been designed with a strong relaxation component which typically consists of varying combinations of techniques.

Tsai & Swanson-Crockett (1993) studied the effects of breathing, imagery and meditation on 68 Chinese nurses in Taiwan who practised these methods regularly for 5 weeks. At the end of this time, the stress scores of the participants were found to be significantly lower than those of the control group members who attended lectures on the theory of nursing. Thus, it seems that relaxation training may have a part to play in the control of occupational stress.

However, research is not marked by consistent findings. The overview of Van der Hek & Plomp (1997) was conducted in the hope of clarifying the picture and singling out the most successful approach. In the event, this proved an impossible task since the different studies had varying targets; for example, it was difficult to compare the effects of a procedure which addressed the individual and her subjective experience of stress with those of a different procedure where the central concern was with attendance rates and productivity levels. Conclusive evidence, therefore, awaits further work.

DIFFERENT FORMS OF RESEARCH

While research is not the only source of evidence for the value of relaxation training, it is the principal one, enabling the health care professional to provide the best treatment. Other sources include clinical experience, expert consensus, reflective practice, patient assessment and patient preferences (Bury & Mead 1998).

Evidence of effectiveness is most valued in the form of the review, which collects and scrutinizes relevant studies. Reviews may vary in terms of scientific rigour, the most respected one being the systematic review. Here, strict criteria are laid down, i.e. the databases employed are to be cited, the years which relate to the search stated, the number of papers involved recorded, the basis on which the selection was made stated and the key words listed. A critical review is also a useful document. It is often described as a narrative review and tends to express the opinion of the researcher. Critical reviews can vary in quality. Another type of review is the overview which is a description of key findings (M. Donaghy 2004, personal communication).

Appendix 4 contains a list of the reviews referred to in the text and includes all three kinds.

Individual studies can also be classified in terms of scientific rigour. Here, the most highly respected form is the randomized controlled trial (RCT). A hypothesis is first formulated and tested, then the data are analysed for statistical significance. A well-designed RCT will fulfil the following criteria. It will:

- contain a control group which does not receive the intervention and acts as a baseline
- adopt a randomized process both for the selection of participants and their assignment to particular groups
- be designed so that the results can be statistically analysed
- consist of a sample large enough to have a chance of reaching statistical significance
- carry a precise description of the intervention so that the study can be replicated
- be free of bias and order effects which may confound the results.

When these criteria are not met the study is said to be methodologically flawed, which means that the results lose some of their credibility. However, it is not always ethical or appropriate to use the randomized controlled trial as a design, and in these situations other forms of trial may be adopted such as non-randomized controlled studies and single system studies. The experiment, however, is not the only way to answer a question in research: a qualitative approach, in which descriptive data are collected, can also provide useful information and may be the method of choice where the function of research is one of exploration (Sim 1999). Interviews can be employed here.

Wherever subtleties in the therapeutic situation are being studied, the qualitative approach has much to offer. It reflects the lived experience of clients (Gibson & Martin 2003). Qualitative methods can also be used to complement the findings of experimental work, thereby building up a more complete picture.

SOME PITFALLS OF RESEARCH IN THIS FIELD

With regard to the different relaxation approaches, research does not show one method to be any more effective than another. Lichstein (1988), reviewing studies on progressive relaxation, autogenic training and meditation, points out that this conclusion may not, for several reasons, reflect the true picture. Research in this area is complicated by a number of factors related to procedural variability (Hillenberg & Collins 1982, Lichstein 1988):

1. different methods of delivery: 'live' or taped
2. different number of training sessions
3. variations in amount of home practice
4. variations in interpretation of the procedure.

1. Different methods of delivery

The procedure may be 'live' or taped. Early research supported the view that a 'live' delivery was more effective than a taped one for reducing tension levels (Paul & Trimble 1970). A more recent study (Sloman et al 1994), however, has demonstrated equal benefit from both 'live' and taped delivery in a hospital oncology ward. The taped delivery has the advantage of standardizing the procedure and, by this means, promoting reliability.

2. Different number of training sessions

Studies offer varying amounts of training. The more lessons a participant receives, the more skilled she is likely to become in the technique under investigation, where results will be influenced accordingly.

3. Variations in amount of home practice

It is believed that home practice is given inadequate attention (Hillenberg & Collins 1983). Reasons which may account for this phenomenon include failure of the therapist or researcher to convey its importance, misunderstanding by the participant of the nature of the technique or disinclination to carry it out. If, however, the technique is practised more frequently, the effect it creates is increased (Borkovec & Mathews 1988). Most writers recommend two practice periods a day, each lasting 15–20 minutes, accompanied by some kind of self-monitoring system to ensure that they are carried out and to record their effect.

4. Variations in interpretation of the procedure

A single technique may be presented in several different ways: for example, progressive relaxation may appear in Jacobson's original form, in Wolpe's, in Bernstein & Borkovec's or in any other derived form. This can lead to confusion.

Further difficulties arise when studies fail to specify the relaxation method used or assume that relaxation is synonymous with progressive relaxation training.

These are some of the points to bear in mind when designing a research project in the field of relaxation training. For further guidance, health care professionals are referred to other works, since the scale of the topic places it outside the scope of this book (see Further reading).

Further reading

Bowling A 1997 Research methods in health: investigating health and health services. OUP, Buckingham

Bury T J, Mead J M (eds) 1998 Evidence-based health care: a practical guide for therapists. Butterworth-Heinemann, Oxford

Crombie I K 2000 The pocket guide to critical appraisal. BMJ Publishing Group, London

Donaghy M, Durward B 2000 A report on the clinical effectiveness of physiotherapy in mental health. Chartered Society of Physiotherapy, London

Everett T, Donaghy M, Feaver S (eds) 2003 Interventions for mental health: an evidence-based approach for physiotherapists and occupational therapists. Butterworth-Heinemann, Oxford

French S, Reynolds F, Swain J 2001 Practical research: a guide for therapists. Butterworth-Heinemann, Oxford

Hammell K W, Carpenter C M, Dyke I 2000 Using qualitative research: a practical introduction for occupational and physical therapists. Churchill Livingstone, Edinburgh

Polgar S, Thomas S A 2000 Introduction to research in the health sciences, 4th edn. Churchill Livingstone, Edinburgh

Chapter 28

Drawing the threads together

This chapter addresses a few topics not so far covered. It begins with a discussion of the similarities among the methods and leads into a description of a general theory of relaxation. This is followed by a consideration of the ways in which techniques can be combined. Finally a few additional techniques are mentioned.

SIMILARITIES AMONG APPROACHES

In an enterprise such as relaxation training where many approaches all lead to the same goal, there are likely to be wide areas of overlap. Some of these have already been pointed out. Lichstein (1988) has identified common threads with respect to meditation, autogenics and progressive relaxation. He finds that dwelling on the breath (as in meditation), reciting phrases (as in autogenic training) and concentrating on muscle sensations (as in progressive relaxation), are activities which resemble one another since they all involve attention-focusing and the reduction of motor activity. Benson (1976) is of the same view in claiming that all three methods are characterized by a monotonous, repetitive stimulus equivalent to the mantra. Thus, the differences between the methods would seem to be more apparent than real; their similarities concealed by their terminology. This might help to explain why the different methods are so often shown to be equally effective when compared with each other.

KOKOSZKA'S GENERAL THEORY OF RELAXATION

The underlying similarities of the above three methods are reflected in the states of consciousness they produce. All three create altered states, which are, however, only slightly altered from the waking state. Eastern meditation and hallucinatory drugs, on the other hand, produce deeply altered states.

An attempt to integrate the major states of consciousness in the context of relaxation and place them on one conceptual canvas has been made by Kokoszka (1987–1988, 1992). He posits four main states of consciousness: ordinary waking states, differentiated waking states, rapid eye movement sleep, and non-rapid eye movement sleep. His model (Fig. 28.1) shows progressive relaxation and autogenic training to lie between the waking state and non-rapid eye movement (non-REM)

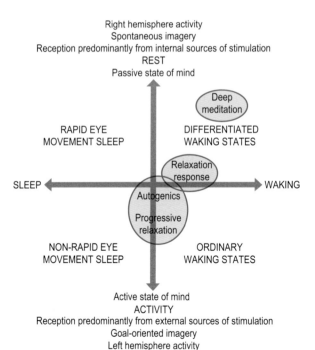

Figure 28.1   Integrated model of the main states of consciousness. (Adapted from Kokoszka A. 1987–1988 Imagination, Cognition and Personality 7: 292, with permission from Baywood Publishing Co., Inc., Amityville, New York and the author.)

sleep. Characterized by mental contact with the body, both progressive relaxation and autogenics have their roots in physiological, goal-oriented, left hemisphere concerns, such as the release of muscle tension, although autogenics in particular, relying on sensory images, reaches into the influence of the right hemisphere. Overlapping the other two, but lying in the waking quadrants, is Benson's relaxation response technique, its passive emphasis placing it predominantly among right hemisphere concerns but not entirely, since its imaginal content is weak.

Deep meditation of a kind that reaches profound spiritual levels is seen as being different in kind from Benson's meditation; Kokoszka calls it an 'ultra consciousness state' and places it firmly in the domain of the right hemisphere, far away from rational ideas and goal-oriented thought.

Moving on to the sleep zones: rapid eye movement sleep is characterized by dreaming and therefore has strong right hemisphere connections; it is distinctly remote from physical and rational concerns. Non-rapid eye movement sleep, however, is far removed from imaginal concerns; the individual is, of course, unaware of her surroundings but the state is accompanied by muscular (albeit weak) activity.

COMBINING APPROACHES

It is not suggested in this book that attention should be systematically given to the methods in turn. The health care professional may take up any method she feels comfortable with. She may, however, wish to take up more than one method and to present them in a single tuition period. This can have advantages. Combinations of different relaxation and stress reduction techniques seem to be more effective than single techniques (Lehrer & Woolfolk 1983, Woolfolk & Lehrer 1984, Poppen 1988, Titlebaum 1988, Davis et al 2000). Lehrer & Woolfolk (1983) found that more powerful effects were produced when techniques were used in combination than when any one technique was used alone.

Ways of combining techniques may be found in *The Relaxation and Stress Reduction Workbook* (Davis et al 2000) from which the following two combinations are drawn. The first is for mental stress, the second is for physical tension.

1. 'Changing channels':
   a. attention-switching (Appendix 1),
   b. guided imagery (Ch. 17, p. 157) and
   c. coping mantra, e.g. 'I am at peace' (Ch. 20, p. 188).
2. 'Stretch and relax':
   a. stretchings (Ch. 13),
   b. abdominal breathing (Ch. 15, p. 132) and
   c. Mitchell's method (Ch. 10).

For groups of people with varied kinds of stress, more general combined programmes can be built. A few examples are given below:

1. Abdominal breathing (Ch. 15, p. 132), tense–release (Ch. 6) and guided imagery (Ch. 17, p. 157).
2. Passive relaxation (Ch. 7), goal-directed visualizations using receptive and programmed components (Ch. 18) and self-statements (Ch. 18, p. 163).
3. Abdominal breathing (Ch. 15, p. 132), warmth and heaviness phrases (Ch. 19) and differential relaxation (Ch. 12).
4. Passive relaxation (Ch. 7), Benson's meditation (Ch. 21) and self-awareness exercises (Ch. 16).
5. Behavioural relaxation training (Ch. 9, p. 77), breathing meditation (Ch. 15, p. 133) and guided imagery (Ch. 17, p. 157).
6. Breathing pouch (Ch. 15, p. 133), eye and tongue muscle work (Ch. 4, p. 38) and meditation on a visual object (Ch. 20, p. 185).

Set patterns will not suit everyone since the needs and preferences of each person are different. Davis et al (2000) urge people to construct their own combination of techniques.

Although client preferences cannot be predicted, it is clear that they exist (Fanning 1988, Kutner & Zahourek 1988, Lichstein 1988, Payne 1989). In the author's experience it is useful to ask the client which techniques best suit her. Involving the client in the choice of technique, as in other aspects of therapy, enriches the treatment. All this, of course, means that therapists may need to learn several methods in order to respond to the client's needs.

EXAMPLE OF A SCRIPT CONTAINING A VARIETY OF APPROACHES

As well as grouping different techniques together, several techniques can be worked into a single passage as shown here.

Please lie down. Get yourself comfortable. Allow your eyelids to grow heavy and eventually to close.

Feel the rest of your body also growing heavy ... feel it sinking into the rug or the upholstery ... compressing the fibres ... sinking down so that more body area comes in contact with it ... let your weight flow out ... feel your body totally freed from its responsibility to hold you up...

Turn your attention to your breathing ... without attempting to alter its rhythm, become aware of the movement of your chest and abdomen ... notice the passage of the air ... the coolness of the air entering your nostrils ... travelling through your nose and down the back of your throat ... notice also, the warm, moist air being exhaled ... next time you breathe out, think the word 'relax' ... continue slowly...

Now, I'd like you to scan your muscle groups one by one, checking them for tension ... adjust your position if you are uncomfortable ... starting with the feet, notice how they rest heavily on the floor ... heavy as lead ... now your legs, imagine them too heavy to lift ... your hips too are lying heavily ... and your shoulders, feel how they are dropped down ... with your arms resting heavily by your sides...

Now, your head, let it sink back, giving its weight to the pillow, making a dent in it ... feel your brow smoothed and your jaw relaxed ... feel your whole body heavy, warm and relaxed ... if tension returns, just let it go ... let it flow out through your fingertips and toes...

Transfer yourself in your mind's eye to a sandy beach ... see yourself lying in the soft sand ... run your fingers through the dry grains ... smell the sea air ... feel the hot sun on your skin ... listen to the waves breaking on the shore ... enjoy the peace ... if disturbing thoughts intrude, accept that they exist ... then let them drift away like clouds passing across the sky ... you'll attend to them later...

When you are ready, let the scene fade ... gradually bring your attention back to the room in which you are lying ... count one ... two ... three ... and slowly open your eyes ... then give your arms and legs a gentle stretch...

OTHER WAYS OF ACHIEVING RELAXATION

There are countless other means by which an individual may achieve relaxation: hypnosis, dance therapy and music therapy, to mention just a few. Many of these require the presence of a therapist to carry out a procedure.

Hobbies also may provide a source of relaxation since creating for sheer pleasure induces undeniable feelings of well-being and fulfilment. In her hobby the individual spontaneously expresses herself and this experience gives her a sense of being at one with herself. Feelings of peace and relaxation are the natural result.

SUMMARY AND CONCLUSION

This chapter has touched on a few questions that a book of this nature might raise: the way methods relate to each other and the possibility of combining techniques.

In the rest of the book, selected methods of relaxation have been presented. The author has tried to convey the essence of each one and, for most approaches, to offer enough detail to enable them to be used by someone previously unfamiliar with them.

Wherever possible, the description has been followed by some kind of evaluation which is based on the research literature. Some methods such as progressive relaxation, autogenics and meditation have received a great deal of attention by researchers, while others such as Mitchell's method and the Alexander technique have been studied very little.

Is there one technique more effective than another? Kerr (2000, p. 87) tells us that in the present state of knowledge that question cannot be answered. No clear picture yet emerges in this regard in spite of the work that has already been carried out. However, it is not easy to draw conclusions because of the problems which beset scientific investigation in this area. A larger body of research is necessary. This research is slowly growing, and it is hoped that data will emerge from future projects which allow firmer conclusions to be drawn.

Further reading

For combinations of techniques

Davis M, Eshelman E, McKay M 2000 The relaxation and stress reduction workbook, 5th edn. New Harbinger, Oakland, California

For other methods of achieving relaxation

Sutcliffe J 1991 The complete book of relaxation techniques. Headline, London

SECTION 5

Appendices, Glossary, References and Index

Appendix 1

Attention switching and thought stopping

Among the many devices for distracting the attention away from disturbing thoughts are the cognitive techniques of attention switching and thought stopping.

ATTENTION SWITCHING

This technique consists of giving attention to particular items for specified lengths of time. The individual spends 15–20 seconds exclusively thinking about a prearranged item, then abruptly switches to another prearranged item for the same length of time. If a stopwatch is not available, she guesses the times. The items range from pleasant to neutral. The next stage is to deliberately introduce the disturbing thought, let it take shape, and as soon as it does, to replace it with a pleasant or neutral thought. The method may be described to the participant as follows:

Make a list of topics that are pleasant (such as hobbies, holidays, happy experiences) or neutral (such as the weather, telephone numbers, geometric shapes); say, 10 examples of each. Take the first one on the list and focus attention on it for 20 seconds. At the end of that time abruptly switch your attention to the next item. Concentrate on this for 20 seconds, then switch to the next item, working your way through the list. The object is to concentrate so firmly on the item that all other thoughts are excluded. It helps if the item is made as vivid as possible, and this is done by bringing out its sensory detail (the sights, sounds, smells, textures, etc.).

Work through the list every day for a week. When you feel you have built up the skill, try deliberately introducing the disturbing thought; give it a moment to take shape, then abruptly replace it with the next item on your list.

In this way you cultivate the ability to control your thoughts. You may not be able to stop uncomfortable thoughts entering your head, but you can decide how much attention you give them.

The ability to control the thoughts is present in every person. Attention switching simply helps to strengthen it. Widely used as a technique, it offers most benefit to people who have a facility for creating visual imagery.

THOUGHT STOPPING

Thought stopping (Quick & Quick 1984) intercepts stress-inducing thoughts and substitutes stress-relieving ones. The technique involves the word 'STOP', spoken or imagined, but in such a way that it momentarily blots out the disturbing thought. This is immediately replaced with an idea or activity which diverts and holds the attention, such as counting games, puzzles or physical exercise.

Appendix 2

Some examples of standardized self-administered outcome measuring tools

extracted from CLEF05, Chartered Society of Physiotherapy (2002), with permission

TO MEASURE MOOD

The Profile of Mood State (McNair et al 1992)
Multiple Affect Adjective Check List (Herron 1969)

TO MEASURE NEGATIVE FEELINGS OF DEPRESSION AND ANXIETY

Goldberg General Health Questionnaire
(Goldberg & Williams 1988)
Spielberger State–Trait Anxiety Inventory
(Spielberger et al 1970)
Beck Depression Inventory 2 (Beck 1988)
Hospital Anxiety and Depression Scale
(Zigmond & Snaith 1983)

TO MEASURE SELF–ESTEEM

Rosenberg Self-Esteem Inventory (Rosenberg 1965)
Physical Self-Perception Profile (Fox &
Corbin 1989)

TO MEASURE QUALITY OF LIFE

SF36 (Ware & Sherbourne 1992)
EQ5D (EuroQuol Group 1990)

Appendix 3

Table of suggested techniques for specific conditions

Method	Major principles	Suggested applications	Relevant chapters
Progressive relaxation	• relaxed musculature is reflected in a relaxed mind • underpinned by unitary theory • physiological principles predominate but there are cognitive elements	anxiety, psychiatric conditions, hypertension, tension headache, asthma, insomnia, chronic pain, ulcerative colitis, pre- and post-surgery, epilepsy, athletic injury, HIV/AIDS, chronic obstructive pulmonary disease, panic, migraine	Chapters 4 and 27
Progressive relaxation training	• similar to progressive relaxation except that the cognitive element is stronger because of the use of suggestion	similar to progressive relaxation	Chapters 5 and 27
Applied relaxation	• built around a core technique of progressive relaxation • addresses the concept of anxiety from cognitive and behavioural as well as physiological standpoints	anxiety, panic attacks, phobia, headache, tinnitus, epilepsy, chronic pain	Chapters 8 and 27
Behavioural relaxation training	• underpinned by behaviourist principles of reinforcement and corrective adjustment • contains physical and cognitive elements	learning difficulties, ataxic tremor	Chapters 9 and 27
Mitchell's method	• based on physiological principles of reciprocal inhibition • has a weak cognitive element	childbirth, hypertension, rheumatoid arthritis	Chapters 10 and 27
Alexander technique	• underpinned by principles of body positioning • is atheoretical	performance stress, motor problems, Parkinson's disease	Chapters 11 and 27

continued

Method	Major principles	Suggested applications	Relevant chapters
Stretchings	• these link into physiological principles • the process of stretching entails a relaxation of the muscles being stretched	physical and psychological stress, generalized anxiety, chronic neck tension	Chapters 13 and 27
Exercise	• essentially a physical approach to relaxation • linked to neurobiological changes, it is underpinned by physiological principles	cardiovascular problems, osteopenia, osteoporosis, depression, chronic fatigue syndrome, drug and alcohol dependence, eating disorders, low self-esteem	Chapters 14 and 27
Breathing	• based on physiological principles which link the method to the autonomic nervous system • slow breathing is associated with parasympathetic dominance • a cognitive feature is represented by the imagery which accompanies some breathing sequences	coronary heart disease, hypertension, panic attacks, chronic pain, occupational stress	Chapters 15 and 27
Self-awareness	• a cognitive approach concerned with the thoughts one has about the self	low self-esteem	Chapters 16 and 27
Imagery	• cognitive principles underlie this approach • image-making is thought to be governed by the right cerebral hemisphere	chronic pain, anxiety, pre- and post-surgery, athletic injury, occupational stress	Chapters 17 and 27
Goal-directed visualizations	• a cognitive approach which uses techniques of imagery and self-suggestion • based on the belief that the body cannot distinguish between the event as imagined and the event as experienced	performance stress, alcohol and substance misuse, eating disorders, smoking abstinence, chronic pain, sport and athletics, phobia and panic attack	Chapters 18 and 27
Autogenics	• based on principles of suggestion, which create a light trance • primarily a cognitive approach, although the sensations of warmth generated by the phrases provide a physiological element • is atheoretical	anxiety, depression, insomnia, drug and alcohol misuse, eating disorders, tension headache, hypertension, coronary heart disease, injury rehabilitation, asthma, HIV/AIDS, different kinds of pain	Chapters 19 and 27
Meditation	• a cognitive activity involving what is considered to be a shift in cerebral hemispherical dominance from left to right	hypertension, coronary heart disease, menopausal symptoms, insomnia, occupational stress, HIV/AIDS	Chapters 20 and 27

Method	Major principles	Suggested applications	Relevant chapters
Benson's method	<ul><li>underpinned by unitary theory</li><li>cognitive principles predominate in the focusing of attention on the mantra</li><li>in diminishing the activity in the sympathetic nervous system, it draws on physiological principles</li></ul>	hypertension, coronary heart disease, psychological stress, irritable bowel syndrome, menopausal problems	Chapters 21 and 27
Cognitive behavioural approaches	<ul><li>these use a variety of techniques drawn from cognitive principles on the one hand, and behavioural principles on the other</li><li>the client is encouraged to adopt a collaborative role in the management of her condition</li></ul>	anxiety, depression, eating disorders, panic disorder, drug and alcohol dependence, hypertension, chronic fatigue syndrome, insomnia, HIV/AIDS, psychiatric disorders, chronic pain	Chapters 22 and 27

Appendix 4

Review articles referred to in the text

Researcher	Area of concern	Nature of the review
Arroll & Beaglehole 1992	blood pressure and exercise	critical view
Blaine & Crocker 1993	self-esteem	integrative review
Borkovec & Sides 1979	progressive relaxation	review
Bowling 1997	measurement scales for health	review
Bowling 2001	measurement scales for disease	review
Carlson & Hoyle 1993	abbreviated progressive relaxation	quantitative review
Carroll & Seers 1998	chronic pain	systematic review
Clum et al 1993	panic disorder	meta-analysis
Cooke & Ernst 2000	aromatherapy	systematic review
Craft & Landers 1998	exercise and depression	meta-analysis
Donaghy & Durward 2000	physiotherapy in mental health	report
Donaghy & Mutrie 1999	exercise and alcohol misuse	critical review
Duckro & Cantwell-Simmons 1989	paediatric headache and relaxation	review
Faulkner & Biddle 1999	schizophrenia	review
Furlan et al 2000	massage for back pain	Cochrane systematic review
Glenister 1996	exercise and mental health	review
Gould et al 1995	panic disorder	meta-analysis
Hardman 1996	hypertension and exercise	review
Herbert & Gabriel 2002	stretching and protection from injury	systematic review
Hillenberg & Collins 1982	relaxation training	review
Huntley et al 2002	asthma and relaxation	systematic review
Kanji & Ernst 2000	autogenic training and anxiety	systematic review
Kerr 2000	progressive relaxation, Mitchell's method, massage, Alexander technique, Benson's method, Yoga	critical review
King et al 2002	meditation and hypertension	review
Kugler et al 1994	anxiety and depression in coronary disease	meta-analysis
Lawler & Hopker 2001	exercise for depression	systematic review
Luskin et al 2000	mind-body therapies	review
Mandle et al 1996	relaxation interventions in different diseases	review
Mutrie 2001	exercise for depression	review
Oliver et al 2001	fibromyalgia	review
Petry 2000	surgery	review

Researcher	Area of concern	Nature of the review
Roth & Fonaghy 1996	psychotherapy	critical review
Scully et al 1998	exercise and well-being	critical review
Seers & Carroll 1998	acute pain	systematic review
Sharma & Alexander 1996	meditation	review
Silagy et al 1994	smoking cessation	systematic review
Sim 2002	fibromyalgia	systematic review
Stetter & Kupper 2002	autogenic training	meta-analysis
Van der Hek & Plomp 1997	occupational stress	overview

Appendix 5

Events and 1995 life change unit (LCU) values for the Recent Life Changes Questionnaire

(Reprinted from Journal of Psychosomatic Research 43(3) Miller MA, Rahe RH 1997 Life changes scaling for the 1990s, pp 291–292)

Life change event	LCU
Health	
An injury or illness which:	
kept you in bed a week or more, or sent you to the hospital	74
was less serious than above	44
Major dental work	26
Major change in eating habits	27
Major change in sleeping habits	26
Major change in your usual type and/or amount of recreation	28
Work	
Change to a new type of work	51
Change in your work hours or conditions	35
Change in your responsibilities at work:	
more responsibilities	29
fewer responsibilities	21
promotion	31
demotion	42
transfer	32
Troubles at work:	
with your boss	29
with co-workers	35
with persons under your supervision	35
other work troubles	28
Major business adjustment	60
Retirement	52
Loss of job:	
laid off from work	68
fired from work	79
Correspondence course to help you in your work	18

Life change event	LCU
Home and family	
Major change in living conditions	42
Change in residence:	
move within the same town or city	25
move to a different town, city or state	47
Change in family get-togethers	25
Major change in health or behaviour of family member	55
Marriage	50
Pregnancy	67
Miscarriage or abortion	65
Gain of a new family member:	
birth of a child	66
adoption of a child	65
a relative moving in with you	59
Spouse beginning or ending work	46
Child leaving home:	
to attend college	41
due to marriage	41
for other reasons	45
Change in arguments with spouse	50
In-law problems	38
Change in the marital status of your parents:	
divorce	59
remarriage	50
Separation from spouse:	
due to work	53
due to marital problems	76
Divorce	96
Birth of grandchild	43
Death of spouse	119

Life change event	LCU
Death of other family member:	
child	123
brother or sister	102
parent	100
Personal and social	
Change in personal habits	26
Beginning or ending school or college	38
Change of school or college	35
Change in political beliefs	24
Change in religious beliefs	29
Change in social activities	27
Vacation	24
New, close, personal relationship	37
Engagement to marry	45
Girlfriend or boyfriend problems	39
Sexual difficulties	44
'Falling out' of a close personal relationship	47

Life change event	LCU
An accident	48
Minor violation of the law	20
Being held in jail	75
Death of a close friend	70
Major decision regarding your immediate	
future	51
Major personal achievement	36
Financial	
Major change in finances:	
increased income	38
decreased income	60
investment and/or credit difficulties	56
Loss or damage of personal property	43
Moderate purchase	20
Major purchase	37
Foreclosure on a mortgage or loan	58

Glossary

Bio–psycho–social   this approach gives weight to psychosocial aspects as well as biological ones.

Blinding   this is a condition built into the study design whereby participants are kept in ignorance of the group they are in: experimental or control. When the researchers are also in ignorance of this fact the situation is called double-blind. Single- and double-blinding are techniques for reducing the risk of bias in the results.

Catecholamines   these include adrenaline, noradrenaline and dopamine. They play an important role as neurotransmitters in the functioning of the autonomic and central nervous systems.

Catharsis   in psychoanalytic theory, this refers to the release of tension which occurs when repressed thoughts are brought into consciousness.

Centring   refers to the focusing of attention on the interior of the self. To achieve this state all external stimuli must be disregarded. The purpose is to find and make contact with the essence of the self.

Clinical depression   is depression that requires clinical intervention. The question is, at what level of severity should this be introduced? Some clinicians define clinical depression as persistent low mood, low enough to interfere with daily life and lasting more than two weeks. Others, including researchers, look for numerical ratings which are obtained through standardized screening devices, such as the Beck Depression Inventory, where the severity of the condition can be classified into mild, medium and severe.

Cognitive behavioural therapy   is an approach which teaches cognitive and behavioural skills to enable individuals to function adaptively. Patient and therapist are engaged in a collaborative effort to address and solve or alleviate the patient's problem. The therapy is of predetermined and short duration and is focused on the patient's current circumstances.

Cognitive restructuring   this involves a re-evaluation of a person's perception of danger or vulnerability and a questioning of the beliefs which underlie it. The technique consists of three stages: identifying negative thoughts, challenging their accuracy and replacing them with constructive alternatives based upon new judgements about the degree of risk.

Confidence interval   is the distance between an upper and a lower point between which the true result lies with a probability of 95%. Presented in this way the result assumes a range of possibilities. A narrow range will indicate a more precise result than a wide one.

Control group   a basic scientific study will consist of two groups, resembling each other in as many ways as possible. One of these is the experimental group. This group receives the intervention; the other group is the control which does not receive the intervention. The control thus provides a baseline against which to measure the effects of the intervention.

Epidemiology   is the study of diseases in populations and is concerned with the cause of the disease and the way the disease is distributed within a given population.

Evidence-based practice   is practice informed by research findings. It consists of procedures which current evidence shows to be the most effective. Thus, it may be referred to as best practice.

Exposure techniques   these are introduced to help individuals face situations which they find anxiety-inducing such as occur in panic and phobia. Exposure generally involves a hierarchy of low-to-high-threat versions of this event. The individual is first presented with the item of lowest threat. With the help of a relaxation technique, she works to overcome her fear at that level. When she succeeds, she moves on to the next level of threat, dealing with it in the same way.

Fear-avoidance   this is behaviour which the individual adopts to avoid situations which give rise to fear. However, by avoiding the situation, the fear attached to it mounts. Avoidance may lead to an immediate sense of relief but creates an increase in anxiety levels on the next occasion of threat. The solution is to face the feared situation.

Generalized anxiety disorder   is characterized by excessive worry, overtense muscles and impairment of function, all of which have persisted for at least 6 months and are not confined to any specific circumstances.

Homeostasis   the process whereby a balanced state is maintained in body systems throughout varying external conditions. An example can be found in the regulation of body temperature during extreme heat and cold.

Hypothesis   this is a statement which acts as a provisional explanation. In science a hypothesis must undergo a test, the findings of which will tell the researcher whether the hypothesis has been supported or whether it should be rejected. The conclusion reached, however, will only apply within the context of the particular piece of research.

Meta-analysis   is a statistical technique which collates and analyses the findings of many different studies and identifies trends in outcome.

Mindfulness   this refers to the experience of being in the here-and-now.

Motor skill   refers to a skill which involves physical movement.

Number needed to treat (NNT)   this represents the number of people who would be needed in an intervention group before one specific outcome occurred. For example, in an experimental group of elderly women wearing hip protectors, the NNT is an estimate of how many participants would be necessary before one hip fracture was avoided. The NNT is one way of presenting the effectiveness of a treatment.

Outcome measuring devices   are tools used for measuring the results of interventions.

Pacing   refers to the way a learning programme is structured to allow for the varying level of skill in the performer. New material is introduced in a gradual and controlled way.

Pre-experimental studies   here, a single system such as a cohort is studied to explore an idea. The exercise helps in formulating a hypothesis which may later be tested.

Quasi-experimental studies   these bear some characteristics of a true experiment but lack the full requirements of a randomized controlled trial. They feature, for example, in research where randomization is not possible.

Randomization   is similar to pulling names out of a hat except that it is done by a computer. In psychosocial terms, it means that every member of the parent population has an equal chance of being selected for the sample. The same method is then used to allocate participants to experimental and control groups. Randomization helps to ensure that the participants are representative of the population being studied.

Randomized controlled trials   these are studies which carry the full rigour of a scientific experiment. Participants are selected by a random process and divided into two or more groups, one of which receives the intervention. The presence of a control is essential but it can take different forms.

Reflective practice   refers to the knowledge gained from one's experience in the past and the creative application of it in unfamiliar situations.

Reinforcement   positive reinforcement is action which increases the likelihood of a certain behaviour, for example, giving a dog a biscuit every time it brings back a ball makes it more likely the dog will bring back the ball next time it is thrown.

Reliability   refers to the consistency of results when the test is repeated, either by the same researcher on different occasions or by different researchers on the same occasion.

Repression   is a psychoanalytical concept in which anxiety-inducing thoughts are prevented from reaching conscious awareness.

Reviews   scientific reviews collate the results of all studies in a particular field. They are the result of extensive literature searches and provide the health care professional with the kind of information needed to form a view of the best treatment.

Schizophrenia   this condition is characterized by symptoms such as hallucinations and thought disturbances. It may also be accompanied by social withdrawal, low self-esteem, reduced motivation, emotional and attentional deficits and other symptoms of depression.

Self–efficacy   is the feeling of having the ability to deal with whatever one is faced with in life. In short, feeling competent.

Skill   this enables a person to achieve a goal with a high level of certainty and an economy of time and energy.

Somatization   this is said to occur when an individual complains of symptoms, such as pain, which cannot be explained in terms of organic disease. It differs from hypochondriasis where the individual is constantly in fear of developing a disease.

Standard deviation (SD)   is a measure of the way the scores are spread about the average score. Range is also a measure of spread but it does not reflect the way the scores are distributed, i.e. whether bunched close to the mean or more spread out. The standard deviation expresses this feature in a single unit.

States of altered consciousness   these are states of mental functioning which are different from the ordinary pattern. Examples are: dreaming, drug-induced states, hypnotism, meditation, daydreaming, deep relaxation, guided imagery.

Statistical significance   means that there is a 95% likelihood that the result of the experiment is due to the manipulations of the experimenter and not to chance factors. Expressed another way: the result achieved in the experiment could only have occurred by chance in fewer than 5 out of 100 cases.

Validity   a test is valid when it measures what it claims to measure. It has internal validity when it is devoid of bias, and external validity when its results can be generalized to other situations. It has content validity when its components are representative of the item to be measured and face validity when it *seems* valid after superficial appraisal.

References

Abromowitz S I, Wieselberg N 1978 Reaction to relaxation and desensitization outcome: five angry treatment failures. American Journal of Psychiatry 135:1418–1419

Achterberg J 1985 Imagery in healing: shamanism and modern medicine. New Science Library, Boston

Ackerman C J, Turkoski B 2000 Using guided imagery to reduce pain and anxiety. Home and Healthcare Nurse 18(8):524–530

ACPIRT 2001 Leaflet advertising reflex therapy training. Association of Chartered Physiotherapists. In: Reflex Therapy, Chartered Society of Physiotherapy, 14 Bedford Row, London

Adams M A, Hutton W C 1985 The effect of posture on the lumbar spine. Journal of Bone and Joint Surgery 67B:625–629

Adams M A, McNally D S, Chinn H, Dolan P 1994 Posture and the compressive strength of the lumbar spine. Clinical Biomechanics 9:5–14

Aganoff J A, Boyle G B 1994 Aerobic exercise, mood states and menstrual cycle symptoms. Journal of Psychosomatic Research 38:183–192

Alberti R, Emmons M 1982 Your perfect right: a guide to assertive living, 4th edn. Impact, San Luis Obispo, California

Alexander F N 1932 The use of the self. Dutton, New York

Allied Dunbar National Fitness Survey 1992 Activity and health research: a report on activity patterns and fitness levels. Sports Council and Health Education Authority

American College of Sports Medicine 1993 Physical activity, physical fitness and hypertension. Medicine and Science in Sports and Exercise 25:i–x

Anand M P 1999 Non-pharmacological management of essential hypertension. Journal of the Indian Medical Association 97(6):220–225

Anderson B 1983 Stretching and sports. In: Appenzeller O, Atkinson R (eds) Sports Medicine, 2nd edn. Urban & Schwarzenberg, Baltimore

Antoni M H, Baggett L, Ironson G, LaPerriere A, August S, Klimas N, Schneiderman N, Fletcher M A 1991 Cognitive-behavioural stress management intervention buffers distress responses and immunologic changes following notification of HIV-1 seropositivity. Journal of Consulting and Clinical Psychology 59:906–915

Apter M 2003 On a certain blindness in modern psychology. The Psychologist 16(9):474–475

Argyle M 1978 The psychology of interpersonal behaviour, 3rd edn. Pelican, Harmondsworth, Middlesex

Arroll B, Beaglehole R 1992 Does physical activity lower blood pressure? A critical view of the clinical trials. Journal of Clinical Epidemiology 45:439–447

Assagioli R 1965 Psychosynthesis. Turnstone Books, London

Atkinson R L, Atkinson R C, Smith E E, Bem D J, Nolen-Hoeksema S 1999 Hilgard's introduction to psychology, 13th edn. Harcourt Brace, Fort Worth

Austin J H M, Ausubel P 1992 Enhanced respiratory muscular function in normal adults after lessons in proprioceptive musculo-skeletal education without exercises. Chest 102(2):486–490

Banquet J 1973 Spectral analysis of the EEG in meditation. Electroencephalography and Clinical Neurophysiology 35:143–151

Barber T X 1969 Hypnosis: a scientific approach. Van Nostrand-Reinhold, New York

Barber T X 1970 LSD, marijuana, yoga and hypnosis. Aldine, Chicago

Barber T X 1984 Hypnosis, deep relaxation and active relaxation: data, theory and clinical applications. In: Woolfolk R L, Lehrer P M (eds) Principles and practice of stress management. Guilford Press, New York

Barber T X, Chauncey H M, Winer R A 1964 The effect of hypnotic and non-hypnotic suggestion on parotid gland response to gustatory stimuli. Psychosomatic Medicine 26:374–380

Barlow W 2001 The Alexander principle. Orion, London

Barnard S, Hartigan G 1998 Clinical audit in physiotherapy: from theory into practice. Butterworth-Heinemann, Oxford

Barnes V A, Treiber F A, Davis H 2001 Impact of transcendental meditation on cardiovascular function at rest and during acute stress in adolescents with high normal blood pressure. Journal of Psychosomatic Research 51(4):597–605

Batson G 1996 Conscious use of the human body in movement: the peripheral neuro-anatomic basis of the Alexander technique. Medical Problems of Performing Artists 11(1):3–11

Beck A T 1976 Cognitive therapy and the emotional disorders. International Universities Press, New York

Beck A T 1984 Cognitive approaches to stress management. In: Woolfolk R L, Lehrer P M (eds) Principles and practice of stress management. Guilford Press, New York

Beck A T 1988 The Beck Depression Inventory. The Psychological Corporation, Sidcup

Beck A T, Ward C H, Mendelson M, Mock J E, Erbaugh J K 1961 An inventory for measuring depression. Archives of General Psychiatry 4:53–63

Beck A T, Rush A J, Shaw B F, Emery G 1979 Cognitive theory of depression. John Wiley, New York

Beiman I, Israel E, Johnson S J 1978 During-training and post-training effects of live and taped extended progressive relaxation, self-relaxation and electromyogram biofeedback. Journal of Consulting and Clinical Psychology 46:314–321

Bell J A, Saltikov J B 2000 Mitchell's relaxation technique: is it effective? Physiotherapy 86(9):473–478

Bendelow W A, Williams S J 1995 Transcending the dualisms: towards a sociology of pain. Sociology of Health and Illness 17(2):139–165

Benson H 1976 The relaxation response. Collins, London

Benson H, Beary J F, Carol M P 1974 The relaxation response. Psychiatry 37:37–46

Beresford-Cooke C 1996 Shiatsu theory and practice: a comprehensive text for the student and professional. Churchill Livingstone, Edinburgh

Berk L S, Tan S A, Nehlsen-Cannarella S L et al 1988 Mirth modulates adrenocorticomedullary activity: suppression of cortisol and epinephrine. Clinical Research 36:121A

Bernstein D A, Borkovec T D 1973 Progressive relaxation training: a manual for the helping professions. Research Press, Champaign, Illinois

Bernstein D A, Given B A 1984 Progressive relaxation: abbreviated methods. In: Woolfolk R L, Lehrer P M (eds) Principles and practice of stress management. Guilford Press, New York

Bethell H J N, Mullee M A 1990 A controlled trial of community-based coronary rehabilitation. British Heart Journal 64:370–375

Biddle S J H, Mutrie N 2001 Psychology of physical activity: determinants, well-being and interventions. Routledge, London, ch 9

Birk T J, Birk C A 1987 Use of ratings of perceived exertion for exercise prescription. Sports Medicine 4:1–8

Blackburn I, Davidson K M 1990 Cognitive therapy for depression and anxiety: a practitioner's guide. Blackwell Scientific Publications, Oxford

Blackburn I-M, Twaddle V 1996 Cognitive therapy in action. Souvenir Press, London

Blaine B, Crocker J 1993 Self-esteem and self-serving biases in reactions to positive and negative events: an integrative review. In: Baumeister R F (ed) Self-esteem: the puzzle of low self-regard. Plenum, New York, pp 55–86

Blair S N, Kohl H W, Gordon N F, Paffenbarger R S Jr 1992 How much physical activity is good for health? Annual Review of Public Health 13:99–126

Blanchard E B, Young L D 1973 Self-control of cardiac functioning: a promise as yet unfulfilled. Psychological Bulletin 79:145–163

Bloom L J, Gonzales A M 1981 Anxiety management with schizophrenic outpatients. Journal of Clinical Psychology 38:280–285

Blumenstein B, Bar-Eli M, Tenenbaum G 1997 A five-step approach to mental training incorporating biofeedback. Sport Psychologist 11:440–453

Bond M 1986 Stress and self-awareness: a guide for nurses. Butterworth-Heinemann, Oxford

Bootzin R R, Perlis M L 1992 Non-pharmacological treatments of insomnia. Journal of Clinical Psychiatry. June 53 Supplement:37–41

Borg G A V 1970 Perceived exertion as an indicator of somatic stress. Scandinavian Journal of Rehabilitation Medicine 2:92–98

Borg G A V 1998 Borg's perceived exertion and pain scales. Human Kinetics, Europe

Borkovec T D, Heide F 1980 Relaxation-induced anxiety: psychophysiological evidence of anxiety enhancement in tense subjects practising relaxation. Paper presented at the Annual Meeting of the Association for the Advancement of Behaviour Therapy, New York

Borkovec T D, Mathews A 1988 Treatment of non-phobic anxiety disorders: a comparison of non-directive cognitive and coping desensitization therapy. Journal of Consulting and Clinical Psychology 56(6):877–884

Borkovec T D, Sides J K 1979 Critical procedural variables related to the physiological effects of progressive relaxation: a review. Behaviour, Research and Therapy 17:119–125

Bowling A 1997 Measuring health: a review of quality of life measurement scales, 2nd edn. Open University Press, Buckingham

Bowling A 2001 Measuring disease: a review of disease-specific quality of life measurement scales, 2nd edn. Open University Press, Buckingham

Brannon L, Feist J 1992 Health psychology: an introduction to behaviour and health, 2nd edn. Wadsworth, New York

Bravo G, Gauthier P, Roy P M et al 1996 Impact of a 12-month exercise programme on the physical and psychological health of osteopenic women. Journal of the American Geriatric Society 44:756–762

Bricklin M 1990 Meditation: the healing silence. In: Bricklin M (ed) Positive living and health. Rodale Press, Emmaus, Pennsylvania

Broms C 1999 Free from stress by autogenic therapy: a relaxation technique yielding peace of mind and self-insight. Lakartidningen 96(6):588–592

Broocks A, Bandelow B, Pekrun G et al 1998 Comparison of aerobic exercise, clomipramine and placebo in the treatment of panic disorder. American Journal of Psychiatry 155(5):603–609

Burke C, Macnish S, Saunders J, Gallini A, Warne L, Downing J 1994 The development of a massage service for cancer patients. Clinical Oncology 6(6):381–384

Burke E J, Collins M S 1984 Using perceived exertion for the prescription of exercise in healthy adults. In: Cantu R C (ed) Clinical sports medicine. The Collamore Press, Lexington

Burnard P 1991 Coping with stress in the health professions: a practical guide. Chapman and Hall, London

Burnard P 1992 Know yourself! self-awareness activities for nurses. Scutari Press, London

Bury T J, Mead J M (eds) 1998 Evidence-based health care: a practical guide for therapists. Butterworth-Heinemann, Oxford

Buxton R St J 1973 Maternal respiration in labour. Nursing Mirror, September 7th, 22–25

Cady S H, Jones G E 1997 Massage therapy as a workplace intervention for reduction of stress. Perceptual and Motor Skills 84(1):157–158

Cantor P H 2003 The therapeutic effects of meditation (Leading article). British Medical Journal 326:1049–1050

Carless D, Fox K R 2003 The physical self. In: Everett T, Donaghy M, Feaver S. Interventions in mental health. Butterworth-Heinemann, Oxford

Carlson C R, Curran S L 1994 Stretch-based relaxation training. Patient Education and Counselling 23:5–12

Carlson C R, Collins F L, Nitz A J, Sturgis E T, Rogers J L 1990 Muscle stretching as an alternative relaxation training procedure. Journal of Behaviour Therapy and Experimental Psychiatry 21(1):29–38

Carlson C R, Hoyle R H 1993 Efficacy of abbreviated progressive muscle relaxation training: a quantitative review of behavioural medicine research. Journal of Consulting and Clinical Psychology 61(6):1059–1067

Carrington P 1984 Modern forms of meditation. In: Woolfolk R L, Lehrer P M (eds) Principles and practice of stress management. Guilford Press, New York

Carroll D, Seers K 1998 Relaxation for the relief of chronic pain: a systematic review. Journal of Advanced Nursing 27(3):476–487

Cassidy T 1999 Stress, cognition and health. Routledge, London

Chandler C, Bodemhamer-Davis E, Holden J M, Evenson T, Bratton S 2001 Enhancing personal wellness in counsellor trainees using biofeedback: an exploratory study. Applied Psychophysiology and Biofeedback 26(1):1–7

Chaouloff F 1989 Physical exercise and brain monoamines: a review. Acta Physiologica Scandinavica 137:1–13

Chartered Society of Physiotherapy 1999 Effectiveness bulletin on mental health. Chartered Society of Physiotherapy 1(3):1–6

Chartered Society of Physiotherapy 2002 Information Paper CLEF05: outcome measures for people with depression. Chartered Society of Physiotherapy, London

Clark D M 1986 A cognitive approach to panic. Behaviour Research and Therapy 24:461–470

Clark D M, Salkovskis P M, Chalkley A J 1985 Respiratory control as a treatment for panic attacks. Journal of Behaviour Therapy and Experimental Psychiatry 16:23–30

Clum G A, Clum G A, Surls R 1993 A meta-analysis of treatments for panic disorder. Journal of Consulting and Clinical Psychology 61(2):317–326

Cochrane A L 1972 Effectiveness and efficiency: random reflections on health services. Nuffield Provincial Hospitals Trust, London

Cohen S, Wills T A 1985 Stress, social support and the buffering hypothesis. Psychological Bulletin 98:310–357

Collier J (ed) 2002 Lifestyle advice for fracture prevention. Drug and Therapeutics Bulletin 40(11):83–86

Conklin C A, Tiffany S T 2001 The impact of imagining personalized versus standardized urge scenarios on cigarette craving and autonomic reactivity. Experimental and Clinical Psychopharmacology 9(4):399–408

Cooke B, Ernst E 2000 Aromatherapy: a systematic review. British Journal of General Practice 50(455):493–496

Cooper C L 1981 The stress check. Prentice-Hall, Spectrum, New Jersey

Cooper C, Dennison E 1997 Osteoporosis: prevention of osteoporotic fractures. Prescribers' Journal 37(2):112–119

Cooper-Patrick L, Ford D E, Mead L A, Chang P P, Klag M J 1997 Exercise and depression in mid-life: a prospective study. American Journal of Public Health 87(4):670–673

Cornbleet M 2001 Research in complementary medicine is essential. British Medical Journal March 24th 322:735

Cowley D S 1987 Hyperventilation and panic disorder. American Journal of Medicine 83:929–937

Cox T 1978 Stress. Macmillan, London

Cox T, Mackay C J 1976 A psychological model of occupational stress. A paper presented to The Medical Research Council. Mental Health in Industry, London (November)

Craft L L, Landers D M 1998 The effect of exercise on clinical depression and depression resulting from mental illness: a meta-analysis. Journal of Sport and Exercise Psychology 20:339–357

Crist D A, Rickard H C 1993 A 'fair' comparison of progressive and imaginal relaxation. Perceptual and Motor Skills 76:691–700

Culverwell G, McKenna J 1988 Aspects of body learning for the childbearing year. In: McKenna J (ed) Obstetrics and Gynaecology. Churchill Livingstone, Edinburgh

Cupal D D, Brewer B W 2001 Effects of relaxation and guided imagery on knee strength, reinjury anxiety and pain following anterior cruciate ligament reconstruction. Rehabilitation and Psychology 46(1):28–43

Dalloway M 1992 Visualization: the master skill in mental training. Optimal Performance Institute, Phoenix, Arizona

Davidson R J, Schwartz G E 1976 The psychobiology of relaxation and related states: a multiprocess theory. In: Mostofsky D I (ed) Behaviour control and modification of physiological activity. Prentice-Hall, Englewood Cliffs, New Jersey

Davis M, Eshelman E, McKay M 1988 The relaxation and stress reduction workbook, 3rd edn. New Harbinger, Oakland, California

Davis M, Eshelman E, McKay M 2000 The relaxation and stress reduction workbook, 5th edn. New Harbinger, Oakland, California

Dawes R M 1994 House of cards: psychology and psychotherapy built on myth. Free Press, New York

De Coverley Veale D M W 1987 Exercise and mental health. Acta Psychiatrica Scandinavica 76:113–120

Department of Health 1994 The evolution of clinical audit. HMSO, London

Dick-Read G D 1942 Childbirth without fear. Heinemann, Oxford

Donaghy M E 1997 An investigation into the effects of exercise as an adjunct to the treatment and rehabilitation of the problem drinker. PhD Thesis, Medical Faculty, Glasgow University

Donaghy M E 2001 A critical approach to physiotherapy in mental health. Workshop Pack. Queen Margaret University College, Edinburgh

Donaghy M E 2003 Models of mental health disorder. In: Everett T, Donaghy M E, Feaver S. Interventions for mental health. Butterworth-Heinemann, Oxford

Donaghy M E, Durward B 2000 A report on the clinical effectiveness of physiotherapy in mental health. Chartered Society of Physiotherapy, London

Donaghy M E, Morss K 2000 Guided reflection. Physiotherapy Theory and Practice 16:3–14

Donaghy M E, Ralston G, Mutrie N 1991 Exercise as a therapeutic adjunct for problem drinkers. Journal of Sports Sciences 9(4):440

Donaghy M E, Mutrie N 1999 Is exercise beneficial in the treatment and rehabilitation of the problem drinker? A critical review. Physical Therapy Reviews 4:153–166

Donovan M I 1980 Relaxation with guided imagery: a useful technique. Cancer Nursing 3:27–32

Dossey B M 1988 Imagery: awakening the inner healer. In: Dossey B M, Keagan L, Guzzetta C E, Kolkmeier L G (eds) Holistic nursing: a handbook for practice. Aspen, Rockville, Maryland

Doyne E J, Ossip-Klein D J, Bowman E D, Osborn K M, McDougall-Wilson I B, Neimeyer R A 1987 Running versus weight lifting in the treatment of depression. Journal of Consulting and Clinical Psychology 55:748–754

Duckro P N, Cantwell-Simmons E 1989 A review of studies evaluating biofeedback and relaxation training in the management of pediatric headache. Headache 29:428–433

Duclos S E, Laird J D, Schneider E, Sexter M, Stern L, Van Lighten O 1989 Emotion-specific effects of facial expressions and postures on emotional experience. Journal of Personality and Social Psychology 57:100–108

Duncan E A S 2003 Cognitive behavioural therapy in physiotherapy and occupational therapy. In: Everett T, Donaghy M E, Feaver S Interventions for mental health: an evidence-based approach for physiotherapists and occupational therapists. Butterworth-Heinemann, Oxford, ch 10

Durham R C, Turvey A A 1987 Cognitive therapy versus behaviour therapy in the treatment of chronic general anxiety. Behaviour Research and Therapy 25:229–234

Edinger J D, Jacobsen R 1982 Incidence and significance of relaxation treatment side effects. The Behaviour Therapist 5:137–138

Eisenberg D M, Delbanco T L, Berkey C S, Kaptchuk T J, Kupelnick B, Kuhl J, Chalmers T C 1993 Cognitive-behavioural techniques for hypertension: are they effective? Annals of Internal Medicine 118(12):964–972

Eisenberg D M, Landsberg L, Allred E N, Saper R B, Delbanco T L 1991 Inability to demonstrate physiologic correlates of subjective improvement among patients taught the relaxation response. Journal of General Internal Medicine 6(1):64–70

Ekman P 1984 Expression and the nature of emotion. In: Scherer K, Ekman P (eds) Approaches to emotion. Laurance Erlbaum, Hillsdale, New Jersey

Ellis A 1962 Reason and emotion in psychotherapy. Lyle Stuart, New York

Ellis A 1976 The biological basis of human irrationality. Journal of Individual Psychology 32:145–168

Erickson M, Rossi E 1979 Hypnotherapy: an exploratory casebook. Irvington, New York

Eriksson E, Nordwall V, Kurlberg G, Rydholm H, Eriksson A 2002 Effects of body awareness therapy in patients with irritable bowel syndrome. Advances in Physiotherapy 4:125–135

Ernst E 2003 Massage treatment for back pain (Leading article). British Medical Journal 326:562–563

Ernst E, Pittler M H, Stevinson C, White A R, Eisenberg D 2001 The desk-top guide to complementary and alternative medicine. Mosby, Edinburgh

Ernst S, Goodison L 1981 In our own hands: a book of self-help therapy. The Women's Press, London

EuroQuol Group 1990 EuroQuol: a new facility for the measurement of health-related quality of life. Health Policy 16:199–208

Everett T 2003 Chronic fatigue syndrome. In: Everett T, Donaghy M E, Feaver S Interventions for mental health. Butterworth-Heinemann, Oxford, p 257

Everly G S, Rosenfeld R 1981 The nature and treatment of the stress response. Plenum Press, New York

Fahrni W H, Trueman G E 1965 Comparative radiological study of the spines of a primitive population with North Americans and Northern Europeans. Journal of Bone and Joint Surgery 47-B:552–555

Fakouri C, Jones P 1987 Relaxation treatment: slow stroke back rub. Journal of Gerontological Nursing 13(2):32–35

Fanning P 1988 Visualization for change. New Harbinger, Oakland, CA

Farmer K U 1995 Biofeedback and visualization for peak performance. Journal of Sport Rehabilitation 4:59–64

Farrell P, Ebert T, Kampine J 1991 Naloxone augments muscle sympathetic nerve activity during isometric exercise in humans. American Journal of Physiology 260:E379–E388

Fasko D, Grueninger R W 2001 T'ai chi ch'uan and physical and psychological health. Clinical Kinesiology 55(1):4–12

Faulkner G, Biddle S 1999 Exercise as an adjunct treatment for schizophrenia: a review of the literature. Journal of Mental Health 8(5):441–457

Fehmi L 1974 The effects of electro-encephalographic biofeedback training on middle management executives. Paper presented at the annual meeting of the Biofeedback Research Society, Colorado Springs, Colorado

Feldmann B M, Richard E 1986 Prevalence of nurse smokers and variables identified with successful and unsuccessful smoking cessation. Research in Nursing and Health 9:131–138

Fenwick P 1987 Meditation and the electroencephalograph. In: West M A (ed) The Psychology of Meditation. Oxford University Press, Oxford

Ferrell-Torry A T, Glick O J 1993 The use of massage as a nursing intervention to modify anxiety and the perception of cancer pain. Cancer Nursing 16(2):93–101

Ferrucci P 1982 What we may be. Mandala, London

Finke R A 1989 Principles of mental imagery. Massachusetts Institute of Technology, Cambridge, Massachusetts

Finlayson J M 1997 The role of exercise in rehabilitation after uncomplicated myocardial infarction. Physiotherapy 83(10):519–524

Fontana D 1991 The elements of meditation. Element, Shaftesbury

Fontana D 1992 The meditator's handbook: a comprehensive guide to eastern and western meditation techniques. Element, Shaftesbury

Fordham F 1966 An introduction to Jung's psychology, 2nd edn. Pelican, London

Fox K R (ed) 1997 The physical self: from motivation to well-being. Human Kinetics, Leeds

Fox K R 2000a Physical activity and mental health promotion: the natural partnership. International Journal of Mental Health Promotion 2:4–12

Fox K R 2000b The effects of exercise on self-perceptions and self-esteem. In: Biddle S J H, Fox K R, Boucher S H (eds) Physical activity and psychological well-being. Routledge, London, pp 88–117

Fox K R 2000c Self-esteem, self-perceptions and exercise. International Journal of Sports Psychology 31:228–240

Fox K R, Corbin C B 1989 The physical self-perception profile: development and preliminary validation. Journal of Sport and Exercise Psychology 11(4):408–430

Fraser J, Kerr J R 1993 Psychophysiological effects of back massage on elderly institutionalized patients. Journal of Advanced Nursing 18:238–245

Freud S 1973 Introductory lectures on psychoanalysis. Translated by James Strachey. Penguin, Harmondsworth

Friedman M, Rosenman R H 1974 Type A behaviour and your heart. Knoft, New York

Frontline 1999 Health and Safety News. Chartered Society of Physiotherapy, London, January 6th, p 10

Fulcher K, White P 1998 Chronic fatigue syndrome: a description of graded exercise treatment. Physiotherapy 84(5):223–226

Fulden S 1989 The handbook of complementary medicine, 2nd edn. Coronet/Hodder & Stoughton, London

Furlan A D, Brosseau L, Welch V, Wong J 2000 Massage for low back pain. Cochrane Database Systematic Reviews 4:CD 001929

Ganster D C, Victor B 1988 The impact of social support on mental and physical health. British Journal of Medical Psychology 61:3–17

Gardner W N 1992 Hyperventilation syndromes. Respiratory Medicine 86:273–275

Gardner W N, Bass C 1989 Hyperventilation in clinical practice. British Journal of Hospital Medicine 41:73–81

Garssen B, De Ruiter C, Van Dyke R 1992 Breathing retraining: a rational placebo? Clinical Psychology Review 12:141–153

Gauvin L, Spence J C 1996 Physical activity and psychological well-being: knowledge base, current issues and caveats. Nutrition Reviews 54(4):S53–S65

Gibson B E, Martin D K 2003 Qualitative research and evidence-based physiotherapy practice. Physiotherapy 89(6):350–358

Gift A G, Moore T, Soeken K 1992 Relaxation to reduce dyspnoea and anxiety in chronic obstructive pulmonary disease. Nursing Research 41(4):242–246

Gilbert C 1999 Yoga and breathing. Journal of Bodywork and Movement Therapies 3(1):44–54

Glenister D 1996 Exercise and mental health: a review. Journal of the Royal Society of Health, February:7–13

Goldberg D, Huxley P 1992 Common mental disorders: a biosocial model. Routledge, London, pp 83–113

Goldberg D P, Williams P 1988 A user's guide to the general health questionnaire. NFER-Nelson, Windsor

Goldfried M R 1971 Systematic desensitization as training in self-control. Journal of Consulting and Clinical Psychology 37:228–234

Goleman D 1996 Emotional intelligence: why it can matter more than IQ. Bloomsbury, London

Good M, Stanton-Hicks M, Grass J A, Anderson G C, Lai H L, Roykulcharoen V, Adler P A 2001 Relaxation and music to reduce post-surgical pain. Journal of Advanced Nursing 33(2):208–215

Gould R A, Otto M W, Pollack M H 1995 A meta-analysis of treatment outcomes for panic disorder. Clinical Psychology Review 15:819–844

Gray J 1990 Your guide to the Alexander technique. Gollancz, London

Grealish L, Lomasney A, Whiteman B 2000 Foot massage: a nursing intervention to modify the distressing symptoms of pain and nausea in patients hospitalized with cancer. Cancer Nurse 23(3):237–243

Greeff A P, Conradie W S 1998 Use of progressive relaxation training for chronic alcoholics with insomnia. Psychological Reports 82(2):407–412

Greenberger D, Padesky C A 1995 Mind over mood. Guilford Press, New York

Gregson M, Roberts I, Amiri M 1996 Absorption and imagery locate immune responses in the body. Biofeedback and Self-Regulation 21:149–165

Guercio J M, Ferguson K E, McMorrow M J 2001 Increasing functional communication through relaxation training and neuromuscular feedback. Brain Injury 15(12):1073–1082

Gyllesten A L, Ekdahl C, Hansson L 1999 Validity of the Body Awareness Scale – health. Scandinavian University Press. ISSN 0283-9318

Haas F, Axen K 1991 Pulmonary therapy and rehabilitation. Williams and Wilkins, London

Hagberg J M, Brown M D 1995 Does exercise training play a role in the treatment of essential hypertension? Journal of Cardiovascular Risk 2(4):296–302

Halpin L S, Speir A M, Capobianco P, Barnett S D 2002 Guided imagery in cardiac surgery. Outcomes Management for Nursing Practice 6(3):137

Hamm B H, O'Flynn A I 1984 Teaching the client to cope through guided imagery. Journal of Community Health Nursing 1:39–45

Han J N, Stegen E, De Valck C, Clement J, Van de Woestijne K P 1996 The influence of breathing therapy on anxiety and breathing patterns in patients with hyperventilation syndrome and anxiety disorders. Journal of Psychosomatic Research 41(5):481–493

Harding V, Watson P 2000 Increasing activity and improving function in chronic pain management. Physiotherapy 86(12):619–630

Hardman A E 1996 Exercise in the prevention of atherosclerotic metabolic and hypertensive diseases: a review. Journal of Sports Sciences 14:201–218

Harkapaa K 1991 Relationships of psychological distress and health locus of control beliefs with use of cognitive and behavioural coping strategies in low back pain patients. Clinical Journal of Pain 7:275–282

Hartland J 1971 Medical and dental hypnosis and its clinical applications, 2nd edn. Baillière Tindall, London

Hassenbring M, Ulrich H W, Hartmann M, Soyka D 1999 The efficacy of a risk factor-based cognitive-behavioural intervention and electromyographic feedback in patients with acute sciatic pain. Spine 24:2525–2535

Hatfield E, Cacioppo J T, Rapson R L 1992 Primitive emotional contagion. In: Clark M S (ed) Emotion and social behaviour. Sage, Newbury Park, California

Health Education Authority 1995 Health update 5: physical activity. Health Education Authority, London

Heatley D G, Leverson G E, McConnell K E, Kille T L 2000 Nasal irrigation for the alleviation of sinonasal symptoms. Paper presented to the American Academy of Otolaryngology, Head and Neck Surgery Foundation Annual Meeting/Oto Expo, Washington DC, September 25th

Heimberg R G 2002 Cognitive-behavioural therapy for social anxiety disorder: current status and future directions. Biological Psychiatry 51:101–108

Heinonen A, Kannus P, Sievanen H et al 1996 Randomized controlled trial of effect of high impact exercise on selected risk factors for osteoporotic fractures. Lancet 348:1343–1347

Hendler C S, Redd W H 1986 Fear of hypnosis: the role of labelling in patients' acceptance of behavioural interventions. Behaviour Therapy 17:2–13

Henry M, De Rivera J L G, Gonzales-Martin I J, Abreu J 1993 Improvement of respiratory function in chronic asthmatic patients with autogenic therapy. Journal of Psychosomatic Research 37:265–270

Heptinstall S T 1995 Relaxation training. In: Everett T, Dennis M, Ricketts E (eds) Physiotherapy in mental health. Butterworth-Heinemann, Oxford, pp 188–208

Herbert R D, Gabriel M 2002 Effects of stretching before and after exercising on muscle soreness and risk of injury: systematic review. British Medical Journal 325: 468–470

Hernandez-Reif M, Field T, Krasnegor J, Theakston H, Hossain Z, Burman I 2000 High blood pressure and associated symptoms were reduced by massage therapy. Journal of Bodywork and Movement Therapy 4(1):31–38

Heron J 1977 Catharsis in human development. Human Potential Research Project, University of Surrey, Guildford

Herron E W 1969 The multiple affect adjective checklist: a critical analysis. Journal of Clinical Psychology 25(1):46–53

Hiebert B, Fox E E 1981 Reactive effects of self-monitoring anxiety. Journal of Counselling Psychology 28:187–193

Hillenberg J B, Collins F L 1982 A procedural analysis and review of relaxation training research. Behaviour Research and Therapy 20:251–260

Hillenberg J B, Collins F L 1983 The importance of home practice for progressive relaxation training. Behaviour Research and Therapy 21:633–642

Hodgkinson L 1987 Smile therapy: how smiling and laughter can change your life. Optima, London

Holmes D S, Solomon S, Cappo B M, Greenberg J L 1983 Effects of transcendental meditation versus resting on physiological and subjective arousal. Journal of Personality and Social Psychology 44:1245–1252

Holmes T H, Rahe R H 1967 The social re-adjustment rating scale. Journal of Psychosomatic Research 11:213–218

Hough A 1991 Physiotherapy in respiratory care: a problem-solving approach to respiratory and cardiac management. Chapman and Hall, London

Hough A 1996 Physiotherapy in respiratory care: a problem-solving approach to respiratory and cardiac management, 2nd edn. Stanley Thornes, Cheltenham

Hough A 2001 Physiotherapy in respiratory care: an evidence-based approach to respiratory and cardiac management, 3rd edn. Nelson Thornes, Cheltenham

Huntley A, White A R, Ernst E 2002 Relaxation therapies for asthma: a systematic review. Thorax 57(2):127–131

Innocenti D M 1983 Chronic hyperventilation syndrome. In: Downie P A (ed) Cash's textbook of chest, heart and vascular disorders for physiotherapists, 3rd edn. Faber and Faber, London

Innocenti D M 2002 Hyperventilation. In: Pryor J A, Prasad S A (eds) Physiotherapy for respiratory and cardiac problems: adults and paediatrics, 3rd edn. Churchill Livingstone, Edinburgh, pp 563–581

Irvin J H, Domar A D, Clark C, Zuttermeister P C, Friedman R 1996 The effects of relaxation response training on menopausal symptoms. Journal of Psychosomatic Obstetrics and Gynaecology 17(4):202–207

Izard C E 1977 Human emotions. Plenum, New York

Jackson T 1991 An evaluation of the Mitchell method of simple physiological relaxation for women with rheumatoid arthritis. British Journal of Occupational Therapy 54:105–107

Jacobson E 1934 Electrical measurements concerning muscular contraction (tonus) and the cultivation of relaxation in man: relaxation times of individuals. American Journal of Physiology 108:573–580

Jacobson E 1938 Progressive relaxation, 2nd edn. University of Chicago Press, Chicago

Jacobson E 1964 Anxiety and tension control. J B Lippincott, Philadelphia

Jacobson E 1970 Modern treatment of tense patients including the neurotic and depressed, with case illustrations, follow-ups and EMG measurements. Charles C Thomas, Springfield, Illinois

Jacobson E 1976 You must relax. Souvenir Press, London

Jakicic J M, Wing R R, Butler B A, Roberson R J 1995 Prescribing exercise in multiple short bouts versus one continuous bout: effects on adherence, cardiorespiratory fitness and weight loss in overweight women. International Journal of Obesity Related to Metabolic Disorders 19(12):893–901

James W 1890/1950 The principles of psychology. Dover, New York

Jefferies W M 1991 Cortisol and immunity. Medical Hypotheses 34:198–208

Johnson U 2000 Short-term psychological intervention: a study of long-term injured competitive athletes. Journal of Sport Rehabilitation 9(3):207–218

Johnstone M, Wright S, Weinman J 1995 Stress, emotion and life events. In: Measures in health psychology: a user's portfolio. NFER-Nelson, Windsor

Johnstone R, Donaghy M, Martin D 2002 A pilot study of a cognitive-behavioural therapy approach to physiotherapy for acute low back pain patients who show signs of developing chronic pain. Advances in Physiotherapy 4(4):182–188

Jones D, Martin D 2003 Chronic pain. In: Everett T, Donaghy M, Feaver S (eds) Interventions in mental health. Butterworth-Heinemann, Oxford

Jung C G 1963 Memories, dreams, reflections. Vintage Books, New York

Kanji N 2000 Management of pain through autogenic training. Complementary Therapy in Nursing and Midwifery 6(3):143–148

Kanji N, Ernst E 2000 Autogenic training for stress and anxiety: a systematic review. Complementary Therapies in Medicine 8:106–110

Kanner A D, Coyne J C, Schaefer C, Lazarus R S 1981 Comparison of two modes of stress management: daily hassles and uplifts versus major life events. Journal of Behavioural Medicine 4:1–3

Kay J A, Carlson C R 1992 The role of stretch-based relaxation in the treatment of chronic neck tension. Behaviour Therapy 23:423–431

Kazarian L 1975 Creep characteristics of the human spinal column. Orthopedic Clinics of North America 6(1):3–15

Keable D 1997 The management of anxiety: a manual for therapists, 2nd edn. Churchill Livingstone, Edinburgh

Keefe F 2003 The Patrick Wall Memorial Lecture. Chartered Society of Physiotherapy Congress, Birmingham

Keefer L, Blanchard E B 2001 The effects of relaxation response meditation on the symptoms of irritable bowel syndrome: results of a controlled treatment study. Behaviour Research and Therapy 39:801–811

Kelly G A 1955 The psychology of personal constructs. Norton, New York

Kelly G A 1969 The psychotherapeutic relationship. In: Maher B (ed) Clinical psychology and personality. Wiley, New York

Kermani K S 1990 Autogenic training. Souvenir Press, London

Kerr G A, Kotynia F, Kolt G S 2002 Feldenkrais awareness-through-movement and state anxiety. Journal of Bodywork and Movement Therapies 6(2):102–107

Kerr K M 2000 Relaxation techniques: a critical review. Critical Reviews in Physical and Rehabilitation Medicine 12:51–89

Khanam A A, Sachdeva U, Guleria R, Deepak K K 1996 Study of pulmonary and autonomic functions of asthma patients after yoga training. Indian Journal of Physiology and Pharmacology 40(4):318–324

King A C, Taylor C, Haskell W L 1993 Effects of differing intensities and formats of 12 months of exercise training on psychological outcomes in older adults. Health Psychology 12(4):292–300

King A C, Oman R F, Brassington C S, Bliwise D L, Haskell W L 1997 Moderate intensity exercise and self-rated quality of sleep in older adults: a randomized controlled trial. Journal of the American Medical Association 277(1):32–37

King J V 1988 A holistic technique to lower anxiety: relaxation with guided imagery. Journal of Holistic Nursing 6(1):16–20

King M S, Carr T, D'Cruz C 2002 Transcendental meditation, hypertension and heart disease: a review. Australian Family Physician 31(2):164–168

King N J, Ollendick T H, Murphy G C, Molloy G N 1998 Utility of relaxation training with children in school settings: a plea for realistic goal setting and evaluation. British Journal of Educational Psychology 68(1):53–66

Kitzinger S 1987 The experience of childbirth. Penguin, Harmondsworth

Kobasa S C 1982 The hardy personality. In: Sanders G, Suls J (eds) The social psychology of health and illness. Lawrence Erlbaum, New Jersey

Kokoszka A 1987–1988 An integrated model of the main states of consciousness. Imagination, Cognition and Personality 7(3):285–294

Kokoszka A 1992 Relaxation as an altered state of consciousness: a rationale for a general theory of relaxation. International Journal of Psychosomatics 39:4–9

Kolt G S, McConville J C 2000 The effects of a Feldenkrais awareness-through-movement program on state anxiety. Journal of Bodywork and Movement Therapies 4(3):216–220

Kosslyn S M 1983 Ghosts in the mind's machine. W W Norton, New York

Kosslyn S M, Ganis G, Thomson W L 2001 Neural foundations of imagery. Nature Reviews: neuroscience 2:635–642

Krall E A, Dawson-Hughes B 1993 Heritable and lifestyle determinants of bone mineral density. Journal of Bone Mineral Research 8:1–10

Kugler J, Seelbach H, Kruskemper G M 1994 Effects of rehabilitation programmes on anxiety and depression in coronary patients: a meta-analysis. British Journal of Clinical Psychology 33(3):401–410

Kurosawa M, Lundeberg T, Agren G, Lund I, Uvnas-Moberg K 1995 Massage-like stroking of the abdomen lowers blood pressure in rats: the influence of oxytoxin. Journal of the Autonomic Nervous System 56:26–30

Kutner G, Zahourek R P 1988 Relaxation/imagery with alcoholics in group treatment. In: Zahourek R P (ed) Relaxation and imagery: tools for therapeutic communication and intervention. W B Saunders, Philadelphia

La Forge R 1995 Exercise-associated mood alteration: a review of interactive neurobiological mechanisms. Medicine, Exercise, Nutrition and Health 4:17–32

Larkin D M 1988 Therapeutic suggestion. In: Zahourek R P (ed) Relaxation and imagery: tools for therapeutic communication and intervention. W B Saunders, Philadelphia

Law M R, Wald N J, Meade T W 1991 Strategies for prevention of osteoporosis and hip fracture. British Medical Journal 303:453–459

Lawler D A, Hopker S W 2001 The effectiveness of exercise as an intervention in the management of depression: systematic review and meta-regression analysis of randomized controlled trials. British Medical Journal 322:763–767

Lazarus R S 1991 Cognition and motivation in emotion. American Psychologist 46:352–367

Lazarus R S, Folkman S 1984 Stress, appraisal and coping. Springer, New York

Lazarus R S, Cohen J B, Folkman S, Kanner A, Schaefer C 1980 Psychological stress and adaptation: some unresolved issues. In: Selye H (ed) Selye's guide to stress research. Van Nostrand-Reinhold, New York, vol 1, pp 90–117

Lee C, Russell A 2003 Effects of physical activity on emotional well-being among older Australian women: cross-sectional and longitudinal analyses. Journal of Psychosomatic Research 54(2):155–160

Lehrer P M 1979 Anxiety and cultivated relaxation: reflections on clinical experiences and psychophysiological research. In: McGuigan F J (ed) Tension control: proceedings of the fifth annual meeting of The American Association for the Advancement of Tension Control, Chicago

Lehrer P M 1982 How to relax and how not to relax: a re-evaluation of the work of Edmund Jacobson. Behaviour Research and Therapy 20:417–428

Lehrer P M 1996 Varieties of relaxation methods and their unique effects. International Journal of Stress Management 3:1–15

Lehrer P M, Woolfolk R L 1983 Are stress reduction techniques interchangeable or do they have specific effects? In: Woolfolk R L, Lehrer P M (eds) Stress reduction techniques. Guilford Press, New York

Lehrer P M, Batey D M, Woolfolk R L, Remde A, Garlick T 1988 The effect of repeated tense–release sequences on EMG and self-report of muscle tension: an evaluation of Jacobsonian and post-Jacobsonian assumptions about progressive relaxation. Psychophysiology 25:562–567

Lehrer P M, Sargunaraj D, Hochron S 1992 Psychological approaches to the treatment of asthma. Journal of Consulting and Clinical Psychology 60(4):639–643

Leibowitz J, Connington B 1990 The Alexander technique. Souvenir Press, London

Ley P, Spelman S 1967 Communicating with the patient. Staples Press, London

Ley R 1988 Panic attacks during relaxation and relaxation-induced anxiety: a hyperventilation interpretation. Journal of Behaviour Therapy and Experimental Psychiatry 19:253–259

Lichstein K L 1983 Ocular relaxation as a treatment for insomnia. Behavioural Counselling and Community Interventions 3:178–185

Lichstein K L 1988 Clinical relaxation strategies. John Wiley, New York

Lichstein K L, Sallis J F, Hill D, Young M C 1981 Psycho-physiological adaptation: an investigation of multiple parameters. Journal of Behavioural Assessment 3:111–121

Lindsay W R, Hood E H 1982 A cognitive anxiety questionnaire. Unpublished, University of Sheffield

Lindsay W R, Morrison F M 1996 The effects of behavioral relaxation on cognitive performance in adults with severe intellectual disabilities. Journal of Intellectual Disability Research 40(4):285–290

Lindsay W R, Pitcaithly D, Geelen N, Buntin L, Broxholme S, Ashby M 1997 A comparison of the effects of four therapy procedures on concentration and responsiveness in people with profound learning disabilities. Journal of Intellectual Disability Research 41(3):201–207

Loew T H, Sohn R, Martus P, Tritt K, Rechlin T 2000 Functional relaxation as a somatopsychotherapeutic intervention: a prospective controlled study. Alternative Therapy In Health and Medicine 6(6):70–75

Loew T H, Tritt K, Siegfried W, Bohmann H, Martus P, Hahn E G 2001 Efficacy of functional relaxation in comparison to terbutaline and a 'placebo relaxation' method in patients with acute asthma: a randomized, prospective, placebo-controlled, cross-over experimental investigation. Psychotherapy and Psychosomatics 70(3):151–157

Long A F, Dixon P, Hall R, Carr-Hill R A, Seldon T A 1993 The outcomes agenda: contribution of the UK clearing house on health outcomes. Quality in Health Care 2:49–52

Looker T, Gregson O 1989 Stresswise: a practical guide for dealing with stress. Hodder and Stoughton, London

Lovas J M, Ashley R C, Raison R L, Weston K M, Segal Y D, Markus M R 2002 The effects of massage therapy on the human immune response in healthy adults. Journal of Bodywork and Movement Therapies 6(3):143–150

Lucic K S, Steffen J J, Harrigan J A, Stuebing R C 1991 Progressive relaxation training: muscle contractions before relaxation? Behaviour Therapy 22:249–256

Lucini D, Covacci G, Milani R, Mela G S, Malliani A, Pagani M 1997 A controlled study of the effects of relaxation on autonomic excitatory responses in healthy subjects. Psychosomatic Medicine 59(5):541–552

Lum L C 1981 Hyperventilation and anxiety state. Journal of the Royal Society of Medicine 74:1–4

Luskin F M, Newell K A, Griffith M, Holmes M, Telles S, Dinucci E, Marvasti F F, Hill M, Pelletier K R, Haskell W L 2000 A review of mind-body therapies in the treatment of musculo-skeletal disorders with implications for the elderly. Alternative Therapies 6(2):46–56

Lutgendorf S K, Antoni M H, Ironson G, Klimas N, Kumar M, Starr K, McCabe P 1997 Cognitive-behavioural stress management decreases dysphoric mood and herpes simplex virus-type 2 antibody titers in symptomatic HIV-seropositive gay men. Journal of Consulting and Clinical Psychology 65(1):31–43

Luthe W (ed) 1965 Autogenic training: psychosomatic correlations. Grune and Stratton, New York

Luthe W 1970 Research and theory. In: Luthe W (ed) Autogenic therapy. Grune and Stratton, New York, vol 4

Lyman B, Bernadin S, Thomas S 1980 Frequency of imagery in emotional experience. Perceptual and Motor Skills 50:1159–1162

Lynn S J, Rhue J W 1977 Hypnosis, imagination and fantasy. Journal of Mental Imagery 11:101–113

McArdle W, Katch F, Katch V 1986 Exercise physiology: energy, nutrition and human performance, 2nd edn. Lea & Febiger, Philadelphia

McCance K, Heuther S 1998 Patho-physiology: the biologic basis for disease in adults and children, 3rd edn. Mosby, St Louis

McCormack G L 1992 The therapeutic benefits of the relaxation response. Occupational Therapy Practice 4(1):51–60

McGuigan F J 1971 Covert linguistic behaviour in deaf subjects during thinking. Journal of Comparative and Physiological Psychology 75:417–420

McGuigan F J 1981 Calm down: a guide for stress and tension control. Prentice-Hall, Englewood Cliffs, New Jersey

McGuigan F J 1984 Progressive relaxation: origins, principles and clinical applications. In: Woolfolk R L, Lehrer P M (eds) Principles and practice of stress management. Guilford Press, New York

McKenna J (ed) 1988 Obstetrics and gynaecology. Churchill Livingstone, Edinburgh

McMurdo M E T, Mole P A, Paterson C R 1997 Controlled trial of weight-bearing exercise in older women in relation to bone density and falls. British Medical Journal 314:569

McNair D M, Lorr N, Droppleman L F I971 Manual for the profile of mood states. Educational and Industrial Testing Service, San Diego, California

McNair D M, Lorr M, Droppleman L F 1992 Manual for the profile of mood states (POMS). Educational and Industrial Testing Services, San Diego, California

Mack C 1980 A theoretical model of psychosomatic illness and an innovative treatment strategy. Journal of Psychology 7:27–43

Madders J 1981 Stress and relaxation: self-help ways to cope with stress and relieve nervous tension, ulcers, insomnia, migraine and high blood pressure, 3rd edn. Martin Dunitz, London

Maisel E 1969 The Alexander technique. Thames & Hudson, London

Malmgren-Olssen E-B, Armelius B-A, Kerstin A 2001 A comparative outcome study of body awareness therapy, Feldenkrais and conventional physiotherapy for patients with non-specific musculo-skeletal disorders: changes in psychological symptoms, pain and self-image. Physiotherapy Theory and Practice 17:77–95

Maltz M 1966 Psycho-cybernetics. Pocket Books, New York

Mandle C L, Jacobs S C, Arcari P M, Domar A D 1996 The efficacy of relaxation response interventions with adult patients: a review of the literature. Journal of Cardiovascular Nursing 10(3):4–26

Mantle J, Haslam J, Polden M 2004 Physiotherapy in obstetrics and gynaecology, 2nd edn. Butterworth-Heinemann, Oxford

Marcus D A, Scharff L, Mercer S, Turk D C 1998 Nonpharmacological treatment for migraine: incremental utility of physical therapy with relaxation and thermal biofeedback. Cephalalgia 18(5):266–272

Marshall S, Turnbull J 1996 Cognitive-behaviour therapy: an introduction to theory and practice. Baillière Tindall, London

Martinsen E W 1990 Physical fitness, anxiety and depression. British Journal of Hospital Medicine 43:194–199

Martinsen E W, Hoffart A, Solbert O 1989 Comparing aerobic and nonaerobic forms of exercise in the treatment of clinical depression: a randomized trial. Comparative Psychiatry 30:324–331

Mattsson M, Wikman M, Dahlgren L, Mattsson B, Armelius K 1998 Body awareness therapy with sexually abused women. Part 2: evaluation of body awareness in a group setting. Journal of Bodywork and Movement Therapies 2(1):38–45

Matsumoto M, Smith J C 2001 Progressive muscle relaxation, breathing exercises and ABC relaxation theory. Journal of Clinical Psychology 57(12): 1551–1557

Mead G H 1934 Mind, self and society. Chicago University Press, Chicago

Meek S S 1993 Effects of slow stroke back massage on relaxation in hospice clients. Journal of Nursing School 25(1):17–21

Meichenbaum D 1977 Cognitive behaviour modification: an integrative approach. Plenum Press, New York

Meichenbaum D, Cameron R 1974 Modifying what clients say to themselves. In: Mahoney M J, Thoresen C E (eds) Self-control: power to the person. Brooks/Cole, Monterey, California

Meichenbaum D, Cameron R 1983 Stress inoculation training. In: Meichenbaum D, Jaremko M E (eds) Stress reduction and prevention. Plenum Press, New York

Melzack R 1975 The McGill pain questionnaire: major properties and scoring methods. Pain 1:277–299

Melzack R, Wall P D 1965 Pain mechanisms: a new theory. Science 150:971–979

Melzack R, Wall P D 1983 The challenge of pain. Penguin, London

Miller K M, Perry P A 1990 Relaxation techniques and post-operative pain in patients undergoing cardiac surgery. Heart and Lung 19(2):136–146

Miller M A, Rahe R H 1997 Life changes scaling for the 1990s. Journal of Psychosomatic Research 43(3):279–292

Mitchell L 1987 Simple relaxation: the Mitchell method for easing tension, 2nd edn. John Murray, London

Morgan W P 1981 Psychophysiology of self-awareness during vigorous physical activity. Research Quarterly for Exercise and Sports 52:385–427

Morris J N, Clayton D G, Everitt M G, Semmence A M, Burgess E H 1990 Exercise in leisure time: coronary attack and death rates. British Heart Journal 63:325–334

Moses J, Steptoe A, Mathews A, Edwards S 1989 The effects of exercise training on mental well-being in the normal population: a controlled trial. Journal of Psychosomatic Research 33:47–61

Mutrie N 1997 The therapeutic effects of exercise on the self. In: Fox K R (ed) The physical self: from motivation to well-being. Human Kinetics, Leeds, pp 287–314

Mutrie N 2001 A review of randomized controlled trials for the use of exercise in clinically defined depression. In: Biddle S J H, Fox K R (eds) A review of the relationship between mental health and exercise. Somerset Health Authority

Mutrie N, Faulkner G 2003 Physical activity and mental health. In: Everett T, Donaghy M, Feaver S (eds) Interventions for mental health. Butterworth-Heinemann, Oxford, ch 7

Neimeyer R A 1985 Personal constructs in clinical practice. In: Kendall P C (ed) Advances in cognitive-behavioural research and therapy. Academic Press, Orlando, vol 4

Niaura R S, Shadel W G, Abrams D B, Monti P M, Rohsenow D J, Sirota A 1998 Individual differences in cue reactivity among smokers trying to quit: effects of gender and cue type. Addictive Behaviours 23:209–224

Noble E 1988 Maternal effort during labour and delivery. In: McKenna J (ed) Obstetrics and gynaecology. Churchill Livingstone, Edinburgh

North T C, McCullagh P, VuTran Z 1990 Effect of exercise on depression. Exercise and Sports Science Review 18:379–415

Norton M, Holm J E, McSherry W C (2nd edn) 1997 Behavioral assessment of relaxation: the validity of a behavioral rating scale. Journal of Behavior Therapy and Experimental Psychiatry 28(2):129–137

O'Brien M 1996 Editorial: osteoporosis and exercise. British Journal of Sports Medicine 30:191

Oliver K, Cronan T A, Walen H R 2001 A review of multidisciplinary interventions for fibromyalgia patients. Where do we go from here? Journal of Musculo-skeletal Pain 9(4):63–80

Olton D S, Noonberg A R 1980 Biofeedback: clinical applications in behavioural medicine. Prentice-Hall, Englewood Cliffs, New Jersey

Öst L-G 1987 Applied relaxation: description of a coping technique and review of controlled studies. Behaviour Research and Therapy 25:397–407

Öst L-G 1988 Applied relaxation versus progressive relaxation in the treatment of panic disorder. Behaviour Research and Therapy 26:13–22

Öst L-G, Breitholtz E 2000 Applied relaxation versus cognitive therapy in the treatment of generalized anxiety disorder. Behaviour Research and Therapy 38(8):777–790

Oyle I 1976 Magic, mysticism and modern medicine. Celestial Arts, Millbrae, California

Paivio A 1985 Cognitive and motivational functions of imagery in human performance. Canadian Journal of Applied Sport Science 10:22S–28S

Paluska S A, Schwenk T L 2000 Physical activity and mental health: current concepts. Sports Medicine 29(3):167–180

Pate R R, Pratt M, Blair S N 1995 Physical activity and public health: a recommendation from the Centers for Disease Control and Prevention and the American College of Sports Medicine. Journal of the American Medical Association 273:402–407

Patel C, Marmot M G 1988 Can general practitioners use training in relaxation and management of stress to reduce mild hypertension? British Medical Journal 296:21–24

Paul G L 1969 Physiological effects of relaxation training and hypnotic suggestion. Journal of Abnormal Psychology 74:425–437

Paul G L, Trimble R W 1970 Recorded versus live relaxation and hypnotic suggestion: comparative effectiveness for reducing physiological arousal and inhibiting stress responses. Behaviour Therapy 1:285–302

Payne R A 1989 Glad to be yourself: a course of practical relaxation and health education talks. Physiotherapy 75:8–9

Penava S J, Otto M W, Maki K M, Pollak M H 1998 Rate of improvement during cognitive-behavioural group treatment for panic disorder. Behaviour Research and Therapy 36(7–8):665–673

Pennebaker J W 1990 Opening up: the healing power of confiding in others. William Morrow, New York

Petry J J 2000 Surgery and complementary therapies: a review. Alternative Therapy in Health and Medicine 6(5):64–76

Peveler R, Carson A, Rodin G 2002 Depression in medical patients. British Medical Journal 325:149–152

Peveler R, Johnston D W 1986 Subjective and cognitive effects of relaxation. Behaviour Research and Therapy 24:413–420

Pinney S, Freeman L J, Nixon P G F 1987 Role of the nurse counsellor in managing patients with the hyperventilation syndrome. Journal of the Royal Society of Medicine 80:216–218

Piret M, Beziers P 1979 La co-ordination motrice. Masson et Cie, Paris

Polden M, Mantle J 1990 Physiotherapy in obstetrics and gynaecology. Butterworth-Heinemann, Oxford

Pope K S, Singer J L 1978 The stream of consciousness: scientific investigations into the flow of human experience. Plenum Publications, New York

Poppen R 1988 Behavioural relaxation training and assessment. Pergamon Press, Oxford

Poppen R, Maurer J 1982 Electromyographic analysis of relaxed postures. Biofeedback and Self-Regulation 7:491–498

Potter M, Grove J R 1999 Mental skills training during rehabilitation: case studies of injured athletes. New Zealand Journal of Physiotherapy 27(2):24–31

Powell K E, Thompson P D, Casperson C W, Kendrick J S 1987 Physical activity and the incidence of coronary heart disease. Annual Review of Public Health 8:253–287

Powell T J 1987 Anxiety management groups in clinical practice: a preliminary report. Behavioural Psychotherapy 15:181–187

Powell T J, Enright S J 1990 Anxiety and stress management. Routledge, London

Price J R, Couper J 2000 Cognitive-behaviour therapy for adults with chronic fatigue syndrome. The Cochrane Library, Issue 2. Update Software, Oxford

Priest J, Schott J 1991 Leading antenatal classes: a practical guide. Butterworth-Heinemann, Oxford

Prins J B, Bleijenberg G, Bazelmans E et al 2001 Cognitive-behaviour therapy for chronic fatigue syndrome: a multicentre randomized controlled trial. Lancet 357:841–847

Puskarich C A, Whitman S, Dell J, Hughes J R, Rosen A J, Hermann B P 1992 Controlled examination of effects of progressive relaxation training on seizure reduction. Epilepsia 33(4):675–680

Quick J C, Quick J D 1984 Organizational stress and preventative management. McGraw-Hill, New York

Rachman J 2003 Eysenck and the development of cognitive-behavioural therapy. The Psychologist 16(11):588–591

Rahe R H 1975 Epidemiological studies of life change and illness. International Journal of Psychiatric Medicine 6:133–146

Rasid Z M, Parish T S 1998 The effects of two types of relaxation training on students' levels of anxiety. Adolescence 33(129):99–101

Read M 1984 Sports medicine: a unique guide to self-diagnosis and rehabilitation. Breslich and Foss, London

Reber A S, Reber E S 2001 The Penguin dictionary of psychology, 3rd edn. Penguin Books, London

Rees B L 1995 Effect of relaxation with guided imagery on anxiety, depression and self-esteem in primiparas. Journal of Holistic Nursing 13(3):255–267

Reid G J, McGrath P J 1996 Psychological treatments for migraine. Biomedical Pharmacotherapy 50(2):58–63

Remocker A J, Storch E T 1992 Action speaks louder: a handbook of structured group techniques, 5th edn. Churchill Livingstone, Edinburgh

Richardson A 1969 Mental imagery. Springer, New York

Richmond J, Berman B M, Docherty J P et al 1996 Integration of behavioral and relaxation approaches into the treatment of chronic pain and insomnia. Journal of the American Medical Association 276(4):313–318

Ritz T 2001 Relaxation therapy in adult asthma: is there new evidence for its effectiveness? Behaviour Modification 25(4):640–666

Rogers C R 1961 On becoming a person: a therapist's view of psychotherapy. Houghton Mifflin, Boston

Romain K 1995 Outcome measurement in physiotherapy practice. Outcomes pack: an introduction to implementing outcomes of care for chartered physiotherapists. Chartered Society of Physiotherapy, London

Rosa K R 1976 Autogenic training. Victor Gollancz, London

Rosenberg M 1965 Society and the adolescent self-image. Princetown University Press, Princetown, New Jersey

Roth A, Fonagy P 1996 What works for whom? A critical review of psychotherapy research. Guilford Press, New York

Rotter J B 1966 Generalized expectancies for internal versus external control of reinforcement. Psychological Monographs 80:609

Rowbottom I 1992 The physiotherapy management of chronic hyperventilation. Journal of the

Association of Chartered Physiotherapists in Respiratory Conditions 21:9–12

Royal College of Physicians of London 1991 Medical aspects of exercise: benefits and risks. Royal College of Physicians, London

Ruuskanen J M, Ruoppila I 1995 Physical activity and psychological well-being among people aged 65–84 years. Age and Ageing 24(4):292–296

Roxendal G 1990 Physiotherapy as an approach in psychiatric care with emphasis on body awareness therapy. In: Hegna T, Sveram M (eds) Psychological and psychosomatic problems. Churchill Livingstone, Edinburgh, pp 75–101

Ryman L 1994 Relaxation and visualization. In: Wells R J, Tschudin V (eds) Wells' supportive therapies in health care. Baillière Tindall, London

Ryman L 1995 Relaxation and visualization. In: Rankin-Box D (ed) The nurses' handbook of complementary therapies. Churchill Livingstone, Edinburgh

Safran M R, Seaber A V, Garrett W E 1989 Warm-up and muscular injury prevention. Sports Medicine 8:239–249

Salt V L, Kerr K M 1997 Mitchell's simple physiological relaxation and Jacobson's progressive relaxation techniques: a comparison. Physiotherapy 83(4):200–207

Samuels M, Samuels N 1975 Seeing with the mind's eye: the history, technique and uses of visualization. Random House, Toronto

Sartory G, Muller B, Metsch J, Pothman R 1998 A comparison of psychological and pharmacological treatment of pediatric migraine. Behavior Research and Therapy 36(12):1155–1170

Schell E J, Allolio B, Schonecke O W 1994 Physiological and psychological effects of Hatha Yoga exercise in healthy women. International Journal of Psychosomatics 41:46–52

Schilling D J, Poppen R 1983 Behavioural relaxation training and assessment. Journal of Behaviour Therapy and Experimental Psychiatry 14:99–107

Schmidt R A 1998 Motor learning and performance: from principles to practice, 3rd edn. Human Kinetics, Champaign, Illinois

Schneider R H, Staggers F, Alexander C N, Sheppard W, Rainforth M, Kondwani K et al 1995 A randomized controlled trial of stress reduction for hypertension in older African Americans. Hypertension 26:820–827

Scholz J, Campbell S 1980 Muscle spindles and the regulation of movement. Physical Therapy 60:1416

Schott J, Priest J 2002 Leading ante-natal classes: a practical guide, 2nd edn. Books for Midwives, Oxford

Schultz J H, Luthe W 1969 Autogenic methods. Grune and Stratton, New York

Schwartz G E, Davidson R J, Goleman D T 1978 Patterning of cognitive and somatic processes in the self-regulation of anxiety: effects of meditation versus exercise. Psychosomatic Medicine 40:321–328

Schwartz J L 1987 Smoking cessation methods: the United States and Canada 1978–1985. National Cancer Institute, National Institutes of Health, Washington DC. NIH Publication number 87:2940

Scully D, Kremer J, Meade M M, Graham R, Dudgeon K 1998 Physical exercise and psychological well-being: a critical review. British Journal of Sports Medicine 32:111–120

Sealey C 1999 Two common pitfalls in clinical audit: failing to complete the audit cycle and confusing audit with research. British Journal of Occupational Therapy 62(6):238–243

Seers K, Carroll D 1998 Relaxation techniques for acute pain management: a systematic review. Journal of Advanced Nursing 27(3):466–475

Seligman M E P 1975 Helplessness. Freeman, San Francisco

Selye H 1956 The stress of life. McGraw-Hill, New York

Selye H 1974 Stress without distress. New American Library of Canada, Scarborough, Canada

Sharma H M, Alexander C N 1996 Maharashi ayurveda: research review. Complementary Medicine International 3(1):21–28

Sharp C, Hurford D P, Allison J, Sparks R, Cameron B P 1997 Facilitation of internal locus of control in adolescent alcoholics through a brief biofeedback-assisted autogenic relaxation training procedure. Journal of Substance Abuse and Treatment 14(1):55–60

Shephard R J 1997 Exercise and relaxation in health promotion. Sports Medicine 23(4):211–217

Sher L 1996 Exercise, well-being and endogenous molecules of mood. Lancet 348:477

Shiffman S 1985 Coping with temptations to smoke. In: Shiffman S, Wills T A (eds) Coping and substance use. Academic Press, New York

Shone R 1982 Autohypnosis: a step by step guide to self-hypnosis. Thorsons, Wellingborough

Shone R 1984 Creative visualization. Thorsons, Wellingborough

Silagy C, Lancaster T, Gray S, Fowler G 1994 Effectiveness of training health professionals to provide smoking cessation interventions. Systematic review of randomized controlled trials. Quality in Health Care 3:193–198

Sim J 1999 Randomized controlled trials. In: Frontline. Clinical effectiveness supplement. Chartered Society of Physiotherapy, London, March, pp 12–13

Sim J 2002 Systematic review of randomized controlled trials of non-pharmacological interventions for fibromyalgia. The Clinical Journal of Pain 18:324–336

Sime W E 1990 Discussion: exercise, fitness and mental health. In: Bouchard C, Shephard R J, Stephens T, Sutton J R, McPherson B D (eds) Exercise, fitness and health: a consensus of current knowledge. Human Kinetics Books, Champaign, Illinois

Simonton O C, Matthews-Simonton S, Creighton J L 1986 Getting well again. Bantam, London

Sinclair V, Wallston K, Dwyer K et al 1998 Effects of a cognitive-behavioural intervention for women with rheumatoid arthritis. Research in Nursing and Health 21:315–326

Singer J L 1975 The inner world of day-dreaming. Harper and Row, New York

Singh N A, Clements K M, Fiatarone M A 1997 A randomized controlled trial of progressive resistance training in depressed elders. Journal of Gerontology Annals in Biological Science and Medical Science 52:M27–35

Skelly M 2003 Stress and mental health. In: Everett T, Donaghy M, Feaver S (eds) Interventions for mental health. Butterworth-Heinemann, Oxford

Skinner B F 1938 The behaviour of organisms. Appleton-Century Crofts, New York

Slaven L, Lee C 1997 Mood and symptom reporting among middle-aged women: the relationship between menopausal status, hormone replacement therapy and exercise participation. Health Psychology 16(3):203–208

Sloman R 2002 Relaxation and guided imagery for anxiety and depression control in community patients with advanced cancer. Cancer Nursing 25(6):432–435

Sloman R, Brown P, Aldana E, Chee E 1994 The use of relaxation for the promotion of comfort and pain relief in persons with advanced cancer. Contemporary Nurse 3(1):6–12

Slonim N B, Hamilton L H 1976 Respiratory physiology, 3rd edn. Mosby, St. Louis

Smeaton J 1995 Exercise and mental health. In: Everett T, Dennis M, Ricketts E (eds) Physiotherapy in mental health. Butterworth-Heinemann, Oxford

Smith E, Wilks N 1988 Meditation. Optima, London

Smith E L 1995 The role of exercise in the prevention and treatment of osteoporosis. Topics in Geriatric Rehabilitation 10(4):55–63

Smith J C 2001 Advances in ABC relaxation: application and inventories. Springer, New York

Smith J C, Amutio A, Anderson J P, Aria L A 1996 Relaxation: mapping an uncharted world. Biofeedback and self-regulation 21(1):63–90

Snow-Harter C, Bouxsein M L, Lewis B T, Carter D, Marcus R 1992 Effects of resistance and endurance exercise on bone mineral status of young women: a randomized exercise intervention trial. Journal of Bone Mineral Research 7:761–769

Snyder M 1985 Independent nursing interventions. John Wiley, New York

Sordoni C, Hall C, Forwell L 2002 The use of imagery in athletic injury rehabilitation and its relationship to self-efficacy. Physiotherapy Canada 54(3):177–185

Spence S H, Sharpe L, Newton-John T, Champion D 1995 Effect of electromyographic biofeedback compared to applied relaxation training with chronic, upper extremity cumulative trauma disorders. Pain 63(2):199–206

Spiegel D, Moore R 1997 Imagery and hypnosis in the treatment of cancer patients. Oncology 11(8):1179–1195

Spielberger C D 1980 Manual for the state–trait anxiety inventory. Consulting Psychologists Press, Palo Alto, California

Spielberger C D, Gorsuch R L, Lushene R E 1970 Manual for the state–trait anxiety inventory. Consulting Psychologists Press, Palo Alto

Spinhoven P, Corry A, Linssen G, Van Dyke R, Zitman F G 1992 Autogenic training and self-hypnosis in the control of tension headache. General Hospital Psychiatry 14:408–415

Stallibrass C, Sissons P, Chalmers C 2002 Randomized controlled trial of the Alexander technique for idiopathic Parkinson's disease. Clinical Rehabilitation 16:705–718

Stenstrom C H, Arge B, Sundbom A 1996 Dynamic training versus relaxation training as home exercise for patients with inflammatory rheumatic diseases: a randomized controlled study. Scandinavian Journal of Rheumatology 25:28–33

Stephens R L 1992 Imagery: a treatment for nursing student anxiety. Journal of Nursing Education 31(7):314–320

Stephenson N L, Weinrich S P, Tavakoli A S 2000 The effects of foot reflexology on anxiety and pain in patients with breast and lung cancer. Oncology Nursing Forum 27(1):67–72

Steptoe A, Butler N 1996 Sports participation and emotional well-being in adolescents. Lancet 347:1789–1792

Stetter F, Kupper S 2002 Autogenic training: a meta-analysis of clinical outcome studies. Applied Psychophysiology and Biofeedback 27(1):45–98

Stevens A, Price J 1996 Evolutionary psychiatry: a new beginning. Routledge, London

Stevens J O 1971 Awareness: exploring, experimenting, experiencing. Real People Press, Moab, Utah

Stevenson C 1995 The role of shiatsu in palliative care. Complementary Therapies in Nursing and Midwifery 1:51–58

Stoyva J M, Anderson C D 1982 A coping–rest model of relaxation and stress management. In: Goldberger L, Breznitz S (eds) Handbook of stress: theoretical and clinical aspects. Free Press, New York

Stradling J 1983 Respiratory physiology in labour. Journal of the Association of Chartered Physiotherapists in Obstetrics and Gynaecology 53:5–7

Strongman K T 1987 The psychology of emotion. John Wiley, Chichester

Sudsuang R, Chentanez V, Veluvan K 1991 Effect of Buddhist meditation on serum cortisol and total protein levels, blood pressure, pulse rate, lung volume and reaction time. Physiology and Behaviour 50:543–548

Takaishi N 2000 A comparative study of autogenic training and progressive relaxation as methods for teaching clients to relax. Sleep and Hypnosis 2(3):132–137

Talmage R V, Stinnett S S, Landwehr J T, Vincent L M, McCartney W H 1986 Age-related loss of bone mineral density in non-athletic and athletic women. Bone Mineral 1:115–125

Tate A K, Petruzzello S J 1995 Varying the intensity of acute exercise: implications for changes in affect. Journal of Sports in Medicine and Physical Fitness 35:1–8

Taylor A H 2000 Physical activity, anxiety and stress. In: Biddle S J H, Fox K R, Boutcher S H (eds) Physical activity and psychological well-being. Routledge, London, pp 10–45

Taylor D N 1995 Effects of a behavioural stress-management programme on anxiety, mood, self-esteem and T-cell count in HIV positive men. Psychological Reports 76(2):451–457

Telles S, Nagarathna R, Nagendra H R, Desiraju T 1993 Physiological changes in sports teachers following three months of training in yoga. Indian Journal of Medical Science 47(10):235–238

Telles S, Reddy S K, Nagendra H R 2000 Oxygen consumption and respiration following two yoga relaxation techniques. Applied Psychophysiology and Biofeedback 25(4):221–227

Titlebaum H 1988 Relaxation. In: Zahourek R P (ed) Relaxation and imagery: tools for therapeutic communication and intervention. W B Saunders, Philadelphia

Trousdale P, Uphoff-Chmielnik A 1997 User perception of the effects of reflexology and counselling: an evaluation of a complementary health care project at Worthing MIND

Tsai S, Swanson-Crockett M 1993 Effects of relaxation training combining imagery and meditation on the stress level of Chinese nurses working in modern hospitals in Taiwan. Issues in Mental Health Nursing 14:51–66

Tschudin V 1991 Beginning with awareness: a learner's handbook. Churchill Livingstone, Edinburgh

Tulkin S, Frank G, Bernstein A et al 1996 Management of chronic benign pain in a prepaid practice. In: Lazarus A (ed) Controversies in managed mental health care. American Psychiatric Press, Washington DC

Turner J A M, Jensen M P 1993 Efficacy of cognitive therapy for chronic low back pain. Pain 52:169–177

Tusek D L, Cwynar R E 2000 Strategies for implementing a guided imagery programme to enhance patient experience. Advanced Practice in Acute and Critical Care 11(1):68–76

Twomey L T 1993 Lumbar biomechanics and physical therapy. Journal of the Organization of Chartered Physiotherapists in Private Practice 70:14–19

Twomey L T, Taylor J R 1987 Physical therapy of the low back. Churchill Livingstone, New York

US Preventive Services Task Force 1989 Exercise counselling. In: Guide to clinical preventive services 49:297–303. Williams and Wilkins, Baltimore

Valentine E R 1993 The effect of lessons in the Alexander technique on music performance in high and low stress situations. Paper given at the 2nd International Conference on Psychology and the Performing Arts, Institute of Psychiatry, London, September

Van der Hek H, Plomp H N 1997 Occupational stress management programmes: a practical overview of published effect studies. Occupational Medicine (Oxford) 47(3):133–141

Van Dixhoorn J 1997 The effect of relaxation training on patients following myocardial infarction. Nederlands Tijdschrift voor Geneeskunde 141(11):530–534

Van Dixhoorn J, Duivenvoorden H J 1985 Efficacy of the Neimegen questionnaire in recognition of the hyperventilation syndrome. Journal of Psychosomatic Research 29(2):199–206

Van Dixhoorn J, Duivenvoorden J A 1989 Breathing awareness as a relaxation method in cardiac rehabilitation. In: Stress and Tension Control 3. Plenum, New York, pp 19–36

Van Doorn P, Colla P, Folgering H 1982 Control of end-tidal PCO_2 in the hyperventilation syndrome: effects of biofeedback and breathing instructions compared. Bulletin Européen de Physiopathologie Respiratoire 18:829–836

Van Hooff J A 1972 A comparative approach to the phylogeny of laughter and smiling. In: Hinde R A (ed) Non-verbal communication. Cambridge University Press, Cambridge

Vansteenkiste J, Rochette M, Demedts M 1991 Diagnostic tests of the hyperventilation syndrome. European Respiratory Journal 4:393–399

Vasterling J, Jenkins R A, Tope D M, Burish T G 1993 Cognitive distraction and relaxation training for the control of side effects due to cancer chemotherapy. Journal of Behavioral Medicine 16(1):65–80

Vazquez M I, Buceta J M 1993 Effectiveness of self-management programmes and relaxation training in the treatment of bronchial asthma: relationships with trait anxiety and emotional attack triggers. Journal of Psychosomatic Research 37(1):71–81

Vissing Y, Burke M 1984 Visualization techniques for health care workers. Journal of Psychosocial Nursing and Mental Health Services 22:29–32

Waddington P J 1983 Basic anatomy. In: Downie P A (ed) Cash's textbook of chest, heart and vascular disorders for physiotherapists, 3rd edn. Faber and Faber, London

Wallace J M 1980 Muscular relaxation. In: Look after yourself. Health Education Authority, London

Wallace K G 1997 Analysis of recent literature concerning relaxation and imagery interventions for cancer pain. Cancer Nursing 20(2):79–87

Ware J E, Sherbourne C D 1992 The MOS 36-item short form health survey (SF-36) 1. Conceptual framework and item selection. Medical Care 30:473–483

Waugh A, Grant A 2001 Ross & Wilson anatomy and physiology in health and illness, 9th edn. Elsevier Science, Edinburgh

Weber S 1996 The effects of relaxation exercises on anxiety levels in psychiatric patients. Journal of Holistic Nursing 14(3):196–205

West M A (ed) 1987 The psychology of meditation. Oxford Science Publications, Oxford

Weyerer S, Kupfer B 1994 Physical exercise and psychological health. Sports Medicine 17(2):108–116

Williamson J, White A, Hart A, Ernst E 2002 Randomized controlled trial of reflexology for menopausal symptoms. British Journal of Obstetrics and Gynaecology 109(9):1050–1055

Wilson K J W 1990 Ross & Wilson anatomy and physiology in health and illness, 7th edn. Churchill Livingstone, Edinburgh

Wishart L R, Lee T D, Ezekiel H J, Marley T L, Lehto N K 2000 Application of motor learning principles: the physiotherapy client as a problem-solver: 1. Concepts. Physiotherapy Canada 52(3):229

Wolpe J 1958 Psychotherapy by reciprocal inhibition. Stanford University Press, Stanford

Wolpe J, Lazarus A A 1966 Behaviour therapy techniques. Pergamon Press, New York

Woolfolk R L, Lehrer P M (eds) 1984 Principles and practice of stress management. Guilford Press, New York

World Health Organization 1994 Assessment of fracture risk and its application to screening for post-menopausal osteoporosis. World Health Organization, Geneva (WHO Technical Report Series 843)

Wynd C A 1989 The use of guided imagery to enhance power for smoking change. Dissertation Abstracts International 50 08B:3408. University microfilms order number QVM 90–02682

Wynd C A 1992 Relaxation imagery used for stress reduction in the prevention of smoking relapse. Journal of Advanced Nursing 17:294–302

Yen L L, Patrick W K, Chie W C 1996 Comparison of relaxation techniques, routine blood pressure measurements and self-learning packages in hypertension control. Preventive Medicine 25(3):339–345

Yucha C B, Clark L, Smith M, Uris P, LaFleur B, Duval S 2001 The effect of biofeedback in hypertension. Applied Nursing Research 14(1):29–35

Yung P, French P, Leung B 2001 Relaxation training as complementary therapy for mild hypertension control and the implications of evidence-based medicine. Complementary Medicine In Nursing and Midwifery 1(2):59–65

Zahourek R P (ed) 1985 Clinical hypnosis and therapeutic suggestion in nursing. Grune and Stratton, Orlando, Florida

Zahourek R P (ed) 1988 Relaxation and imagery: tools for therapeutic communication and intervention. W B Saunders, Philadelphia

Zigmond A S, Snaith R P 1983 The hospital anxiety and depression scale. Acta Psychiatrica Scandinavica 67:361–370

Index